2020

国家儿童肿瘤监测年报

National Pediatric Cancer Surveillance Annual Report

顾问委员会　阮长耿　孙　燕　张金哲　陆道培
　　　　　　陈赛娟　程书钧　焦雅辉　赫　捷
名誉主编　张金哲　胡亚美
主　　编　倪　鑫
副主编　李　哲　徐　新

U0199854

人民卫生出版社
·北京·

图书在版编目（CIP）数据

国家儿童肿瘤监测年报 / 倪鑫主编 . —北京：人
民卫生出版社，2021.2
　ISBN 978-7-117-31242-4

　Ⅰ.①国…　Ⅱ.①倪…　Ⅲ.①小儿疾病—肿瘤—卫生
监测—中国—年报　Ⅳ.①R73-54

　中国版本图书馆 CIP 数据核字（2021）第 025395 号

人卫智网　**www.ipmph.com**	医学教育、学术、考试、健康， 购书智慧智能综合服务平台
人卫官网　**www.pmph.com**	人卫官方资讯发布平台

审图号　GS（2021）300 号

国家儿童肿瘤监测年报

Guojia Ertong Zhongliu Jiance Nianbao

主　　编：倪　鑫
出版发行：人民卫生出版社（中继线 010-59780011）
地　　址：北京市朝阳区潘家园南里 19 号
邮　　编：100021
E - mail：pmph @ pmph.com
购书热线：010-59787592　010-59787584　010-65264830
印　　刷：北京盛通印刷股份有限公司
经　　销：新华书店
开　　本：889×1194　1/16　　印张：31
字　　数：917 千字
版　　次：2021 年 2 月第 1 版
印　　次：2021 年 2 月第 1 次印刷
标准书号：ISBN 978-7-117-31242-4
定　　价：197.00 元

打击盗版举报电话：**010-59787491**　E-mail：WQ @ pmph.com
质量问题联系电话：**010-59787234**　E-mail：zhiliang @ pmph.com

顾问委员会 阮长耿 孙 燕 张金哲 陆道培 陈赛娟 程书钧 焦雅辉 赫 捷

名誉主编 张金哲 胡亚美

主 编 倪 鑫

副主编 李 哲 徐 新

专家委员会（以姓氏笔画为序）

马晓莉 王天有 王焕民 方建培 冯国双 吕善根 汤静燕 李 哲

吴晔明 吴润晖 吴敏媛 陈 静 竺晓凡 郑荣寿 郑胡镛 赵 强

贾晨光 倪 鑫 徐 新 黄晓军 董岿然 曾跃萍 翟晓文

编 委（以姓氏笔画为序）

丁百静 丁岩冰 丁雅明 于亚滨 于红梅 马 东 马立旭 马先莹

马晓莉 马涌霞 马瑞霞 马颖霞 丰东蒙 王平（北京） 王平（昆明）

王 荣 王 勇 王 莉 王 倩 王 健 王 琛 王天有 王丹波

王文君 王世中 王占祥 王生才 王宁玲 王成伟 王伟林 王军辉

王忠民 王金湖 王学伟 王桂秀 王曼莉 王焕民 王晶桐 王献民

韦建瑞 毛静远 仇 杰 方建培 尹 勇 尹传高 巴桑次仁

邓英虎 石春和 龙 莉 龙思哲 叶 舟 叶丁剑 田 龙 田 剑

田 魁 田娇妮 代 艳 白元松 冯 梅 冯国双 尼 玛 邢泉生

达其伟 成保胜 吕沐瀚 吕善根 朱利明 乔晓红 任建林 华 飞

向 华 庄树铨 庄德义 刘 冰 刘 超 刘 磊 刘文平 刘玉林

刘正霞 刘加明 刘光华 刘先胜 刘伟光 刘江玲 刘安生 刘远飞

刘志宇 刘连新 刘青光 刘卓炜 刘昌明 刘祖国 刘原虎 刘培敏

刘福云 闫 勇 关小倩 米 阳 汤静燕 汤黎明 安鲁毅 许 敏

许志扬 许爱东 孙兴昌 孙安平 孙琛贤 孙艳丽 严 辉 严 媚

严友德 苏学峰 杜金林 李 兵 李 卓 李 凯 李 哲 李 晖

3

儿童是人类的未来,是整个社会可持续发展的重要资源,其健康直接关系到国家的发展和民族的希望。提高儿童的整体素质,促进儿童的身心健康和全面发展,是世界各国政府孜孜不倦的奋斗目标。然而,随着社会节奏的日益加快和人类生存环境的不断改变,恶性肿瘤已成为威胁儿童和青少年生命健康最主要的疾病之一,成为我国儿童因病致残和家庭因病致贫的重要原因。

国家儿童医学中心充分发挥儿科医学高地作用,在国家卫生健康委员会的指导下,开展儿童血液病、恶性肿瘤救治保障相关工作。2019年国家卫生健康委员会批复成立国家儿童肿瘤监测中心,依托国家儿童医学中心(北京)开展全国儿童肿瘤监测工作,建立国家儿童肿瘤监测体系,为实现肿瘤患儿诊疗和救治的信息监测和全程管理奠定重要基础。此项工作的成功开展,对儿童肿瘤防治工作意义重大,对促进诊疗随访以及全程管理的规范化水平、推动开展相关领域科学研究发挥了积极作用,同时能够为卫生健康行政部门实施精细化管理提供有力的科学数据支撑。

《国家儿童肿瘤监测年报》是基于全国监测数据的儿童肿瘤研究报告,作为我国儿童肿瘤监测工作的标志性成果之一,对促进儿童肿瘤流行病学、临床医学以及卫生经济学等方面的发展具有里程碑意义。

希望国家儿童肿瘤监测中心继续做好病例登记管理和数据统计分析工作,加强儿童肿瘤的科学研究,进一步完善监测体系。希望各地卫生健康行政部门和各医疗机构借鉴先进地区经验,推动优化儿童肿瘤医疗资源配置,调整完善相关政策,为提高我国乃至全球儿童健康水平做出更大的贡献。

中国工程院院士
首都医科大学附属北京儿童医院　教授
2020 年 12 月

Preface

Children are the future of mankind and an important resource for sustainable social development, whose health bears directly on the development and future of a country. Governments around the world are working tirelessly to improve children's mental and physical health and promote their overall development. However, as the pace of society fastens and mankind's living environment constantly changes, cancer has become one of the major diseases threatening the lives and health of children and adolescents, and a leading cause of child disability and family poverty in China.

Under the guidance of the National Health Commission, the National Center for Children's Health has given full play to its leading role in pediatrics to provide and secure the treatment of pediatric hematological diseases and cancers. In 2019, the National Center for Pediatric Cancer Surveillance has been established with the approval of the National Health Commission, aiming to carry out national pediatric cancer surveillance based in the National Center for Children's Health (Beijing). By setting up a pediatric cancer surveillance system, it has laid a solid foundation for information mornitoring and whole-process management of pediatric cancer diagnosis and treatment. The success of this work bears great significance to pediatric cancer prevention and treatment, plays an active role in the standardization of follow-up treatment and whole-process management and in the development of research in relevant fields, and supports fine management by health administrators with a strong data basis.

National Pediatric Cancer Surveillance Annual Report is a research report on children's cancer based on national surveillance data. As one of the landmark achievements of children's cancer surveillance in China, it has milestone significance in promoting the development of epidemiology, clinical medicine and health economics of pediatric cancer.

Hopefully, the National Center for Pediatric Cancer Surveillance will continue to do a good job in case registration management and data collection and analysis, strengthen research on pediatric cancer, and further improve the surveillance system. It is also hoped that local health administrators and medical institutions will learn from the experience of advanced regions to optimize their resource allocation for pediatric cancer and adjust and improve relevant policies, so as to contribute more to children's health in China and across the world.

Dr. Zhang Jinzhe

Academician, the Chinese Academy of Engineering

Professor, Beijing Children's Hospital, Capital Medical University

December, 2020

　　儿童健康受到党和政府及全社会的高度关注。习近平总书记多次就儿童健康作出重要指示批示；李克强总理多次深入调研，推动儿童重大疾病诊疗和保障工作；孙春兰副总理专题研究儿童血液病、恶性肿瘤医疗救治及保障制度建设工作。2019年，国家卫生健康委员会将儿童血液病、恶性肿瘤救治保障工作，作为落实党中央"不忘初心、牢记使命"主题教育的重要内容，进一步建立健全工作机制并全面部署实施。

　　为落实党和国家对儿童肿瘤防治工作部署要求，了解并掌握我国儿童肿瘤的流行现状及变化趋势，在国家卫生健康委员会的领导下，国家儿童医学中心（北京）首都医科大学附属北京儿童医院于2019年成立国家儿童肿瘤监测中心，在全国范围建立儿童肿瘤登记与监测体系，开展以医院为基础的儿童肿瘤实时动态监测工作。该项工作的持续推进与不断完善，将为国家制定儿童肿瘤相关卫生政策和防控策略提供全面、科学的数据依据；同时为儿童肿瘤流行病学、临床规范化诊疗和药物创新等研究奠定基础。

　　在各级卫生健康行政部门支持及各儿童肿瘤监测点的积极配合下，国家儿童肿瘤监测中心首次编写《国家儿童肿瘤监测年报》。本年报共收集了全国31个省（自治区、直辖市）及新疆生产建设兵团的313家儿童肿瘤监测点数据，展示了2017—2018年我国儿童肿瘤相关信息。诚然，受编者水平及时间所限，本书难免存在疏漏或不足，恳请医疗卫生行业同僚、学界专家及各方读者提出宝贵意见。

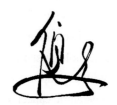

国家儿童医学中心（北京）、国家儿童肿瘤监测中心　主任
首都医科大学附属北京儿童医院　院长
2020 年 12 月

Foreword

Children's health is highly valued by the Party, the government and society. General Secretary Xi Jinping has made important instructions on children's health. Premier Li Keqiang has conducted several in-depth investigations on the work of promoting the treatment and security of major pediatric diseases. And Vice Premier Sun Chunlan has done themed research on building the system for the treatment and security of pediatric hematological diseases and cancers. In 2019, the National Health Commission has further improved the working mechanisms and comprehensively deployed and implemented the treatment and security of pediatric hematological diseases and cancers, as an important endeavor to roll out the Party Central Committee's education campaign themed "remaining true to our original aspiration and keeping our mission firmly in mind".

In order to meet the deployment requirements of pediatric cancer prevention and treatment by the Party and the State, and keep abreast of the current situation and trends of pediatric cancer in China, the National Center for Pediatric Cancer Surveillance has been established in 2019 under the guidance of the National Health Commission by the National Center for Children's Health (Beijing), Beijing Children's Hospital, Capital Medical University. The National Center for Pediatric Cancer Surveillance serves to build a pediatric cancer registration and surveillance system to carry out pediatric cancer surveillance that is hospital-based, real-time, and dynamic. The continuous progress and development of the work will provide comprehensive, scientific data for the country to formulate health policies and prevention and control strategies concerning pediatric cancer. It will also lay a solid foundation for research in the epidemiology, standardized clinical treatment, and medicine innovation of pediatric cancer.

With the support from the National Health Commission and local health commissions as well as the cooperation of pediatric cancer surveillance sites, the National Center for Pediatric Cancer Surveillance compiles the National Pediatric Cancer Surveillance Annual Report for the first time. The report collects data from 313 pediatric surveillance sites in 31 provinces (autonomous regions, municipalities directly under the central government), and Xinjiang Production and Construction Corps, and provides information on pediatric cancer in China between 2017 and 2018. Admittedly, constraints of knowledge and time inevitably lead to omissions and deficiencies. We sincerely invite valuable suggestions from colleagues and experts in the medical and health industry and readers from all sides.

Dr. Ni Xin

Director, National Center for Children's Health (Beijing)

and National Center for Pediatric Cancer Surveillance

President, Beijing Children's Hospital, Capital Medical University

December, 2020

致　谢

《国家儿童肿瘤监测年报》凝聚着全国各儿童肿瘤监测点相关工作人员、国家儿童肿瘤监测平台建设人员和年报编写组成员的辛勤劳动,在此衷心感谢大家为本年报编写给予的大力支持和帮助!

儿童肿瘤监测点和儿童肿瘤监测平台建设人员名单

省（自治区、直辖市）和新疆生产建设兵团	机构名称	主要参与人员
北京	北京大学第一医院	刘 斯　刘辰龙　张 岩　洪 颖
	北京大学人民医院	王 立　张 霞　张晓红　侯晓漫
	首都儿科研究所附属儿童医院	刘一豪　李 盈　崔 英
	首都医科大学附属北京儿童医院	邓 卓　吕亚奇　宋 菲　奚 悦
	首都医科大学附属北京世纪坛医院	李 苗　吴玉萍　黄 俊
	首都医科大学附属北京天坛医院	朱晓东　关 欣　李潇潇　杨 姝　陈佳龙
	首都医科大学附属北京同仁医院	赵莉丽　倪如旸　陶怡聆
	中国医学科学院北京协和医院	李 卓　肖 娟　张占杰　庞 成
天津	天津市儿童医院	刘婷婕　米丽艳　许爱东　吴 斌　林 宏
	天津市肿瘤医院	王丹凝　卢 培　付 鑫　何菁华　陈培翠
	天津中医药大学第一附属医院	夏睦谊　柴恭敏　郭从容
	中国医学科学院血液病医院	王津雨　张晓斌　赵 芊
河北	安新县医院	刘 欢　陈晓宁　金克军
	保定市儿童医院	李尚育　宋马立　庞微微　夏明倩
	承德市医学院附属医院	吉 洁　殷 畅　高菲菲　黄慧洁
	河北北方学院附属第一医院	李 伟　林 昊　赵丽娟　路继航
	河北省儿童医院	吕丽格　李子涛　张仕乔　耿江桥　高明月
	河北省人民医院	王晶晶　计阿丹　赵慧智
	河北省眼科医院	师景顺　赵克鹏
	河北省中医院	何 芳　夏 芳　高雪亮　韩长辉
	河北医科大学第二医院	王炜杰　刘瑞瑞　吴端阳　谢 洋
	河北医科大学第三医院	王纯玲　孔令伟　孙蕴茹
	河北医科大学第四医院	吕 卓　李书梅　赵孝先　段晓瑾
	河北医科大学第一医院	刘笑伟　李爱林　张林泽
	河北中西医结合儿童医院	徐晓东
	廊坊市中医医院	刘 震　张大勇　徐 杨　曾 玲
	石家庄市藁城人民医院	甘秀丽　申彦丽　陈 辉
	石家庄市藁城中西医结合医院	程永信
	无极人和医院	吕月珍　纪亚青　赵军强

省(自治区、直辖市)和新疆生产建设兵团	机构名称	主要参与人员					
	无极血康中医医院	袁军清	袁晓磊	曹庆智			
	新乐市医院	李新虎	张会宾	周彦坤	封英杰		
	邢台市第一医院	孙胜辉	李一丹	杨德志	曹志芳		
	邢台市人民医院	马春燕	王军辉	刘淑娴			
	塞北管理区医院	张 玥	黄文华				
山西	国药同煤总医院	王 娟	赵铃方				
	大同市第一人民医院	王 鹏	史向峰	张树斌	武建平	侯 芳	黄 淼
	大同市第三人民医院	石丽峰	孙雪松	吴继颖	崔英华		
	晋城市人民医院	王淑靖	刘 芳	李 霞	郭燕超	裴杨婷	
	晋中市第一人民医院	许建勋	范云珠	温变珍			
	临汾市人民医院	冯晓飞	成 晶	刘晓剑	李 斌	张银虎	赵 敏
	吕梁市人民医院	王新芳	乔婷婷	李燕军	赵巧锋		
	山西白求恩医院	刘晓红	陈 芳	遆 刚			
	晋城大医院	刘 珊	李雪琴	宋魏魏	张 云	赵洪壮	
	大同市第五人民医院	丁鹏飞	王一楠	任秀花	程 昊		
	山西省儿童医院	王丽燕	王慧丽	李 波	南 晶	高 莉	
	临汾市中心医院	赵娟娟	崔欣宏	梁晓慧			
	山西省人民医院	戎 杰	赵 智	穆璟丽			
	山西省眼科医院	田娇妮	韩媛媛				
	山西省运城市中心医院	杜秋璞	杨 晓	谷一峰	姚 晔		
	山西省肿瘤医院	白文启	张振君	曹元元	童亚兰		
	山西医科大学第二医院	王希英	杜惠丽	梁泽峰	蒋 敏		
	山西医科大学第一医院	王欣欣	李 娜	张 琳	褚云生		
	太原钢铁(集团)有限公司总医院	孙晓玉	张丹阳	武亚倩	周建刚	胡振伟	
	五寨县第一人民医院	王文娟	杜永红	徐莉娟			
	运城市第一医院	仝俊芳	刘海萍	胡瑞英			
	长治市人民医院	李丹丹	张 毅	郭 萍			
	长治医学院附属和平医院	王宇江	李韶霞	降凌燕			
内蒙古	包钢集团第三职工医院	尹诗琦	周静华	樊 波			
	包头市第四医院	王晓宇	张红梅	封 红			
	赤峰市医院	史 赢	周生福	盖 冬	璐 然		
	赤峰学院附属医院	王丽君	王艳军	杨建玲	林 囡		

续表

省（自治区、直辖市）和新疆生产建设兵团	机构名称	主要参与人员
	鄂尔多斯市东胜区人民医院	王　明　呼桂梅　康　凯
	鄂尔多斯市中心医院	王明霞　李思雨　徐冬蕊
	呼伦贝尔市人民医院	钱　程　徐鑫巍　董秀琴
	呼和浩特市第一医院	陈　艳　陈素珍　金　峰
	内蒙古科技大学包头医学院第一附属医院	王惠娟　云　雁　李飞飞　梁　爽
	内蒙古医科大学附属医院	张哲林　张晓燕　周志云
	内蒙古自治区妇幼保健院	王晓琴　包长军　杜　鉴　陈晓梅　武小兰　郭　健
	内蒙古自治区国际蒙医医院	宋颖林　张艳辉　高哈斯宝力高　曹林娟
	内蒙古自治区人民医院	王向文　赵彩霞　郝智慧　唐广飞
	内蒙古自治区中医医院	王丽娜　冯小静　任国华　杨　新
	通辽市医院	王　欢　李　鹰　郝　赫　程　岩
	乌兰浩特市人民医院	冷冰洋　赵小壮
	兴安盟人民医院	白　涛　包银萍　殷金鑫
	准格尔旗大路医院	刘志文　贺　亮
	准格尔旗人民医院	王　丽　王小娟　董永军　魏　云
	准格尔旗中心医院	王生有　刘海波　杨国芳　薛正茹
辽宁	本溪市中心医院	刘　鑫　刘春春　孙传柱　徐玉玲
	朝阳市第二医院	马　丽　卢俞任　李立伟　林鸿峰
	大连市儿童医院	方浩男　牟荟瞳　李　荔　李皆欣　迟　磊　张文闻
	大连市妇女儿童医疗中心	邢文洁　孙　旭　张世恒
	大连医科大学附属第二医院	马志晖　王淑静　王颖洁　李德壮
	锦州市妇婴医院	刘　阳　尚敏捷　薛　政
	锦州医科大学附属第一医院	刘永伟　姬　斯　彭春辉
	辽宁省健康产业集团抚矿总医院	王偲羽　苏艳琦　李　雪
	辽宁省肿瘤医院	王玉名　王忱玉　孙　婷　张一凡
	沈阳市儿童医院	平　丹　李　玢　杨　柳　谢镇玲
	中国医科大学附属第一医院	王　湘　兰　震　迟卫军　徐云伟
	中国医科大学附属盛京医院	王汝南　石　锋　李　宁　赵萌萌　薛满全
吉林	公主岭市中心医院	张笑言　苗星宇　崔嘉麟
	吉林大学第二医院	王江华　王春玲　周艳婷　赵希海
	吉林大学第一医院	王　玥　王　颖　王洪亮　尤海龙　李艳春　潘　峰
	吉林大学中日联谊医院	王宗强　肖博晗　赵小勇　崔永亮

续表

省（自治区、直辖市）和新疆生产建设兵团	机构名称	主要参与人员					
	松原市中西医结合医院	王　宇	李　妍	李媛媛	杨丽新		
	吉林省一汽总医院	王　珏	关鑫磊	栾　珺			
	吉林省肿瘤医院	王　冰	刘雯舒	陈忠民	赵思宇		
	吉林市儿童医院	于明玉	米　果	张　强			
	梅河口市中心医院	刘向春	米　贺	陈　雷	董　帆		
	松原市中心医院	付珊珊	肖俊凤	何欣泽	郭新宇		
	延边大学附属医院	于　丽	李香淑	张锦玉			
	长春市儿童医院	方宝柱	刘　颖	李北岩	陈兆明	陈海霞	魏　葳
	长春中医药大学附属医院	王　巍	王永吉	张雪莲	梁凤珍		
黑龙江	哈尔滨市儿童医院	于纯淼	尤　佳	李恒新	魏红燕		
	哈尔滨市第一医院	李瑞南	邱海英	郝文鹏	解云兴		
	哈尔滨医科大学附属第二医院	李瑞波	张泽鹏				
	哈尔滨医科大学附属肿瘤医院	周婷婷	姜　欢	郭相楠	韩　爽		
	伊春林业管理局中心医院	李子健	姜东旭	姚　帅			
上海	复旦大学附属儿科医院	马　晴	刘枭雄	孙孝恺	劳怡敏	柳龚堡	葛小玲
	上海长海医院	周雁萍	姜治仲	蒋　玲	雷　蕾		
	上海交通大学医学院附属新华医院	沈鸿楼	潘伟华	潘曙明	穆嘉盛		
	上海市同济医院	王　洁	徐　惠	颜梁莉			
	上海交通大学医学院附属上海儿童医学中心	张　悦	周　敏	黄　璐	蔡娇阳		
	上海交通大学医学院附属瑞金医院	孙　木	强佳萍	魏凌云			
江苏	南京医科大学附属常州第二人民医院	孔志君	刘　樾	李敏慧			
	常州市第一人民医院	邱　慧	钟瑞颖	陶　源	曹冬梅		
	常州市儿童医院	邢凤军	李亚民	张　艳	金　晶		
	东南大学附属中大医院	丁佳丽	孙耘玉	姜玲凌			
	淮安市第二人民医院	李江南	肖　坤	张佳龙			
	江苏省妇幼保健院	孙月鑫	陈　亮	徐　露	濮亚宁		
	淮安市第一人民医院	朱海艳	庄　菲	祁海啸	杜　静	高　健	谈　进
	淮安市妇幼保健院	王金锐	吴素梅	高子波			
	苏北人民医院	吴文靖	吴红星	宋　慧	赵　曼		
	镇江市第一人民医院	吴　洁	赵　楠	顾　炜	韩秋君		
	江苏省肿瘤医院	丁　晖	任雨杨	张　敏	席　玮		
	连云港市第一人民医院	刘伟伟	刘燃峰	张红刚	周国辉		

省（自治区、直辖市）和新疆生产建设兵团	机构名称	主要参与人员
	南京鼓楼医院	于成功　华履春　吴植茆　屈　峰
	南京医科大学附属儿童医院	孔　日　田　曼　李承益　张婷婷
	南京医科大学第二附属医院	卞胜军　朱晨成　唐　越
	南通大学附属医院	严卫萍　沙震宇　翟　林
	苏州大学附属第一医院	周明元　徐　洁　郭海铭　程思明
	苏州大学附属儿童医院	孙文静　李建琴　张兵兵　魏　颖
	泰州市人民医院	臧如金
	宿迁市第一人民医院	严友德　张　成　张新静
	宿迁市儿童医院	刘　宏　李小慧　金志琴
	宿迁市人民医院	史　瑞　李运红　吴光启　黄红梅
	徐州医科大学第二附属医院	王　宏　叶晓娜　张兰胜
	徐州市儿童医院	张岫秀　欧兆霏　赵文婧　蒋　宏
	徐州市肿瘤医院	曹　咪　戚　峰　董广辉
	扬州大学附属医院	朱锦丽　徐亚红　魏筱静
	江苏省人民医院	史晓凤　傅　亮　鲁　磊
浙江	杭州市儿童医院	李才学　吴　颖　曹莉君
	浙江大学医学院附属金华医院	何国斌　徐敏慧　蒋国坚
	温州医科大学附属第二医院	张　波　林　巍　黄　珍　谢作楷
	浙江大学医学院附属第二医院	朱晓华　徐　莉　蔡　栋　潘胜东
	浙江大学医学院附属第一医院	何剑琴　徐　周　殷　希　黄　炯
	浙江大学医学院附属儿童医院	李哲明　汪　伟　陈飞波　俞　刚　梁建凤　童鑫发
	中国科学院大学附属肿瘤医院	李方印　吴友妹　胡　曼　袁波英
安徽	安徽省第二人民医院	王文君　周　琳　郑国甫
	安徽省儿童医院	尹传高　郑新芝　郑慧敏　陶亮亮
	安徽省黄山市休宁县总医院	俞芳君　洪巧英　鲍　君
	霍邱县第一人民医院	汪宏才　周　斌　周明佳　周康俊
	中国科学技术大学附属第一医院	王　浩　汪　楠　赵德胜　曾　杨　翟　飞
	芜湖市第一人民医院	王　仲　包爱枝　李芳心
	安徽医科大学第二附属医院	叶　珺　胡胜英　耿　敏　谢志伟
	安徽医科大学第一附属医院	杨小英　汪安勇　张　岩　胡　鹏
	蚌埠市第三人民医院	王胜利　胡建明　程　爽
	蚌埠医学院第一附属医院	方鑫磊　张　超
	当涂县人民医院	许子凡　苏　莓　夏永伟

省（自治区、直辖市）和新疆生产建设兵团	机构名称	主要参与人员
	阜阳市妇女儿童医院	刘达伟　杨芹芹　谭凤萍
	黄山市第三人民医院	叶双双　朱超迪　曹春华
	来安县人民医院	王　庆　杜永洋　张沛霖　周德伟
	马鞍山市人民医院	代恒辉　缪　莉　樊　琴
	南京鼓楼医院集团安庆市石化医院	张小为　操海宝
	祁门县人民医院	王玉霞　叶春俊　程祁波
	全椒县人民医院	马　敏　陈玉秀　苗　静
	太和县中医院	王　辉　刘　磊　路冰莹
	天长市人民医院	李乡兵　张永盛　房　森
	铜陵市人民医院	邓英虎　倪世峰　戚　鑫
	皖南医学院第一附属医院	马丽娟　陈　希　陈珍初
	安徽省望江县医院	朱腊春　陈　波
	岳西县医院	刘绍灿　杨志兵
福建	福鼎市医院	陈岱旺　谢建春　谢莲妹
	福建省福州儿童医院	刘美舟　吴小霞　吴雪梅　陈继何　林　洁
	福建省妇幼保健院	王金吉　林彬彬　曾金浪
	福建省立医院	肖智祥　吴雄伟　陈吴凡　林　梅
	福建省南平市第一医院	朱俊民　何权辉　范云海　雷春燕
	福建省平潭综合实验区医院	杨　庚　薛理花
	三明市第一医院	吴倩鹏　陈德旭　葛孝川　魏　宏
	漳州市医院	李　悦　周继光　黄清华　蔡晓露
	福建医科大学附属第二医院	许丽英　巫应全　李雅辰　陈文亮　郑朝晖　郭宝创
	福建医科大学附属第一医院	叶世岳　林　如　周　梅
	福建医科大学附属协和医院	林永花　涂晓贤　谢贤宇
	福州市第二医院	范义东　林尘艳　钟姬琴
	福州市第一医院	王阿铃　江燕彬　安鲁毅
	福建省龙岩市第一医院	方　勇　张　燕　林梦真　谢艳梅
	宁德市闽东医院	刘清平　陈香斌　高惠仔　郭佺良
	宁德师范学院附属宁德市医院	朱忠寿　杨　晶　陆燕燕　熊莲莲
	莆田市第一医院	方　平　关　军　苏志群　陈淑兴
	莆田学院附属医院	陈　芳　陈希望
	泉州市第一医院	王友羲　江信榕　何巧玲　郭孟玲

省(自治区、直辖市)和新疆生产建设兵团	机构名称	主要参与人员
	泉州市儿童医院	吴旖薇　何文谦　柯若荣
	厦门大学附属第一医院	许云晓　陈幼芬　曾文菁
	厦门大学附属中山医院	孙安琪　钟新迎　覃伟初
	厦门市儿童医院	杨分发　陈　浩
江西	赣南医学院第一附属医院	王　丽　王井妹　李　辉　钟贵鑫　祖国亮
	江西省赣州市人民医院	杨运海　钟春阳　黄雅立
	江西省儿童医院	冯　姗　吴华平　郑小宏　黄文剑
	江西省人民医院	刘　宇　杜云艳　李维康　洪卫祥
	江西省肿瘤医院	万　波　邓春宏　邹　浩　敖惠萍
	南昌大学第二附属医院	龙　莉　何水才　金春莲　康　蘋　熊科亮
	南昌大学第一附属医院	伍姗姗　张连军　胡苏群　蓝淳愉
山东	聊城市人民医院	马　磊　兰　菲　李晓丽　肖启民　韩　丽　韩月芹
	临沂市人民医院	丁相梅　邱世彦　曹　雅
	临沂市中心医院	田　伟　肖云霞　张敬进
	临沂市肿瘤医院	刘　欢　李　绘　周建中
	青岛大学附属医院	万　斌　孙谟健　郭振清
	青岛市妇女儿童医院	王丽燕　孙兆国　查玉龙　隋　砚　温　伟　黎　强
	青岛市中心医院	王　玲　刘全敏　苏天慧
	济南市儿童医院	丁　鑫　冯国红　张　宁　胡令江
	山东大学齐鲁医院	张鲁燕　陈甜甜　孟迎旭　董　阳
	山东省立医院	王　冬　刘瑞红　张喜雨　张晴晴
	山东第一医科大学第一附属医院	王红美　陈国强　顾　艳　廉　颖
	山东省肿瘤医院	刘利妍　李锡瑞　徐　姗
	烟台毓璜顶医院	马先莹　杨　蕾　徐　旭　徐　靖
河南	河南科技大学第一附属医院	乔建超　岳玉桃　郭柯磊
	河南省儿童医院	马　琳　王建设　朱明宇　汤友喜　周一博　孟变红
	河南省人民医院	陈春晓　罗慧中　和　融　程剑剑
	河南省肿瘤医院	李　曦　唐现策
	河南中医药大学第一附属医院	朱　贺　刘　启　徐进杰
	新乡医学院第一附属医院	王　楠　王新建　吉丹霞　吴天赐　赵春晓　郭　峰
	郑州大学第二附属医院	刘正霞　宋红玉　宋美霞
	郑州大学第三附属医院	王　芳　李新霞　陈　晨　程志伟

省(自治区、直辖市)和新疆生产建设兵团	机构名称	主要参与人员
	郑州大学第一附属医院	王春杰　刘新奎　赵哲祎　黄　凯
湖北	湖北省妇幼保健院	刘祎昕　黄自明　鲁新峰
	荆门市第一人民医院	毛　强　郑大成　谢金元
	湖北省肿瘤医院	吴克智　曾　辉
	华中科技大学同济医学院附属同济医院	吴剑宏　张　艾　周文庆
	华中科技大学同济医学院附属协和医院	王莉霞　孙　扬　胡　赛　徐守荣
	荆门市第二人民医院	李　华　陈小军　赵蓉芝　熊　俊
	荆州市第一人民医院	李珍妮　张　欣
	荆州市妇幼保健院	田春霞
	武汉大学人民医院	周　涛　贺　华　夏利平　颜利晶
	武汉大学中南医院	苏义武　李　飞　杨奇盛
	武汉儿童医院	王育继　严春香　余盛军
	应城市人民医院	王林风　徐曲荣　韩　银
湖南	湖南省儿童医院	龙美元　屈　芳　胡外光　胡珊珊　段鹭茜　徐　晓
	湖南省人民医院	王　叶　王　星
	湖南省肿瘤医院	盛　露　梁　英
	南华大学附属第二医院	宁文锋　姜良艳　黎　俊
	南华大学附属第一医院	朱　柱　陈香兰　袁晓芸　唐再丽
	中南大学湘雅二医院	李　妍　周　薇　徐　维
	中南大学湘雅三医院	于姗姗　刘　琳　邱　琳　张　简
	郴州市第一人民医院	许　斌　张紫翠　彭　珍　雷　军
	中南大学湘雅医院	张　静　陈金彪　金　敏
广东	广东省妇幼保健院	李　晖　李玉萍　彭武江　谢靖懿
	广州市妇女儿童医疗中心	丁春光　韦晓燕　李丽娟　林　旭　曹晓均　廖淑仪
	南方医科大学第三附属医院	伍伟健　刘　锋　关小倩　李　云
	南方医科大学南方医院	朱灼新　杜依蔓　何俊崴　陈莉雅
	深圳市儿童医院	李佳曦　陈西蓉　林荣枢
	中山大学附属第一医院	王禹尧　刘　洋　刘骏峰
	中山大学孙逸仙纪念医院	王明乐　叶青晓　伍耀豪　杨宏橼　杨奕帆　谢丽莎
	中山大学中山眼科中心	方　浩　孙建明　容　莹
	中山大学肿瘤防治中心	王永杰　韦　玮　赵雁梨

省（自治区、直辖市）和新疆生产建设兵团	机构名称	主要参与人员
广西	广西医科大学第一附属医院	邓添薪　尚丽明　莫芳兰　虞丽霞　廖　宁
	广西壮族自治区妇幼保健院	甘杰泽　叶丁剑　李佳霖　陈语中　容丽媚　黄　敏
	广西壮族自治区人民医院	代　艳　何治琛　谭玲玲
	梧州市红十字会医院	汤伟文　苏阳红　黄金菊
	柳州市妇幼保健院	韦青宇　刘　冲　杨　磊　张　玉　覃　陈　温雪婷
	柳州市人民医院	王晓龙　苏俊杰　谭　娟　潘艳芳
	钦州市第一人民医院	叶海林　吴东彦　何振波　钟　蔚
海南	海南省妇女儿童医学中心	杨全略　欧阳珊红　魏陈红
	海南省人民医院	陈小芳　罗文龙　符祥敏
	海南省眼科医院	王　磐　陈秋香　林爱香
	海南省肿瘤医院	于　冰　王煜奋　赵　莉
	解放军总医院海南医院	吕钟琪　邱　禹　梁允兴
	海南省三亚市人民医院	王佳斌　罗丽萍　钟　静
	海南省第三人民医院	李　玮　张春燕　符国宏　廖雅各
重庆	陆军军医大学第二附属医院	杨莉莉　张　萍　陈　雨
	重庆大学附属肿瘤医院	刘煜民　李　琳　汪　刚
	重庆大学附属三峡医院	何友俊　张　娜　钟　胜
	重庆医科大学附属第二医院	王玉廷　刘　仪　周小兰　董　霄
	重庆医科大学附属儿童医院	王壮成　吴启帆　佘　颖　宋　萍　欧阳禾嘉　徐仕宝
	重庆医科大学附属永川医院	叶　流　周昌龙　程　笛
四川	成都市妇女儿童中心医院	肖　藜　陈富琴　姚海波
	四川大学华西第二医院	孙静静　李　黎　何　伟　高　举
	四川大学华西医院	帅冰星　张　睿　赵一洋　赵晓龙
	四川省妇幼保健院	皮光环　刘雪梅　郑姝娟
	四川省人民医院	李钦慧　冷　艳　徐　川
	四川省肿瘤医院	向明飞　杨　颖　康盛伟　熊中华
	西南医科大学附属医院	杨长皓　汪何畏
贵州	贵阳市妇幼保健院	干书汉　朱孝明　何庆红　张绍逸　陈晓云　周晓明
	贵州省人民医院	杨秀林　陈　英　聂　钊　戴石元
	贵州医科大学附属医院	龙先芝　吕　锐　郑明凤
	遵义医科大学附属医院	朱　刚　刘仕方　李成梅　张　骏　赵楷岩　黄　新
云南	昆明市儿童医院	宋　蓉　张文俊　张鸿青
	昆明医科大学第二附属医院	他　卉　李　涛　吴　鹏

省(自治区、直辖市)和新疆生产建设兵团	机构名称	主要参与人员
	昆明医科大学第一附属医院	张绍峰　陈广梅　郭如丽
	云南省第二人民医院	吕　平　李双艳　杨冬平　段兆修
	云南省第一人民医院	李　波　杨寿叶　陈　媛　郭　雨
	云南省肿瘤医院	张锦平　周　海　袁中琴　梅泽超
西藏	阿里地区人民医院	拉姆次仁　原　勇　钱铭艳　程淑芳
	拉萨市人民医院	闫春蕾　周贤贤　胡志强
	浪卡子县卫生服务中心	王立群　白玛卓嘎　张宏伟
	林芝市人民医院	王　蓉　吴丽莎　顾锡英
	日喀则市人民医院	巴桑丹增　边巴多吉　普　琼
	山南市人民医院	达　娃　吴晓莉　荆　浩
	昌都市人民医院	古桑拉姆　时仁龙　容文辉　黄　宇
	西藏自治区人民医院	李几幂　梁　娜　曾燕波
陕西	汉中市中心医院	王正伟　杨宏伟　骆　毅
	岚皋县人民医院	王　敏　宋春先　陈　刚
	留坝县医院	文　莉　曾　瑶
	三二〇一医院	王　勇　冯　蓉　刘　春
	陕西省人民医院	马文霞　苏亚妮　李　婷　董　睿
	西乡县中医医院	田　芳　孙　洁　杨　洋　梅　丹
	旬阳县中医院	王永刚　吴　媛　陈　昱
	石泉县医院	刘春阳　李　兵　吴小勇
	铜川市人民医院	马　悦　李　程　吴慧锋
	西安交通大学第二附属医院	张超黎　陈　毓　高　亚
	西安交通大学第一附属医院	李晓亮　杨静怡　周　铭　康　娅　彭　蓉　蔡宏伟
	西安市儿童医院	卢　萌　白　莹　师军利　李　静
	西北妇女儿童医院	王丽娟　米　阳　施　姣　贺崇慧　高　鹏　葛文利
	渭南市中心医院	刘　韬　刘舒眉　曹　蕾
	咸阳市中心医院	田治海　苏凯悦　杨　荣
甘肃	定西市第二人民医院	张小霞　赵晓娜
	定西市人民医院	孙艳丽　魏煜亚
	甘肃宝石花医院	朱　燕　任芳晖　张　斌　郭俊贤
	甘肃省第二人民医院	丰　晖　张丽丽　魏洪涛
	甘肃省妇幼保健院	达振强　李　玮　韩玉真

续表

省（自治区、直辖市）和新疆生产建设兵团	机构名称	主要参与人员
	嘉峪关市第一人民医院	邓福仓　尚颜萍　周　莹
	甘肃省人民医院	石育春　贠小燕　杨　燕　周　蕾
	文县第一人民医院	任亚峰　张　越　张　瑞
	甘肃省武威肿瘤医院	白永萍　刘玉华　李强华　范　琳
	甘肃省中医院	赵永强　黎媛媛
	河西学院附属张掖人民医院	严翠兰　杨发英　张建平　周　晨
	兰州大学第二医院	史晓媛　苏　明　吴小璐　陈静丽
	兰州大学第一医院	陆贞贞　赵　越　赵正斌　崔　琦
	两当县人民医院	王金林　林　琳
	甘肃省临夏回族自治州人民医院	马　莉　王桂秀　宗　雪　蒋玉红
	民勤县人民医院	王　甫　常建萍
	天水市第一人民医院	王素霞　刘　婷　李晶文　赵　丽
	武威市人民医院	王永柱　徐燕润　高万琦
	张掖市第二人民医院	冯玉婷　张西柳　徐步轩
青海	青海大学附属医院	孙　艺　程　珲
	青海省第五人民医院	马生祥　邓雯君　刘维彦　杜　斓
	青海省妇女儿童医院	阮连军　罗妍祺　洪　军
	青海省人民医院	王爱兵　张丽婷　董海波
宁夏	宁夏回族自治区妇幼保健院	王　萍　许继宝　耿雨慧
	宁夏回族自治区人民医院	马立旭　刘尚红　梁沛枫
	宁夏医科大学总医院	王学伟　方　浩　龚爱红
	银川市第一人民医院	陈　静　贺红丽　徐海洋
	中卫市人民医院	马忠义　吕　苗　严淑珍
新疆	阿克苏地区第二人民医院	古海克孜·沙伊丁　张大平　高飞凌
	阿克苏地区第一人民医院	宋　军　张荣民　莫合特尔·阿布力米提　蒲伟娟
	阿勒泰地区人民医院	刘翠瑛　杨瑞丽
	巴音郭楞蒙古自治州人民医院	方娅鑫　李淑红　唐　琳
	博尔塔拉州博州人民医院	王艳红　兰　花　娜仁吐亚
	昌吉回族自治州人民医院	邢瀚文　杨蓓蕾　张朝晖　帕热沙提·杰恩思　胡晨国　贾惠莉
	哈密市第二人民医院	范　敏　校卫东
	哈密市中心医院	王怡然　毛苏伟　蒲永亮
	和田地区人民医院	王晓样　阿曼古·艾则孜　楚文川　樊春信

省(自治区、直辖市)和新疆生产建设兵团	机构名称	主要参与人员
	喀什地区第二人民医院	张　青　张素丽　阿不都外力·吾守尔　苑江波
	喀什地区第一人民医院	买日阿巴·赛麦提　李亚东　张璟文　阿布都克尤木·阿布拉
	克拉玛依市中心医院	王　敏　钱丽娟　董　琳　鲁晓蕾
	克孜勒苏柯尔克孜自治州人民医院	肖滨增　帕提姑丽·阿不都克热木　徐祥贵
	伊犁哈萨克自治州塔城地区人民医院	叶静波　刘艳芳
	吐鲁番市人民医院	李学萍　杨　青　杨建丰　杨新琴　魏雪莲
	乌鲁木齐市第一人民医院	马丽娟　吾木提·阿不都热依木　阿尔达可·纳汗　陈　婕　谢　萍
	乌鲁木齐市友谊医院	丁　利　杜春瑾　迪力福扎·乌司慢
	独山子人民医院	达春梅　秦东强　康小媛
	新疆维吾尔自治区儿童医院	王　静　王春梅　吾斯曼·买买提　陈　燕　摆　静
	新疆维吾尔自治区人民医院	向伟荣　吴　岚　潘宜敏
	新疆维吾尔自治区中医医院	周　斌　娄鹏威　梅　琳　潘　静
	新疆医科大学第二附属医院	古丽白合热木·阿巴拜克热　潘候梅
	新疆医科大学第七附属医院	吴　芳　范　青　赵海燕
	新疆医科大学第五附属医院	毛　英　孙李丽　杨淑梅
	新疆医科大学第一附属医院	卢武红　刘才华　李　丞　肖明森　陈　曲　阎景红
	伊犁哈萨克自治州奎屯市人民医院	孙英莲　肖　真　陈　莉　贾静茹
	伊犁哈萨克自治州新华医院	冯云霞　加孜拉·沙吾提　格日丽·新巴依尔　唐努尔·艾克木哈孜
	伊犁哈萨克自治州友谊医院	朱　楠　李　飞　李　娟　佟志坚
	新疆医科大学附属肿瘤医院	付爱玲　张　旭　赵　婷　贾慧民
兵团	石河子大学医学院第一附属医院	王　静　伏云峰　韩　瑞
	石河子市人民医院	刘明珠　陈　静　姜新华
	铁门关市人民医院	周晓龙　贾战疆　谭小彦
	新疆生产建设兵团第二师库尔勒医院	白春玲　张凯琪　唐　娟
	新疆生产建设兵团第九师医院	刘　飞　胡咏泉　颜士家
	新疆生产建设兵团第六师医院	王新军　费文婧　黄　婷
	新疆生产建设兵团第七师医院	李素梅　周智斌　赵晨成
	新疆生产建设兵团第三师医院	王丽英　玛依拉·买买提明　肖　岚
	新疆生产建设兵团第十三师红星医院	安谱光　赵言玲　蒋　丽
	新疆生产建设兵团第十师北屯医院	孙金霞　李娟娟　邵　晶

续表

省(自治区、直辖市)和新疆生产建设兵团	机构名称	主要参与人员					
	新疆生产建设兵团第四师医院	李晓玲	张惠萍	郝思婷			
	新疆生产建设兵团第一师阿拉尔医院	王志强	李　莉				
	新疆生产建设兵团第一师医院	王启伟	卢建华	李　峰			
	新疆生产建设兵团医院	王　丽	宋　宇	张　楠	赵　霞	钱　喜	
北京	北京儿童医院童缘网络科技发展有限公司	王文韬	田艳培	史颖莉	李　志	李月娇	李金芝　徐　君
北京	北京启迪区块链科技发展有限公司	王　鼎　王承馨　卢微微　田成权　田聚宝　付宇杰　吕国财　刘昊哲　李　飞　李亚朴　杨平安　时李爽　吴晓华　余子寒　宋　健　胡　迪　胡国君　段　炜　高云鹏　蔡雪飞　熊小尾　薛　云						

Acknowledgement

National Pediatric Cancer Surveillance Annual Report embodies the hard work of the relevant staff of the surveillance sites, the developers of the national pediatric cancer surveillance platform, and the members of the writing team. We would like to express our sincerest gratitude to them all for their support and assistance in the preparation of this report.

List of the pediatric cancer surveillance sites and the developers of the pediatric cancer surveillance platform

provinces (autonomous regions, municipalities directly under the central government) and Xinjiang Production and Construction Corps	Name of institutions	Main participants
Beijing	Peking University First Hospital	LIU Si LIU Chenlong ZHANG Yan HONG Ying
	Peking University People's Hospital	WANG Li ZHANG Xia ZHANG Xiaohong HOU Xiaoman
	Children's Hospital Capital Institute of Pediatrics	LIU Yihao LI Ying CUI Ying
	Beijing Children's Hospital, Capital Medical University	DENG Zhuo LYU Yaqi SONG Fei XI Yue
	Beijing Shijitan Hospital Affiliated to Capital Medical University	LI Miao WU Yuping HUANG Jun
	Beijing Tiantan Hospital, Capital Medical University	ZHU Xiaodong GUAN Xin LI Xiaoxiao YANG Shu CHEN Jialong
	Beijing Tongren Hospital, Capital Medical University	ZHAO Lili NI Ruyang TAO Yiling
	Peking Union Medical College Hospital, Peking Union Medical College and Chinese Academy of Medical Sciences	LI Zhuo XIAO Juan ZHANG Zhanjie PANG Cheng
Tianjin	Tianjin Children's Hospital	LIU Tingjie MI Liyan XU Aidong WU Bin LIN Hong
	Tianjin Cancer Hospital	WANG Danning LU Pei FU Xin HE Jinghua CHEN Peicui
	First Teaching Hospital of Tianjin University of Traditional Chinese Medicine	XIA Muyi CHAI Gongmin GUO Congrong
	Institute of Hematology & Blood Diseases Hospital, Chinese Academy of Medical Sciences & Peking Union Medical College	WANG Jinyu ZHANG Xiaobin ZHAO Qian
Hebei	Anxin County Hospital	LIU Huan CHEN Xiaoning JIN Kejun
	Baoding Children's Hospital	LI Shangyu SONG Mali PANG Weiwei XIA Mingqian
	Affiliated Hospital of Chengde Medical University	JI Jie YIN Chang GAO Feifei HUANG Huijie
	the First Affiliated Hospital of Hebei North University	LI Wei LIN Hao ZHAO Lijuan LU Jihang

Table (Continued)

provinces (autonomous regions, municipalities directly under the central government) and Xinjiang Production and Construction Corps	Name of institutions	Main participants
	Hebei Children's Hospital	LYU Lige LI Zitao ZHANG Shiqiao GENG Jiangqiao GAO Mingyue
	Hebei General Hospital	WANG Jingjing JI Adan ZHAO Huizhi
	Hebei Eye Hospital	SHI Jingshun ZHAO Kepeng
	Traditional Chinese Medicine Hospital of Hebei Province	HE Fang XIA Fang GAO Xueliang HAN Changhui
	the Second Hospital of Hebei Medical University	WANG Weijie LIU Ruirui WU Duanyang XIE Yang
	the Third Hospital of Hebei Medical University	WANG Chunling KONG Lingwei SUN Yunru
	the Fourth Hospital of Hebei Medical Univercity	LYU Zhuo LI Shumei ZHAO Xiaoxian DUAN Xiaojin
	the First Hospital of Hebei Medical University	LIU Xiaowei LI Ailin ZHANG Linze
	Hebei Children's Hospital of Integrated Traditional Chinese and Western Medicine	XU Xiaodong
	Langfang Traditional Chinese Medicine Hospital	LIU Zhen ZHANG Dayong XU Yang ZENG Ling
	Shijiazhuang Gaocheng People's Hospital	GAN Xiuli SHEN Yanli CHEN Hui
	Shijiazhuang Gaocheng Integrated Traditional Chinese and Western Medicine Hospital	CHENG Yongxin
	Wuji Renhe Hospital	LYU Yuezhen JI Yaqing ZHAO Junqiang
	Wuji Xuekang Hospital of Traditional Chinese Medicine	YUAN Junqing YUAN Xiaolei CAO Qingzhi
	Xinle City Hospital	LI Xinhu ZHANG Huibin ZHOU Yankun FENG Yingjie
	the First Hospital of Xingtai	SUN Shenghui LI Yidan YANG Dezhi CAO Zhifang
	Xingtai People's Hospital	MA Chunyan WANG Junhui LIU Shuxian
	Saibei County Hospital	ZHANG Yue HUANG Wenhua
Shanxi	Sinopharm Tongmei General Hospital	WANG Juan ZHAO Lingfang
	the First People's Hospital of Datong	WANG Peng SHI Xiangfeng ZHANG Shubin WU Jianping HOU Fang HUANG Miao

Table(Continued)

provinces (autonomous regions, municipalities directly under the central government) and Xinjiang Production and Construction Corps	Name of institutions	Main participants
	the Third People's Hospital of Datong	SHI Lifeng SUN Xuesong WU Jiying CUI Yinghua
	Jincheng People's Hospital	WANG Shujing LIU Fang LI Xia GUO Yanchao PEI Yangting
	the First People's Hospital of Jinzhong	XU Jianxun FAN Yunzhu WEN Bianzhen
	Linfen People's Hospital	FENG Xiaofei CHENG Jing LIU Xiaojian LI Bin ZHANG Yinhu ZHAO Min
	Lvliang People's Hospital	WANG Xinfang QIAO Tingting LI Yanjun ZHAO Qiaofeng
	Shanxi Bethune Hospital	LIU Xiaohong CHEN Fang TI Gang
	Jincheng General Hospital	LIU Shan LI Xueqin SONG Weiwei ZHANG Yun ZHAO Hongzhuang
	the Fifth People's Hospital of Datong	DING Pengfei WANG Yinan REN Xiuhua CHENG Hao
	Children's Hospital of Shanxi	WANG Liyan WANG Huili LI Bo NAN Jing GAO Li
	Linfen Central Hospital	ZHAO Juanjuan CUI Xinhong LIANG Xiaohui
	Shanxi Provincial People's Hospital	RONG Jie ZHAO Zhi MU Jingli
	Shanxi Eye Hospital	TIAN Jiaoni HAN Yuanyuan
	Yuncheng Central Hospital	DU Qiupu YANG Xiao GU Yifeng YAO Ye
	Shanxi Cancer Hospital	BAI Wenqi ZHANG Zhenjun CAO Yuanyuan TONG Yalan
	the Second Hospital of Shanxi Medical University	WANG Xiying DU Huili LIANG Zefeng JIANG Min
	First Hospital of Shanxi Medical University	WANG Xinxin LI Na ZHANG Lin CHU Yunsheng
	General Hospital of Taiyuan Iron & Steel (Group) Co. LTD	SUN Xiaoyu ZHANG Danyang WU Yaqian ZHOU Jiangang HU Zhenwei
	Wuzhai County First People's Hospital	WANG Wenjuan DU Yonghong XU Lijuan
	Yuncheng First Hospital	TONG Junfang LIU Haiping HU Ruiying
	Changzhi People's Hospital	LI Dandan ZHANG Yi GUO Ping
	Heping Hospital Affiliated to Changzhi Medical College	WANG Yujiang LI Shaoxia JIANG Lingyan

provinces (autonomous regions, municipalities directly under the central government) and Xinjiang Production and Construction Corps	Name of institutions	Main participants
Inner Mongolia	the Third Hostipal of Baogang Group	YIN Shiqi ZHOU Jinghua FAN Bo
	the Fourth Hospital of Baotou	WANG Xiaoyu ZHANG Hongmei FENG Hong
	Chifeng Municipal Hospital	SHI Ying ZHOU Shengfu GAI Dong LU Ran
	Affiliated Hospital of Chifeng University	WANG Lijun WANG Yanjun YANG Jianling LIN Nan
	Dongsheng People's Hospital	WANG Ming HU Guimei KANG Kai
	Ordos Central Hospital	WANG Mingxia LI Siyu XU Dongrui
	Hulunbeir People's Hospital	QIAN Cheng XU Xinwei DONG Xiuqin
	Huhhot First Hospital	CHEN Yan CHEN Suzhen JIN Feng
	the First Affiliated Hospital of Baotou Medical College, Inner Mongolia University of Science and Technology	WANG Huijuan YUN Yan LI Feifei LIANG Shuang
	the Affiliated Hospital of Inner Mongolia Medical University	ZHANG Zhelin ZHANG Xiaoyan ZHOU Zhiyun
	Inner Mongolia Maternity and Child Health Care Hospital	WANG Xiaoqin BAO Changjun DU Jian CHEN Xiaomei WU Xiaolan GUO Jian
	Inner Mongolia International Mongolian Hospital	SONG Yinglin ZHANG Yanhui GAO Hasibaoligao CAO Linjuan
	Inner Mongolia People's Hospital	WANG Xiangwen ZHAO Caixia HAO Zhihui TANG Guangfei
	Inner Mongolia Hospital of Traditional Chinese Medicine	WANG Lina FENG Xiaojing REN Guohua YANG Xin
	Tongliao City Hospital	WANG Huan LI Ying HAO He CHENG Yan
	Ulanhot People's Hospital	LENG Bingyang ZHAO Xiaozhuang
	Xing'an League People's Hospital	BAI Tao BAO Yinping YIN Jinxin
	Zhungeer Qi Dalu Hospital	LIU Zhiwen HE Liang
	Zhungeer Qi People's Hospital	WANG Li WANG Xiaojuan DONG Yongjun WEI Yun
	Zhungeer Qi Central Hospital	WANG Shengyou LIU Haibo YANG Guofang XUE Zhengru
Liaoning	Benxi Central Hospital	LIU Xin LIU Chunchun SUN Chuanzhu XU Yuling
	the Second Hospital of Chaoyang	MA Li LU Yuren LI Liwei LIN Hongfeng

Table (Continued)

provinces (autonomous regions, municipalities directly under the central government) and Xinjiang Production and Construction Corps	Name of institutions	Main participants
	Dalian Children's Hospital	FANG Haonan MU Huitong LI Li LI Jiexin CHI Lei ZHANG Wenwen
	Dalian Municipal Women and Children's Medical Center	XING Wenjie SUN Xu ZHANG Shiheng
	the Second Hospital of Dalian Medical University	MA Zhihui WANG Shujing WANG Yingjie LI Dezhuang
	Women and Children's Hospital of Jinzhou	LIU Yang SHANG Minjie XUE Zheng
	the First Affiliated Hospital of Jinzhou Medical University	LIU Yongwei JI Si PENG Chunhui
	Fukuang General Hospital of Liaoning Health Industry Group	WANG Siyu SU Yanqi LI Xue
	Liaoning Cancer Hospital & Institute	WANG Yuming WANG Chenyu SUN Ting ZHANG Yifan
	Shenyang Children's Hospital	PING Dan LI Bin YANG Liu XIE Zhenling
	the First Hospital of China Medical University	WANG Xiang LAN Zhen CHI Weijun XU Yunwei
	Shengjing Hospital of China Medical University	WANG Runan SHI Feng LI Ning ZHAO Mengmeng XUE Manquan
Jilin	Gongzhuling Center Hospital	ZHANG Xiaoyan MIAO Xingyu CUI Jialin
	the Second Hospital of Jilin University	WANG Jianghua WANG Chunling ZHOU Yanting ZHAO Xihai
	the First Hospital of Jilin University	WANG Yue WANG Ying WANG Hongliang YOU Hailong LI Yanchun PAN Feng
	China-Japan Union Hospital of Jilin University	WANG Zongqiang XIAO Bohan ZHAO Xiaoyong CUI Yongliang
	Songyuan Integrated Traditional Chinese and Western Medicine Hospital	WANG Yu LI Yan LI Yuanyuan YANG Lixin
	Jilin Province FAW General Hospital	WANG Jue GUAN Xinlei LUAN Jun
	Jilin Cancer Hospital	WANG Bing LIU Wenshu CHEN Zhongmin ZHAO Siyu
	Children's Hospital of Jilin	YU Mingyu MI Guo ZHANG Qiang
	Meihekou Central Hospital	LIU Xiangchun MI He CHEN Lei DONG Fan
	Songyuan Central Hospital	FU Shanshan XIAO Junfeng HE Xinze GUO Xinyu

Table (Continued)

provinces (autonomous regions, municipalities directly under the central government) and Xinjiang Production and Construction Corps	Name of institutions	Main participants
	Yanbian University Hospital	YU Li LI Xiangshu ZHANG Jinyu
	Changchun Children's Hospital	FANG Baozhu LIU Ying LI Beiyan CHEN Zhaoming CHEN Haixia WEI Wei
	the Affiliated Hospital to Changchun University of Chinese Medicine	WANG Wei WANG Yongji ZHANG Xuelian LIANG Fengzhen
Heilongjiang	Harbin Children's Hospital	YU Chunmiao YOU Jia LI Hengxin WEI Hongyan
	Harbin the First Hospital	LI Ruinan QIU Haiying HAO Wenpeng XIE Yunxing
	the 2nd Affiliated Hospital of Harbin Medical University	LI Ruibo ZHANG Zepeng
	Harbin Medical University Cancer Hospital	ZHOU Tingting JIANG Huan GUO Xiangnan HAN Shuang
	Central Hospital of Yichun Forestry Administration	LI Zijian JIANG Dongxu YAO Shuai
Shanghai	the Children's Hospital of Fudan University	MA Qing LIU Xiaoxiong SUN Xiaokai LAO Yimin LIU Gongbao GE Xiaoling
	Changhai Hospital of Shanghai	ZHOU Yanping JIANG Zhizhong JIANG Ling LEI Lei
	Xinhua Hospital Affiliated to Shanghai Jiao Tong University School of Medicine	SHEN Honglou PAN Weihua PAN Shuming MU Jiasheng
	Shanghai Tongji Hospital	WANG Jie XU Hui YAN Liangli
	Shanghai Children's Medical Center, Shanghai Jiao Tong University School of Medicine	ZHANG Yue ZHOU Min HUANG Lu CAI Jiaoyang
	Ruijin Hospital Affiliated to Shanghai Jiao Tong University School of Medicine	SUN Mu QIANG Jiaping WEI Lingyun
Jiangsu	the Affiliated Changzhou No.2 People's Hospital of Nanjing Medical University	KONG Zhijun LIU Yue LI Minhui
	the First People's Hospital of Changzhou	QIU Hui ZHONG Ruiying TAO Yuan CAO Dongmei
	Changzhou Children's Hospital	XING Fengjun LI Yamin ZHANG Yan JIN Jing
	Zhongda Hospital Southeast University	DING Jiali SUN Yunyu JIANG Lingling
	Huai'an Second People's Hospital	LI Jiangnan XIAO Kun ZHANG Jialong

Table (Continued)

provinces (autonomous regions, municipalities directly under the central government) and Xinjiang Production and Construction Corps	Name of institutions	Main participants
	Jiangsu Women and Children Health Hospital	SUN Yuexin CHEN Liang XU Lu PU Yaning
	Huai'an First People's Hospital	ZHU Haiyan ZHUANG Fei QI Haixiao DU Jing GAO Jian TAN Jin
	Huai'an Maternal and Child Health Care Hospital	WANG Jinrui WU Sumei GAO Zibo
	Northern Jiangsu People's Hospital	WU Wenjing WU Hongxing SONG Hui ZHAO Man
	Zhenjiang First People's Hospital	WU Jie ZHAO Nan GU Wei HAN Qiujun
	Jiangsu Cancer Hospital	DING Ye REN Yuyang ZHANG Min XI Wei
	the First People's Hospital of Lianyungang	LIU Weiwei LIU Ranfeng ZHANG Honggang ZHOU Guohui
	Affiliated Drum Tower Hospital, Medical School of Nanjing University	YU Chenggong HUA Lüchun WU Zhimao QU Feng
	Children's Hospital of Nanjing Medical University	KONG Ri TIAN Man LI Chengyi ZHANG Tingting
	the Second Affiliated Hospital of Nanjing Medical University	BIAN Shengjun ZHU Chencheng TANG Yue
	Affiliated Hospital of Nantong University	YAN Weiping SHA Zhenyu ZHAI Lin
	the First Affiliated Hospital of Soochow University	ZHOU Mingyuan XU Jie GUO Haiming CHENG Siming
	Children's Hospital of Soochow University	SUN Wenjing LI Jianqin ZHANG Bingbing WEI Ying
	Jiangsu Taizhou People's Hospital	ZANG Rujin
	Suqian First People's Hospital	YAN Youde ZHANG Cheng ZHANG Xinjing
	Suqian Children's Hospital	LIU Hong LI Xiaohui JIN Zhiqin
	Suqian People's Hospital of Nanjing Drum-Tower Hospital Group	SHI Rui LI Yunhong WU Guangqi HUANG Hongmei
	the Second Affiliated Hospital of Xuzhou Medical Hospital	WANG Hong YE Xiaona ZHANG Lansheng
	Xuzhou Children's Hospital	ZHANG Xiuxiu OU Zhaofei ZHAO Wenjing JIANG Hong
	Xuzhou Cancer Hospital	CAO Mi QI Feng DONG Guanghui

Table (Continued)

provinces (autonomous regions, municipalities directly under the central government) and Xinjiang Production and Construction Corps	Name of institutions	Main participants
	Affiliated Hospital of Yangzhou University	ZHU Jinli XU Yahong WEI Xiaojing
	Jiangsu Province Hospital	SHI Xiaofeng FU Liang LU Lei
Zhejiang	Hangzhou Children's Hospital	LI Caixue WU Ying CAO Lijun
	Affiliated Jinhua Hospital, Zhejiang University School of Medicine	HE Guobin XU Minhui JIANG Guojian
	the Second Affiliated Hospital of Wenzhou Medical University	ZHANG Bo LIN Wei HUANG Zhen XIE Zuokai
	the Second Affiliated Hospital, Zhejiang University School of Medicine	ZHU Xiaohua XU Li CAI Dong PAN Shengdong
	the First Affiliated Hospital, Zhejiang University School of Medicine	HE Jianqin XU Zhou YIN Xi HUANG Jiong
	the Children's Hospital of Zhejiang University School of Medicine	LI Zheming WANG Wei CHEN Feibo YU Gang LIANG Jianfeng TONG Xinfa
	Cancer Hospital of the University of Chinese Academy of Sciences	LI Fangyin WU Youmei HU Man YUAN Boying
Anhui	Anhui No.2 Provincial People's Hospital	WANG Wenjun ZHOU Lin ZHENG Guofu
	Anhui Children's Hospital	YIN Chuangao ZHENG Xinzhi ZHENG Huimin TAO Liangliang
	Xiuning County General Hospital, Huangshan City, Anhui Province	YU Fangjun HONG Qiaoying BAO Jun
	Huoqiu County First People's Hospital	WANG Hongcai ZHOU Bin ZHOU Mingjia ZHOU Kangjun
	the First Affiliated Hospital of University of Science and Technology of China	WANG Hao WANG Nan ZHAO Desheng ZENG Yang ZHAI Fei
	Wuhu No. 1 People's Hospital	WANG Zhong BAO Aizhi LI Fangxin
	the Second Hospital of Anhui Medical University	YE Jun HU Shengying GENG Min XIE Zhiwei
	the First Affiliated Hospital of Anhui Medical University	YANG Xiaoying WANG Anyong ZHANG Yan HU Peng
	the Third People's Hospital of Bengbu	WANG Shengli HU Jianming CHENG Shuang

Table (Continued)

provinces (autonomous regions, municipalities directly under the central government) and Xinjiang Production and Construction Corps	Name of institutions	Main participants
	the First Affiliated Hospital of Bengbu Medical College	FANG Xinlei ZHANG Chao
	Dangtu County People's Hospital	XU Zifan SU Mei XIA Yongwei
	Fuyang Women and Children's Hospital	LIU Dawei YANG Qinqin TAN Fengping
	the Third People's Hospital of Huangshan	YE Shuangshuang ZHU Chaodi CAO Chunhua
	Lai An County People's Hospital	WANG Qing DU Yongyang ZHANG Peilin ZHOU Dewei
	Maanshan People's Hospital	DAI Henghui MIAO Li FAN Qin
	Anqing Shihua Hosptial of Nanjing Drum-Tower Hospital Group	ZHANG Xiaowei CAO Haibao
	Qimen County People's Hospital	WANG Yuxia YE Chunjun CHENG Qibo
	Quanjiao County People's Hospital	MA Min CHEN Yuxiu MIAO Jing
	Traditional Chinese Medical Hospital of Taihe County	WANG Hui LIU Lei LU Bingying
	Tianchang City People's Hospital	LI Xiangbing ZHANG Yongsheng FANG Sen
	Tongling People's Hospital	DENG Yinghu NI Shifeng QI Xin
	the First Affiliated Hospital of Wannan Medical College	MA Lijuan CHEN Xi CHEN Zhenchu
	Wangjiang County Hospital, Anhui Province	ZHU Lachun CHEN Bo
	Yuexi County Hospital	LIU Shaocan YANG Zhibing
Fujian	Fuding Hospital	CHEN Daiwang XIE Jianchun XIE Lianmei
	Fuzhou Children's Hospital of Fujian Province	LIU Meizhou WU Xiaoxia WU Xuemei CHEN Jihe LIN Jie
	Fujian Maternity and Child Health Hospital	WANG Jinji LIN Binbin ZENG Jinlang
	Fujian Provincial Hospital	XIAO Zhixiang WU Xiongwei CHEN Wufan LIN Mei
	the First Hospital of Fujian Nanping	ZHU Junmin HE Quanhui FAN Yunhai LEI Chunyan
	Pingtan Comprehensive Experimental Area Hospital of Fujian Province	YANG Geng XUE Lihua
	Sanming First Hospital	WU Qianpeng CHEN Dexu GE Xiaochuan WEI Hong

Table（Continued）

provinces (autonomous regions, municipalities directly under the central government) and Xinjiang Production and Construction Corps	Name of institutions	Main participants
	Zhangzhou Municipal Hospital	LI Yue ZHOU Jiguang HUANG Qinghua CAI Xiaolu
	the Second Affiliated Hospital of Fujian Medical University	XU Liying WU Yingquan LI Yachen CHEN Wenliang ZHENG Zhaohui GUO Baochuang
	Fujian Medical University Union Hospital	YE Shiyue LIN Ru ZHOU Mei
	The Affiliated Union Hospital of Fujian Medical University	LIN Yonghua TU Xiaoxian XIE Xianyu
	Fuzhou Second Hospital	FAN Yidong LIN Chenyan ZHONG Jiqin
	the First Hospital of Fuzhou	WANG Aling JIANG Yanbin AN Luyi
	Longyan First Hospital	FANG Yong ZHANG Yan LIN Mengzhen XIE Yanmei
	Mindong Hospital of Ningde City	LIU Qingping CHEN Xiangbin GAO Huizi GUO Quanliang
	Ningde Municipal Hospital of Ningde Normal University	ZHU Zhongshou YANG Jing LU Yanyan XIONG Lianlian
	the First Hospital of Putian City	FANG Ping GUAN Jun SU Zhiqun CHEN Shuxing
	the Affiliated Hospital Putian University	CHEN Fang CHEN Xiwang
	Quanzhou First Hospital, Fujian	WANG Youxi JIANG Xinrong HE Qiaoling GUO Mengling
	Quan Zhou Women's and Children's Hospital	WU Yiwei HE Wenqian KE Ruorong
	the First Affiliated Hospital of Xiamen University	XU Yunxiao CHEN Youfen ZENG Wenjing
	Zhongshan Hospital Affiliated to Xiamen University	SUN Anqi ZHONG Xinying QIN Weichu
	Xiamen Children's Hospital	YANG Fenfa CHEN Hao
Jiangxi	First Affiliated Hospital of Gannan Medical University	WANG Li WANG Jingmei LI Hui ZHONG Guixin ZU Guoliang
	Ganzhou People's Hospital	YANG Yunhai ZHONG Chunyang HUANG Yali
	Jiangxi Provincial Children's Hospital	FENG Shan WU Huaping ZHENG Xiaohong HUANG Wenjian
	Jiangxi Provincial People's Hospital	LIU Yu DU Yunyan LI Weikang HONG Weixiang
	Jiangxi Cancer Hospital	WAN Bo DENG Chunhong ZOU Hao AO Huiping

Table (Continued)

provinces (autonomous regions, municipalities directly under the central government) and Xinjiang Production and Construction Corps	Name of institutions	Main participants
	the Second Affiliated Hospital of Nanchang University	LONG Li HE Shuicai JIN Chunlian KANG Ping XIONG Keliang
	the First Affiliated Hospital of Nanchang University	WU Shanshan ZHANG Lianjun HU Suqun LAN Chunyu
Shandong	Liaocheng People's Hospital	MA Lei LAN Fei LI Xiaoli XIAO Qimin HAN Li HAN Yueqin
	Linyi People's Hospital	DING Xiangmei QIU Shiyan CAO Ya
	Linyi Central Hospital	TIAN Wei XIAO Yunxia ZHANG Jingjin
	Linyi Cancer Hospital	LIU Huan LI Hui ZHOU Jianzhong
	the Affiliated Hospital of Qingdao University	WAN Bin SUN Mojian GUO Zhenqing
	Qingdao Women and Children's Hospital	WANG Liyan SUN Zhaoguo ZHA Yulong SUI Yan WEN Wei LI Qiang
	Qingdao Central Hospital	WANG Ling LIU Quanmin SU Tianhui
	Jinan Children's Hospital	DING Xin FENG Guohong ZHANG Ning HU Lingjiang
	Qilu Hospital of Shandong University	ZHANG Luyan CHEN Tiantian MENG Yingxu DONG Yang
	Shandong Provincial Hospital	WANG Dong LIU Ruihong ZHANG Xiyu ZHANG Qingqing
	the First Affiliated Hospital of Shandong First Medical University	WANG Hongmei CHEN Guoqiang GU Yan LIAN Ying
	Shandong Cancer Hospital and Institute	LIU Liyan LI Xirui XU Shan
	Yantai Yuhuangding Hospital	MA Xianying YANG Lei XU Xu XU Jing
Henan	the First Affiliated Hospital of Henan University of Science & Technology	QIAO Jianchao YUE Yutao GUO Kelei
	Henan Children's Hospital	MA Lin WANG Jianshe ZHU Mingyu TANG Youxi ZHOU Yibo MENG Bianhong
	Henan Provincial People's Hospital	CHEN Chunxiao LUO Huizhong HE Rong CHENG Jianjian
	Henan Cancer Hospital	LI Xi TANG Xiance
	the First Affiliated Hospital of Henan University of CM	ZHU He LIU Qi XU Jinjie

Table（Continued）

provinces (autonomous regions, municipalities directly under the central government) and Xinjiang Production and Construction Corps	Name of institutions	Main participants
	the First Affiliated Hospital of Xinxiang Medical University	WANG Nan　WANG Xinjian　JI Danxia　WU Tianci　ZHAO Chunxiao　GUO Feng
	the Second Affiliated Hospital of Zhengzhou University	LIU Zhengxia　SONG Hongyu　SONG Meixia
	the Third Affiliated Hospital of Zhengzhou University	WANG Fang　LI Xinxia　CHEN Chen　CHENG Zhiwei
	the First Affiliated Hospital of Zhengzhou University	WANG Chunjie　LIU Xinkui　ZHAO Zheyi　HUANG Kai
Hubei	Hubei Maternal and Child Health Hospital	LIU Yixin　HUANG Ziming　LU Xinfeng
	Jingmen No. 1 People's Hospital	MAO Qiang　ZHENG Dacheng　XIE Jinyuan
	Hubei Cancer Hospital	WU Kezhi　ZENG Hui
	Tongji Hospital, Tongji Medical College of Huazhong University of Science and Technology	WU Jianhong　ZHANG Ai　ZHOU Wenqing
	Union Hospital, Tongji Medical College of Huazhong University of Science and Technology	WANG Lixia　SUN Yang　HU Sai　XU Shourong
	Jingmen No. 2 People's Hospital	LI Hua　CHEN Xiaojun　ZHAO Rongzhi　XIONG Jun
	the First People's Hospital of Jingzhou	LI Zhenni　ZHANG Xin
	Jingzhou Maternal and Child Health Hospital	TIAN Chunxia
	Renmin Hospital of Wuhan University	ZHOU Tao　HE Hua　XIA Liping　YAN Lijing
	Zhongnan Hospital of Wuhan University	SU Yiwu　LI Fei　YANG Qisheng
	Wuhan Children's Hospital	WANG Yuji　YAN Chunxiang　YU Shengjun
	Yingcheng People's Hospital	WANG Linfeng　XU Qurong　HAN Yin
Hunan	Hunan Children's Hospital	LONG Meiyuan　QU Fang　HU Waiguang　HU Shanshan　DUAN Luxi　XU Xiao
	Hunan Provincial People's Hospital	WANG Ye　WANG Xing
	Hunan Cancer Hospital	SHENG Lu　LIANG Ying

provinces (autonomous regions, municipalities directly under the central government) and Xinjiang Production and Construction Corps	Name of institutions	Main participants
	the Second Hospital, University of South China	NING Wenfeng　JIANG Liangyan　LI Jun
	the First Affiliated Hospital of University of South China	ZHU Zhu　CHEN Xianglan　YUAN Xiaoyun TANG Zaili
	the Second Xiangya Hospital of Central South University	LI Yan　ZHOU Wei　XU Wei
	the Third Xiangya Hospital of Central South University	YU Shanshan　LIU Lin　QIU Lin　ZHANG Jian
	Chenzhou First People's Hospital	XU Bin　ZHANG Zicui　PENG Zhen　LEI Jun
	Xiangya Hospital Central South University	ZHANG Jing　CHEN Jinbiao　JIN Min
Guangdong	Guangdong Women and Children's Hospital	LI Hui　LI Yuping　PENG Wujiang　XIE Jingyi
	Guangzhou Women and Children's Medical Center	DING Chunguang　WEI Xiaoyan　LI Lijuan LIN Xu　CAO Xiaojun　LIAO Shuyi
	the Third Affiliated Hospital of Southern Medical University	WU Weijian　LIU Feng　GUAN Xiaoqian　LI Yun
	Nanfang Hospital, Southern Medical University	ZHU Zhuoxin　DU Yiman　HE Junwei　CHEN Liya
	Shenzhen Children's Hospital	LI Jiaxi　CHEN Xirong　LIN Rongshu
	the First Affiliated Hospital of Sun Yat-Sen University	WANG Yuyao　LIU Yang　LIU Junfeng
	Sun Yat-Sen Memorial Hospital, Sun Yat-Sen University	WANG Mingle　YE Qingxiao　WU Yaohao YANG Hongyuan　YANG Yifan　XIE Lisha
	Zhongshan Ophthalmic Center, Sun Yat-Sen University	FANG Hao　SUN Jianming　RONG Ying
	Sun Yat-Sen University Cancer Center	WANG Yongjie　WEI Wei　ZHAO Yanli
Guangxi	the First Affiliated Hospital of Guangxi Medical University	DENG Tianxin　SHANG Liming　MO Fanglan YU Lixia　LIAO Ning
	Maternity and Child Health Care of Guangxi Zhuang Autonomous Region	GAN Jieze　YE Dingjian　LI Jialin　CHEN Yuzhong RONG Limei　HUANG Min
	the People's Hospital of Guangxi Zhuang Autonomous Region	DAI Yan　HE Zhichen　TAN Lingling

Table (Continued)

provinces (autonomous regions, municipalities directly under the central government) and Xinjiang Production and Construction Corps	Name of institutions	Main participants
	Wuzhou Red Cross Hospital	TANG Weiwen SU Yanghong HUANG Jinju
	Liuzhou Maternity and Child Health-care Hospital	WEI Qingyu LIU Chong YANG Lei ZHANG Yu QIN Chen WEN Xueting
	Liuzhou People's Hospital	WANG Xiaolong SU Junjie TAN Juan PAN Yanfang
	the First People's Hospital of Qin-zhou	YE Hailin WU Dongyan HE Zhenbo ZHONG Wei
Hainan	Hainan Maternal and Children's Medical Center	YANG Quanlüe OUYANG Shanhong WEI Chenhong
	Hainan General Hospital	CHEN Xiaofang LUO Wenlong FU Xiangmin
	Eye Hospital of Hainan Province	WANG Pan CHEN Qiuxiang LIN Aixiang
	Hainan Cancer Hospital	YU Bing WANG Yufen ZHAO Li
	Hainan Hospital of PLA General Hospital	LYU Zhongqi QIU Yu LIANG Yunxing
	Sanya People's Hospital	WANG Jiabin LUO Liping ZHONG Jing
	Hainan Third People's Hospital	LI Wei ZHANG Chunyan FU Guohong LIAO Yage
Chongqing	the Second Affiliated Hospital of Army Medical University	YANG Lili ZHANG Ping CHEN Yu
	Chongqing University Cancer Hospital	LIU Yumin LI Lin WANG Gang
	Chongqing University Three Gorges Hospital	HE Youjun ZHANG Na ZHONG Sheng
	the Second Affiliated Hospital of Chongqing Medical University	WANG Yuting LIU Yi ZHOU Xiaolan DONG Xiao
	Children's Hospital of Chongqing Medical University	WANG Zhuangcheng WU Qifan SHE Ying SONG Ping OUYANG Hejia XU Shibao
	Yongchuan Hospital of Chongqing Medical University	YE Liu ZHOU Changlong CHENG Di
Sichuan	Chengdu Women's and Children's Central Hospital	XIAO Li CHEN Fuqin YAO Haibo
	West China Second University Hospital, Sichuan University	SUN Jingjing LI Li HE Wei GAO Ju
	West China Hospital of Sichuan University	SHUAI Bingxing ZHANG Rui ZHAO Yiyang ZHAO Xiaolong

Table（Continued）

provinces (autonomous regions, municipalities directly under the central government) and Xinjiang Production and Construction Corps	Name of institutions	Main participants
	Sichuan Provincial Maternity and Child Health Care Hospital	PI Guanghuan LIU Xuemei ZHENG Shujuan
	Sichuan Provincial People's Hospital	LI Qinhui LENG Yan XU Chuan
	Sichuan Cancer Hospital	XIANG Mingfei YANG Ying KANG Shengwei XIONG Zhonghua
	the Affiliated Hospital of Southwest Medical University	YANG Changhao WANG Hewei
Guizhou	Guiyang Maternal and Child Health Care Hospital	GAN Shuhan ZHU Xiaoming HE Qinghong ZHANG Shaoyi CHEN Xiaoyun ZHOU Xiaoming
	Guizhou Provincial People's Hospital	YANG Xiulin CHEN Ying NIE Zhao DAI Shiyuan
	the Affiliated Hospital of Guizhou Medical University	LONG Xianzhi LYU Rui ZHENG Mingfeng
	Affiliated Hospital of Zunyi Medical University	ZHU Gang LIU Shifang LI Chengmei ZHANG Jun ZHAO Kaiyan HUANG Xin
Yunan	Kunming Children's Hospital	SONG Rong ZHANG Wenjun ZHANG Hongqing
	the Second Affiliated Hospital of Kunming Medical University	TA Hui LI Tao WU Peng
	First Affiliated Hospital of Kunming Medical University	ZHANG Shaofeng CHEN Guangmei GUO Ruli
	the Second People's Hospital of Yunnan Province	LYU Ping LI Shuangyan YANG Dongping DUAN Zhaoxiu
	the First People's Hospital of Yunnan Province	LI Bo YANG Shouye CHEN Yuan GUO Yu
	Yunnan Cancer Hospital	ZHANG Jinping ZHOU Hai YUAN Zhongqin MEI Zechao
Xizang	Ngari Perfecture People's Hospital	Lamuciren YUAN Yong QIAN Mingyan CHENG Shufang
	Lhasa People's Hospital	YAN Chunlei ZHOU Xianxian HU Zhiqiang
	Langkazi County Health Service Center, Tibet	WANG Liqun Baimazhuoga ZHANG Hongwei
	Linzhi People's Hospital	WANG Rong WU Lisha GU Xiying
	Xigaze People's Hospital	Basangdanzeng Bianbaduoji Puqiong
	Shannan People's Hospital	Dawa WU Xiaoli JING Hao
	Changdu People's Hospital	Gusanglamu SHI Renlong RONG Wenhui HUANG Yu

Table（Continued）

provinces (autonomous regions, municipalities directly under the central government) and Xinjiang Production and Construction Corps	Name of institutions	Main participants
	Tibet Autonomous Region People's Hospital	LI Jimi LIANG Na ZENG Yanbo
Shaanxi	Hanzhong Central Hospital	WANG Zhengwei YANG Hongwei LUO Yi
	Langao County People's Hospital	WANG Min SONG Chunxian CHEN Gang
	Liuba County Hospital	WEN Li ZENG Yao
	3201 Hospital	WANG Yong FENG Rong LIU Chun
	Shaanxi Provincial People's Hospital	MA Wenxia SU Yani LI Ting DONG Rui
	Xixiang Traditional Chinese Medicine Hospital	TIAN Fang SUN Jie YANG Yang MEI Dan
	Xunyang Traditional Chinese Medicine Hospital	WANG Yonggang WU Yuan CHEN Yu
	Shiquan County Hospital	LIU Chunyang LI Bing WU Xiaoyong
	People's Hospital of Tongchuan	MA Yue LI Cheng WU Huifeng
	the Second Affiliated Hospital of Xi'an Jiaotong University	ZHANG Chaoli CHEN Yu GAO Ya
	the First Affiliated Hospital of Xi'an Jiaotong University	LI Xiaoliang YANG Jingyi ZHOU Ming KANG Ya PENG Rong CAI Hongwei
	Xi'an Children's Hospital	LU Meng BAI Ying SHI Junli LI Jing
	Northwest Women's and Children's Hospital	WANG Lijuan MI Yang SHI Jiao HE Chonghui GAO Peng GE Wenli
	Weinan Central Hospital	LIU Tao LIU Shumei CAO Lei
	Xian Yang Central Hospital	TIAN Zhihai SU Kaiyue YANG Rong
Gansu	Dingxi Second People's Hospital	ZHANG Xiaoxia ZHAO Xiaona
	Dingxi People's Hospital	SUN Yanli WEI Yuya
	Gansu Gem Flower Hospital	ZHU Yan REN Fanghui ZHANG Bin GUO Junxian
	Second Provincial People's Hospital of Gansu	FENG Hui ZHANG Lili WEI Hongtao
	Gansu Provincial Maternity and Child-Care Hospital	DA Zhenqiang LI Wei HAN Yuzhen
	Jiayuguan First People's Hospital	DENG Fucang SHANG Yanping ZHOU Ying
	Gansu Provincial Hospital	SHI Yuchun YUN Xiaoyan YANG Yan ZHOU Lei
	Wen County First People's Hospital	REN Yafeng ZHANG Yue ZHANG Rui
	Gansu Wuwei Tumour Hospital	BAI Yongping LIU Yuhua LI Qianghua FAN Lin

Table (Continued)

provinces (autonomous regions, municipalities directly under the central government) and Xinjiang Production and Construction Corps	Name of institutions	Main participants
	Gansu Provincial Hospital of Traditional Chinese Medicine	ZHAO Yongqiang LI Yuanyuan
	Zhang Ye People's Hospital Affiliated to Hexi University	YAN Cuilan YANG Faying ZHANG Jianping ZHOU Chen
	Lanzhou University Second Hospital	SHI Xiaoyuan SU Ming WU Xiaolu CHEN Jingli
	the First Hospital of Lanzhou University	LU Zhenzhen ZHAO Yue ZHAO Zhengbin CUI Qi
	Liangdang County People's Hospital	WANG Jinlin LIN Lin
	the People's Hospital of Linxia Hui Autonomous Prefecture	MA Li WANG Guixiu ZONG Xue JIANG Yuhong
	Minqin County People's Hospital	WANG Fu CHANG Jianping
	First People's Hospital of Tianshui	WANG Suxia LIU Ting LI Jingwen ZHAO Li
	Wuwei People's Hospital	WANG Yongzhu XU Yanrun GAO Wanqi
	Zhangye Second People's Hospital	FENG Yuting ZHANG Xiliu XU Buxuan
Qinghai	Qinghai University Affiliated Hospital	SUN Yi CHENG Hui
	the Fifth People's Hospital of Qinghai Province	MA Shengxiang DENG Wenjun LIU Weiyan DU Lan
	Qinghai Women and Children's Hospital	RUAN Lianjun LUO Yanqi HONG Jun
	Qinghai Provincial People's Hospital	WANG Aibing ZHANG Liting DONG Haibo
Ningxia	Maternal and Child Health Care Hospital of Ningxia Hui Autonomous Region	WANG Ping XU Jibao GENG Yuhui
	People's Hospital of Ningxia Hui Autonomous Region	MA Lixu LIU Shanghong LIANG Peifeng
	General Hospital of Ningxia Medical University	WANG Xuewei FANG Hao GONG Aihong
	the First People's Hospital of Yinchuan	CHEN Jing HE Hongli XU Haiyang
	People's Hospital of Zhongwei	MA Zhongyi LYU Miao YAN Shuzhen
Xinjiang	the Second People's Hospital of Aksu Prefecture	Guhaikezi SHAYIDING ZHANG Daping GAO Feiling
	the First People's Hospital of Aksu Prefecture	SONG Jun ZHANG Rongmin Moheteer ABULIMITI PU Weijuan

Table (Continued)

provinces (autonomous regions, municipalities directly under the central government) and Xinjiang Production and Construction Corps	Name of institutions	Main participants
	Altay Region People's Hospital	LIU Cuiying YANG Ruili
	Bayingol Mongolian Autonomous Prefecture People's Hospital	FANG Yaxin LI Shuhong TANG Lin
	Bozhou People's Hospital, Boltala Prefecture	WANG Yanhong Lanhua Narentuya
	People's Hospital of Changji Hui Autonomous Prefecture	XING Hanwen YANG Beilei ZHANG Chaohui Pareshati JIEENSI HU Chenguo JIA Huili
	the Second People's Hospital of Hami City	FAN Min XIAO Weidong
	Hami Central Hospital	WANG Yiran MAO Suwei PU Yongliang
	Hetian District People's Hospital	WANG Xiaoyang Amangu AIZEZI CHU Wenchuan FAN Chunxin
	Kashgar Prefecture Second People's Hospital	ZHANG Qing ZHANG Suli Abuduwaili WUSHOUER YUAN Jiangbo
	First People's Hospital of Kashgar	Mairiaba SAIMAITI LI Yadong ZHANG Jingwen Abudukeyoumu ABULA
	Karamay Central Hospital	WANG Min QIAN Lijuan DONG Lin LU Xiaolei
	Kizilsu Kirgiz Autonomous Prefecture People's Hospital	XIAO Binzeng Patiguli ABUDUKEREMU XU Xianggui
	Yili Kazakh Autonomous Prefecture Tacheng District People's Hospital	YE Jingbo LIU Yanfang
	Turpan People's Hospital	LI Xueping YANG Qing YANG Jianfeng YANG Xinqin WEI Xuelian
	the First People's Hospital of Urumqi	MA Lijuan Wumuti ABUDUREYIMU Aerdake HANNA CHEN Jie XIE Ping
	Urumqi Friendship Hospital	DING Li DU Chunjin Dilifuzha WUSIMAN
	Dushanzi People's Hospital	DA Chunmei QIN Dongqiang KANG Xiaoyuan
	Xinjiang Children's Hospital	WANG Jing WANG Chunmei Wusiman MAIMAITI CHEN Yan BAI Jing
	People's Hospital of Xinjiang Uygur Autonomous Region	XIANG Weirong WU Lan PAN Yimin
	Traditional Chinese Medical Hospital of Xinjiang Uygur Autonomous Region	ZHOU Bin LOU Pengwei MEI Lin PAN Jing

Table(Continued)

provinces (autonomous regions, municipalities directly under the central government) and Xinjiang Production and Construction Corps	Name of institutions	Main participants
	the Second Affiliated Hospital of Xinjiang Medical University	Gulibaiheremu ABABAIKERE PAN Houmei
	the Seventh Affiliated Hospital of Xinjiang Medical University	WU Fang FAN Qing ZHAO Haiyan
	the Fifth Affiliated Hospital of Xinjiang Medical University	MAO Ying SUN Lili YANG Shumei
	the First Affiliated Hospital of Xinjiang Medical University	LU Wuhong LIU Caihua LI Cheng XIAO Mingsen CHEN Qu YAN Jinghong
	Kuitun People's Hospital of Yili Kazakh Autonomous Prefecture	SUN Yinglian XIAO Zhen CHEN Li JIA Jingru
	Xinhua Hospital of Yili Kazakh Autonomous Prefecture	FENG Yunxia Jiazila SHAWUTI Gerili XINBAYIER Tangnuer AIKEMUHAZI
	Yili Friendship Hospital	ZHU Nan LI Fei LI Juan TONG Zhijian
	the Affiliated Cancer Hospital of Xinjiang Medical University	FU Ailing ZHANG Xu ZHAO Ting JIA Huimin
Crops	First Affiliated Hospital, School of Medicine, Shihezi University	WANG Jing FU Yunfeng HAN Rui
	Shihezi City People's Hospital	LIU Mingzhu CHEN Jing JIANG Xinhua
	Tiemenguan City People's Hospital	ZHOU Xiaolong JIA Zhanjiang TAN Xiaoyan
	Korla Hospital of Second Division of Xinjiang Production and Construction Corps	BAI Chunling ZHANG Kaiqi TANG Juan
	the Ninth Division Hospital of Xinjiang Production and Construction Corps	LIU Fei HU Yongquan YAN Shijia
	the Sixth Division Hospital of Xingjiang Production and Construction Corps	WANG Xinjun FEI Wenjing HUANG Ting
	the Seventh Division Hospital of Xinjiang Production and Construction Corps	LI Sumei ZHOU Zhibin ZHAO Chencheng
	the Third Division Hospital of Xinjiang Production and Construction Corps	WANG Liying Mayila MAIMAITIMING XIAO Lan

Table (Continued)

provinces (autonomous regions, municipalities directly under the central government) and Xinjiang Production and Construction Corps	Name of institutions	Main participants
	Xinjiang Production and Construction Corps 13 Division Red Star Hospital	AN Puguang ZHAO Yanling JIANG Li
	XPCC Tenth Division Beitun Hospital	SUN Jinxia LI Juanjuan SHAO Jing
	the Fourth Division Hospital of Xinjiang Production and Construction Corps	LI Xiaoling ZHANG Huiping HAO Siting
	Alar Hospital of the First Division of Xinjiang Production and Construction Crops	WANG Zhiqiang LI Li
	the First Division Hospital of Xinjiang Production and Construction Corps	WANG Qiwei LU Jianhua LI Feng
	Hospital of Xinjiang Production and Construction Corps	WANG Li SONG Yu ZHANG Nan ZHAO Xia QIAN Xi
Beijing	BCH Tongyuan network CO. LTD	WANG Wentao TIAN Yanpei SHI Yingli LI Zhi LI Yuejiao LI Jinzhi XU Jun
Beijing	Beijing Tus Data Asset Co., Ltd.	WANG Ding WANG Chengxin LU Weiwei TIAN Chengquan TIAN Jubao FU Yujie LYU Guocai LIU Haozhe LI Fei LI Yapu YANG Pingan SHI Lishuang WU Xiaohua YU Zihan SONG Jian HU Di HU Guojun DUAN Wei GAO Yunpeng CAI Xuefei XIONG Xiaowei XUE Yun

目 录

Contents

第一章

国家儿童肿瘤监测工作政策背景、目标与任务

Chapter 1

Policy background, objectives and tasks of National Pediatric Cancer Surveillance

1 国家儿童肿瘤监测工作的政策背景

癌症是严重威胁我国居民健康的重要疾病，目前位居我国居民死亡原因的首位。党中央、国务院高度重视癌症防治工作，习近平总书记就癌症防治工作做出重要指示和批示要求；李克强总理在 2019 年政府工作报告中指出：我国受癌症困扰的家庭以千万计，要实施癌症防治行动，推进预防筛查、早诊早治和科研攻关。2019 年 2 月，国务院常务会议部署癌症防治重点工作中提出："要强化癌症早期筛查和早诊早治工作，建立健全癌症诊疗体系，加大癌症防治用药保障力度；下一步要健全肿瘤登记报告制度、加快推进癌症早期筛查和早诊早治、提升基层专业能力、加大防癌抗癌科普宣传；特别强调推动儿童肿瘤学科的发展，加强相关专业人力资源的配备，全面提高肿瘤诊疗各相关学科能力。"

1 Policy background of National Pediatric Cancer Surveillance

Cancer is a serious disease that greatly threatens Chinese people's health, and it is currently the leading cause of death among the Chinese people. The Central Committee of the Communist Party of China and the State Council attach great importance to cancer prevention and control, on which General Secretary Xi Jinping has made important instructions and requirement. Premier Li Keqiang pointed out in the 2019 Government Work Report: tens of thousands of families in China have been affected by cancer. It is necessary to carry out cancer prevention and screening, early diagnosis and early treatment, and scientific research to tackle relevant critical problems. It was proposed at the executive meeting of the State Council in February 2019 concerning the vital work of cancer prevention and treatment: "it is necessary to strengthen early screening and early diagnosis and treatment of cancer, establish and improve the system of diagnosis and treatment of cancer, and strengthen the protection of drugs for prevention and treatment of cancer. The next step is to improve the cancer registration and reporting system, speed up the promotion of early screening and early diagnosis and treatment of cancer, enhance the professional capacity at the primary level, and increase the publicity of anti-cancer science. Particular emphasis is placed on promoting pediatric oncology, strengthening the allocation of relevant professional human resources, and comprehensively improving the ability of various disciplines related to cancer diagnosis and treatment."

2019年6月12日，国家卫生健康委员会（以下简称国家卫生健康委）批复国家儿童医学中心（北京）首都医科大学附属北京儿童医院成立国家儿童肿瘤监测中心（以下简称监测中心），建立儿童肿瘤监测体系，开展全国儿童肿瘤监测工作。2019年7月31日，国家卫生健康委等五部委联合发布《关于开展儿童血液病、恶性肿瘤医疗救治及保障管理工作的通知》（国卫医发〔2019〕50号），明确提出"完善诊疗体系，提高救治管理水平；完善药品供应和综合保障制度"。2019年9月17日，国家卫生健康委办公厅发布《关于做好儿童血液病、恶性肿瘤诊疗信息登记管理工作的通知》（国卫办医函〔2019〕737号），提出"高度重视信息登记工作，积极推进监测平台与全民健康信息平台及医疗机构院内信息系统的对接"。2020年1月14日，国家卫生健康委办公厅发布《关于进一步做好儿童重大疾病救治管理工作的通知》（国卫办医函〔2020〕22号），明确提出"持续推进做好信息登记工作，明确信息登记责任主体，加强对登记数据信息的利用"。

On June 12, 2019, the National Health Commission (hereinafter referred to as the NHC) approved the National Center for Children's Health (Beijing), Beijing Children's Hospital, Capital Medical University to establish the National Center for Pediatric Cancer Surveillance (hereinafter referred to as the NCPCS) that serves to build a children's cancer surveillance system and carry out national child cancer surveillance. On July 31, 2019, the NHC and other five ministries jointly issued *The Notice on the Medical Treatment and Security Management of Children's Hematological Diseases and Cancers* (Medical Letter No.50 of the NHC [2019]), clearly put forward "improve the diagnostics and therapeutics, improve the management and treatment level; improve the drug supply and comprehensive security system." On September 17, 2019, the General Office of the NHC issued *The Circular on the Registration and Management of Diagnostic and Therapeutic Information of Children's Hematological Diseases and Cancers* (Medical Letter No. 737 of the NHC [2019]), which proposed that "great attention should be paid to the work of information registration. The surveillance platform's docking with the universal health information platform and medical institutions'hospital information system should be actively promoted." On January 14, 2020, the General Office of the NHC issued *The Notice on Doing a Better Job in the Treatment and Management of Major Pediatric Diseases* (Medical Letter No. 22 of the NHC [2020]), clearly proposing to "continue to promote information registration, clarify the main body of responsibility for information registration, and strengthen the use of registration data and information."

2 国家儿童肿瘤监测工作的总目标

国家儿童肿瘤监测工作是以医院为基础,以儿童肿瘤诊疗机构为儿童肿瘤监测点(以下简称监测点),开展监测点直报监测中心的两级病例信息登记,逐步建立国家儿童肿瘤监测数据库,完善与人群死因、癌症等相关监测系统的信息互通和共享机制,为国家儿童肿瘤防控工作提供全面、科学、精准的数据支撑(图 1-2-1)。

2 The overall goal of National Pediatric Cancer Surveillance

The national pediatric cancer surveillance is hospital-based, with pediatric cancer medical institutions as pediatric cancer surveillance sites (hereinafter referred to as the surveillance sites). The surveillance sites directly report to the NCPCS for two-level case information registration. A national children's cancer surveillance database is gradually established, and a mechanism is improved for information exchange and sharing of the cause of death and cancer, together with other related monitoring systems, thus providing comprehensive, scientific, and accurate data support for national children's cancer prevention and control work (Figure 1-2-1).

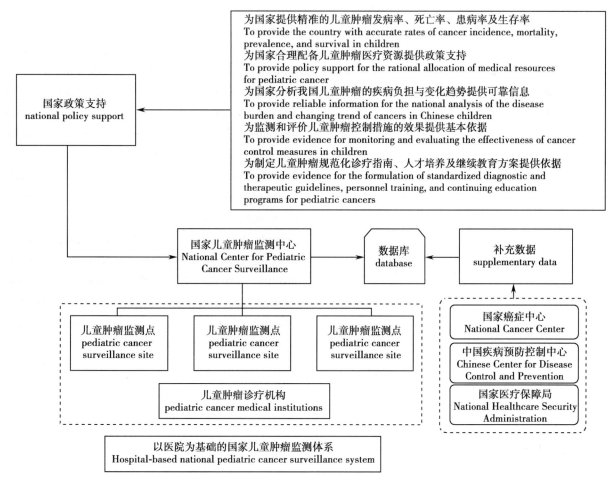

图 1-2-1　国家儿童肿瘤监测体系

Figure 1-2-1　National Pediatric Cancer Surveillance System

3　国家儿童肿瘤监测工作的主要任务

为国家提供儿童肿瘤的发病率、死亡率、患病率及生存率等指标，以及诊断信息、治疗方法、效果评价、不良反应、生存信息等内容，掌握我国儿童肿瘤的疾病负担与变化趋势。

为国家提供区域内诊疗机构儿童肿瘤就诊患儿的概况和动态，向国家提出合理调配儿童肿瘤医疗资源如人员、病床和相关设施的依据与建议，提升区域内儿童肿瘤诊疗、护理的可及性。

为国家提供诊疗机构对肿瘤患儿的诊治和护理状况、水平及效果；对医院开展的新技术、新方法进行追踪随访，科学评估其开展情况及效果，为监测和评价儿童肿瘤控制措施的效果提供基本依据。

为儿童肿瘤临床数据分析研究、大型队列研究、早诊早治工作等奠定基础；为儿童肿瘤病因、临床诊疗、预后、预防等研究提供数据基础；为制定儿童肿瘤规范化诊疗指南、专科人才培养及继续教育方案提供数据支撑。

3　The main tasks of National Pediatric Cancer Surveillance

To provide the country with indicators such as incidence, mortality, prevalence, and survival rate of children with cancer, as well as diagnostic information, therapeutic methods, effect evaluation, adverse reactions, survival information, and help understand the disease burden and changing trends of pediatric cancers in China.

To provide the general situation and developments of children with cancer of medical institutions in the region, to put forward the basis and suggestions for the rational medical resources allocation against pediatric cancer, such as medical personnel, hospital beds, and other related facilities, and to improve the accessibility of cancer diagnosis, treatment and care for children in the region.

To provide the diagnosis, treatment and nursing situation, quality and effect of diagnosis and treatment institutions for children with cancer; to follow up the new technologies and methods carried out by hospitals, scientifically evaluate their development and effect, and provide evidence for monitoring and evaluating the effect of control measures of pediatric cancer.

To lay a foundation for clinical data analysis, large-scale cohort study, as well as early diagnosis and early treatment of pediatric cancer, and to provide data for etiology, clinical diagnosis, treatment, prognosis and prevention of pediatric cancer; to provide data support for the formulation of standardized guidelines for diagnosis and treatment of pediatric cancer, training for specialized talents, and continuing education programs.

第二章

国家儿童肿瘤监测工作方法与内容

1 设立儿童肿瘤监测点

儿童肿瘤监测点设立在开展儿童肿瘤诊疗业务的医疗机构。在国家卫生健康委的政策支持下，全国 31 个省（自治区、直辖市）及新疆生产建设兵团共计 384 家监测点纳入儿童肿瘤监测体系。按照监测点是否为国家儿童血液病、恶性肿瘤定点救治机构划分为定点机构（199 家）、非定点机构（185 家）；按照机构性质划分为综合性医院（295 家）、儿童专科及妇幼保健院（57 家）、肿瘤专科医院（21 家）、其他（11 家）；按照机构等级划分为三级医院（338 家）、二级医院（43 家）、其他（3 家）（图 2-1-1）。

Chapter 2

Methods and contents of National Pediatric Cancer Surveillance

1 Establishment of pediatric cancer surveillance sites

Pediatric cancer surveillance sites are set up in medical institutions that carry out diagnosis and treatment of children's cancer. With the policy support of the NHC, a total of 384 surveillance sites in 31 provinces（autonomous regions, municipalities directly under the central government）and Xinjiang Production and Construction Corps have been included in the pediatric cancer surveillance system. The surveillance sites are divided into 199 designated institutions and 185 non-designated institutions according to whether the surveillance sites are national treatment institutions designated for child hematopathy and cancers. According to their specialties, the institutions are divided into 295 general hospitals, 57 children's hospitals, child and maternal healthcare institutions, 21 cancer hospitals and 11 others. They are divided into 338 tertiary hospitals, 43 secondary hospitals and 3 others by institutional level (Figure 2-1-1).

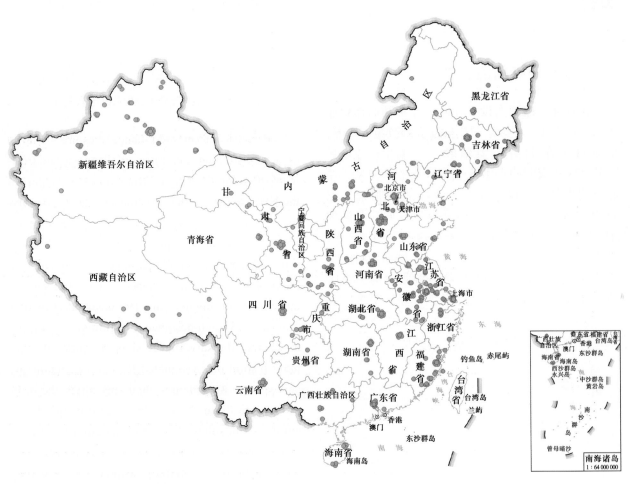

图 2-1-1 全国儿童肿瘤监测点分布

Figure 2-1-1 Distribution of pediatric cancer surveillance sites in China

2　监测信息收集方法

2.1　监测工作的组织实施

国家卫生健康委负责指导全国儿童肿瘤监测体系的建设,组织协调和监督全国儿童肿瘤监测工作。监测中心负责全国儿童肿瘤监测工作的具体实施和推进,对监测资料进行汇总、核查、分析和评价。各省、自治区、直辖市卫生健康委员会负责协调本辖区的儿童肿瘤诊疗机构积极纳入监测体系,监督并定期通报本辖区监测点工作开展情况。监测点负责每月儿童肿瘤病例报告卡(以下简称报告卡)的登记与上报工作。

2.2　监测工作的开展方式

2.2.1　信息上报形式

儿童肿瘤病例登记工作采取网络直报的形式进行。监测中心搭建国家儿童肿瘤监测平台(以下简称监测平台),监测点通过该平台直接上报至监测中心。

2.2.2　信息上报方式

病例登记与上报支持手工填报、文件导入、端口对接三种方式。监测点根据国家卫生健康委的要求并结合实际情况选择任意方式开展工作。

2　Collection methods of surveillance information

2.1　Organization and implementation of surveillance work

The NHC is responsible for guiding the establishment of the national pediatric cancer surveillance system, organizing, coordinating, and supervising national pediatric cancer surveillance. The NCPCS is responsible for the implementation and promotion of pediatric cancer surveillance nationwide, which collects, checks, analyzes and evaluates the surveillance data. The health commissions of provinces, autonomous regions, and municipalities directly under the central government are responsible for coordinating medical institutions for pediatric cancer to actively integrate themselves into the surveillance system in their respective districts, and supervising and regularly reporting the work of surveillance sites in their respective districts. Surveillance sites are responsible for the registration and reporting of the pediatric cancer case report cards (hereinafter referred to as the report cards) every month.

2.2　Implementation methods of surveillance work

2.2.1　Form of information reporting

The registration of pediatric cancer cases is carried out in the form of direct online reporting. The NCPCS has established the National Platform for Pediatric Cancer Surveillance (hereinafter referred to as the surveillance platform), through which the surveillance sites directly report their information to the surveillance center.

2.2.2　Methods of information reporting

Case registration and reporting can be carried out through three methods: manual filling, file import, and port docking. The surveillance sites can choose any method (s) to carry out the work according to the requirements of the NHC and their actual situation.

2.2.3 信息上报部门

国家卫生健康委办公厅发布《关于进一步做好儿童重大疾病救治管理工作的通知》(国卫办医函〔2020〕22号),提出"相关医疗机构分管负责同志是信息报送工作的主要责任人,病案管理部门负责信息登记录入及数据质量管理工作,病案管理部门要商信息管理部门推进信息系统端口对接"。监测点需按要求配备相关负责人开展报告卡登记与上报工作。

2.2.4 信息上报流程

监测点设置报告卡录入员和审核员。录入员负责报告卡导入、补录和提交;审核员负责报告卡审核并上报至监测中心。监测中心负责报告卡的质控、统计等工作,并定期撰写报告、发布统计结果(图2-2-1)。

2.2.3 Department of information reporting

According to *The Notice on Better Treatment and Management of Major Pediatric Diseases* (Medical Letter No. 22 of the NHC [2020]) issued by the General Office of the NHC, "Persons in charge of relevant medical institutions are the main responsible persons for information submission. The medical record management department is responsible for information registration and data quality management, and should cooperate with the information management department to promote the port docking of information system." Surveillance sites shall be equipped with relevant persons in charge to carry out registration and reporting of report cards as required.

2.2.4 Process of information reporting

The surveillance sites are equipped with registrars and reviewers of report cards. Registrars are responsible for importing, refilling, and submitting the report cards. Reviewers are responsible for reviewing the report cards and submitting them to the NCPCS. The surveillance center is responsible for the quality control and data collection of the report cards, as well as the regular writing of reports and release of statistical results (Figure 2-2-1).

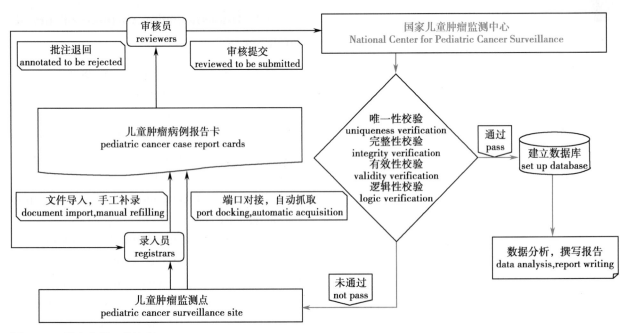

图 2-2-1 信息上报工作流程

Figure 2-2-1 Information reporting process

3　监测信息收集内容

3.1　纳入标准

3.1.1　监测对象

0~19周岁肿瘤出院患儿。

3.1.2　监测疾病

全部恶性肿瘤、良性肿瘤、原位癌、动态未定或未知的肿瘤,以及第一批国家救治病种,包括再生障碍性贫血、免疫性血小板减少症、血友病、噬血细胞综合征。归档后住院病例主诊断或其他诊断的疾病编码(ICD-10)前三位"解剖学部位"符合监测疾病范围(附录)。

3.2　登记变量

监测点根据报告卡进行病例登记和信息上报。报告卡的内容主要包括基本信息、入出院信息、诊断信息、治疗信息、住院费用信息等(表2-3-1)。

3　Collection contents of surveillance information

3.1　Inclusion criteria

3.1.1　Objects under surveillance

Children aged between 0 and 19 with cancer discharged from hospital.

3.1.2　Diseases under surveillance

All cancers, benign tumors, carcinoma *in situ*, dynamic undetermined or unknown tumor, as well as the first batch of nationally treated diseases, including aplastic anemia, immune thrombocytopenia, hemophilia, and hemophagocytic syndrome; the first three ICD-10 digits of the main or other diagnosed diseases of archived hospitalized cases represent anatomical sites within the scope of surveillance (Appendix).

3.2　Registering variables

The surveillance sites register and report the cases according to the report cards. The report cards mainly include basic information and information about admission and discharge, diagnosis, treatment, and hospitalization expenses, etc.(Table 2-3-1).

表 2-3-1 儿童肿瘤病例报告卡主要登记变量

Table 2-3-1 Primary registering variables of pediatric cancer case report cards

主要内容 Main content	变量 Variable
基本信息 basic information	姓名 name
	性别 gender
	出生日期 date of birth
	国籍 nationality
	民族 ethnicity
	身份证号码 ID card No.
	户口地址 registered household address
	联系人姓名 name of contact
	联系人关系 relationship with contact
	联系人电话 phone number of contact
	医疗付费方式 medical payment methods
入出院信息 hospital admission and discharge information	组织机构代码 organization code
	医疗机构名称 medical institution name
	病案号 medical record No.
	入院时间 admission time
	出院时间 discharge time
	离院方式 way of leaving hospital
诊断信息 diagnosis information	出院主要诊断编码 main diagnosis code upon discharge from hospital
	出院主要诊断名称 main diagnosis name upon discharge from hospital
	出院其他诊断编码 codes of other diagnoses upon discharge from hospital
	出院其他诊断名称 names of other diagnoses upon discharge from hospital
	病理诊断编码 pathological diagnosis code
	病理诊断名称 pathological diagnosis name
	ICD-O 编码 ICD-O code
治疗信息 treatment information	主要手术操作编码 code of main operation
	主要手术操作名称 name of main operation
	主要手术操作日期 date of main operation
	放化疗记录 record of chemoradiotherapy
住院费用信息 hospitalization expenses information	总费用 total hospitalization expenses
	自付费用 out of pocket expenses
	分项费用 expenses of each item

注：ICD-O，国际肿瘤学疾病编码（International Classification of Disease for Oncology）

第三章

国家儿童肿瘤监测工作质量控制

Chapter 3

Quality control for work of National Pediatric Cancer Surveillance

1 资料收集阶段

1.1 设置病例报告卡双重审核流程

儿童肿瘤监测点录入员及审核员的设置需符合《关于进一步做好儿童重大疾病救治管理工作的通知》(国卫办医函〔2020〕22号)中"病案管理部门负责信息登记录入及数据质量管理工作"的专业人员要求。由两名专业人员共同配合完成登记及上报工作,录入员在完成报告卡录入或导入后,需通过监测平台的系统校验后提交至审核员,由审核员审核通过后上报至监测中心。此外,通过信息端口对接实现自动推送病例信息的监测点,需配备专业开发人员与录入员、审核员共同完成报告卡的抽查、审核及上报工作。

1 Data collection stage

1.1 Setting up a double-review process of report cards

The employment of registrars and reviewers in pediatric cancer surveillance sites should meet the professional requirements in *The Notice on Better Treatment and Management of Major Pediatric Diseases* (Medical Letter No. 22 of the NHC [2020]), that "Medical record management departments are responsible for information registration and import and data quality management". Two professionals will work together to complete the registration and reporting. After the report cards are filled or imported, the registrar shall submit them to the reviewer after passing the verification of the surveillance platform, who will then report them to the surveillance center after they pass the review. In addition, the surveillance sites that have realized the automatic reporting of case information through the docking of the information port shall be equipped with professional developers to jointly complete the spot check, review and reporting of the report cards with registrars and reviewers.

1.2　开展病例报告卡登记与上报培训

监测中心对监测点相关人员进行病例登记与上报的业务培训、操作培训等。主要包括对录入员和审核员进行平台应用和操作培训,如文件导入的模板整理、版本兼容调试以及审核上报等用户端操作流程。对监测点端口对接的开发工作以及工程师提供技术支持,包括端口对接工作流程、技术要点、开发注意事项以及开发过程遇到的问题。

1.3　明确病例报告卡登记变量与标准

监测中心对报告卡的登记内容和变量制定填报规则和标准,主要包括必填项和条件必填项的填报规则,关键变量的填写标准等。如规定疾病诊断名称及编码使用《疾病分类代码国家临床版 2.0》疾病诊断编码(ICD-10),病理诊断编码及名称使用《疾病分类代码国家临床版 2.0》肿瘤形态学编码(M 码),手术操作编码及名称使用《手术操作分类代码国家临床版 2.0(ICD-9-CM3)》。

2　资料整理阶段

监测中心分别对上报中和上报后的报告卡进行质量控制,主要包括:唯一性校验、完整性校验、一致性校验和逻辑性校验。

1.2　Training on report card registration and reporting

The NCPCS provides professional and operational training on case registration and reporting to relevant personnel at the surveillance sites. It mainly includes in-platform application and operation training for registrars and reviewers, such as template sorting of document import, version compatibility debugging, review and reporting, and other user-end operations. Technical support will be provided for developers and engineers responsible for port docking at surveillance sites, including on port docking process, key technicalities, matters needing attention in development, and problems likely to arise during development.

1.3　Variables and standards of report card registration

The NCPCS has established reporting rules and standards for the contents and variables to be registered in report cards. They mainly include filling rules of compulsory items and conditional compulsory items, filling criteria of key variables, etc. For example, disease diagnosis name and code are based on *International Classification of Diseases National Clinical Edition 2.0* (ICD-10). Pathological diagnosis code and name are based on the cancer morphology code (M code) of the *International Classification of Diseases National Clinical Edition 2.0*. Operation code and name are in accordance with the *International Classification of Diseases, Ninth Revision, Clinical Modification, National Clinical Edition 2.0* (ICD-9-CM3).

2　Data collation stage

The NCPCS carries out quality control of report cards during and after reporting, which mainly includes verification of their uniqueness, integrity, validity, and logic.

2.1　唯一性校验

保证报告卡具有唯一识别编号。根据报告卡的组织机构代码、病案号以及出院时间三项信息，建立报告卡的唯一识别编号。如果三项信息完全相等，由监测点及监测中心专业人员进行识别，决定对其剔除或合并，从而对报告卡进行唯一性校验。

2.2　完整性校验

保证报告卡的关键信息完整无缺失。报告卡设置有必填项变量（如性别、主诊断编码及名称等）、条件必填项变量（如病理诊断编码及名称、死亡原因及编码等）以及其他变量。如报告卡在上报中缺失必填项变量，监测平台即时提醒录入员补充完整后再次上报。

2.3　有效性校验

保证报告卡的关键信息准确、可靠。例如，首先采用身份证号码编码规则及校验位校验算法对身份证号码进行校验，其次对身份证号码与出生日期、性别及疾病诊断的一致性进行校验，对未通过校验的身份证号码进行核查或剔除。如根据出生日期与入院时间计算患儿年龄，对不满足 0~19 周岁的报告卡进行核查或剔除。再如对患儿户口地所在省份进行有效性校验，无法识别患儿户口地所在省份的报告卡退回至监测点，由录入员核查修改后再次上报。

2.1　Uniqueness verification

Every report card must have a unique identification number, composed of the organization code, medical record number, and discharge time. If the three items of information are identical, staff at the surveillance sites and the NCPCS will identify them and decide whether to delete or merge them, thereby verifying the uniqueness of the report cards.

2.2　Integrity verification

Key information of the report cards must be complete. The report cards are set with compulsory variables (such as gender, main diagnosis code and name), conditional compulsory variables (such as pathological diagnosis code and name, cause of death and code, etc.), and other variables. If any compulsory variable is left unfilled on the report cards, the surveillance platform will immediately remind registrars to refill and then report again.

2.3　Validity verification

Key information of case report cards must be accurate and reliable. For example, the ID number will be verified by ID number encoding rules and the parity bit checking algorithm. Secondly, the consistency between the ID number, date of birth, gender, and disease diagnosis will be verified. ID numbers that fail to pass verification will be reexamined or eliminated. For example, the age of children will be calculated according to their date of birth and admission time. Those who are not aged between 0 and 19 will be reexamined or eliminated. Validity verification is also performed on children's provincial-level regions of residence. Those whose provincial-level regions are not identifiable will be returned to the surveillance sites, and submitted again after verification and modification by registrars.

2.4 逻辑性校验

保证报告卡信息的前后一致性和真实性。例如,按照《疾病分类代码国家临床版 2.0》,对疾病诊断名称和编码的一致性进行校验。如对性别与疾病诊断进行校验,包括男病女患校验和女病男患校验。再如对住院费用信息进行一致性校验,主要包括医疗付费方式与自付费用的一致性校验、总费用与分项费用之和关系的校验等。此外,时间逻辑校验主要包括入院时间与出生日期、入院时间与出院时间以及出院时间与手术操作日期等。对未通过逻辑校验规则的报告卡退回至监测点,由录入员核查修改后再次上报。

2.4 Logic verification

Information on report cards must be consistent and authentic. For example, consistency of disease diagnosis name and code will be verified according to the *International Classification of Diseases National Clinical Edition 2.0*. Consistency between gender and disease, i. e. whether a male disease has been diagnosed for a female, or vice versa, will also be verified. Consistency verification of hospitalization expenses information mainly includes the consistency between medical payment methods and out-of-pocket expenses, and expenses of each item. Besides, chronological consistency will also be verified, including between admission time and date of birth, between admission and discharge time, and discharge time and date of operation. If report cards fail to pass verification, they shall be returned to the surveillance sites and submitted again after verification and modification by registrars.

第四章
统计分类与指标

Chapter 4
Statistical classification and indicators

1 统计分类方法

1 Statistical classification method

1.1 按疾病分类

本年报仅纳入恶性肿瘤,中枢神经系统良性肿瘤的报告卡。参照国际上常用的癌症分类方法(ICD-10),按照 ICD-10 前三位"C"类编码,将儿童恶性肿瘤、中枢神经系统良性肿瘤分为 26 大类。其中,骨髓增生异常综合征(D46)、淋巴、造血和有关组织动态未定或动态未知的其他肿瘤(D47)归入白血病(C91-95)(表 4-1-1)。

1.1 Classification by disease

This annual report only includes report cards for cancers and benign tumors of the central nervous system. Referring to the commonly used International Cancer Classification Method (ICD-10), children's cancers and benign tumors of the central nervous system are classified into 26 categories according to the first three "C" digits of the ICD-10 code. Among them, myelodysplastic syndromes (D46) and other neoplasms of uncertain or unknown behaviour of lymphoid, haematopoietic and related tissue (D47) are classified as leukemia (C91-95) (Table 4-1-1).

表 4-1-1 恶性肿瘤分类表
Table 4-1-1 Classification of cancers

部位 Names of sites	部位简称 Shortened names of sites	ICD-10	疾病简称 Shortened names of diseases
口腔和咽喉(除外鼻咽) oral cavity and pharynx except nasopharynx	口腔 oral cavity and pharynx	C00-10, C12-14	口腔癌 oral cancer
鼻咽 nasopharynx	鼻咽 nasopharynx	C11	鼻咽癌 nasopharyngeal cancer
食管 esophagus	食管 esophagus	C15	食管癌 esophageal cancer
胃 stomach	胃 stomach	C16	胃癌 gastric cancer
结直肠肛门 colon, rectum and anus	结直肠 colon-rectum	C18-21	结直肠癌 colorectal cancer
肝脏 liver	肝 liver	C22	肝癌 liver cancer

部位 Names of sites	部位简称 Shortened names of sites	ICD-10	疾病简称 Shortened names of diseases
胆囊及其他 gallbladder etc.	胆囊 gallbladder	C23-24	胆囊癌 gallbladder cancer
胰腺 pancreas	胰腺 pancreas	C25	胰腺癌 pancreatic cancer
喉 larynx	喉 larynx	C32	喉癌 laryngeal cancer
气管、支气管、肺 trachea，bronchus and lung	肺 lung	C33-34	肺癌 lung cancer
其他胸腔器官 other thoracic organs	其他胸腔器官 other thoracic organs	C37-38	其他的胸腔器官癌 other thoracic organ cancer
骨 bone	骨 bone	C40-41	骨肿瘤 bone cancer
皮肤黑色素瘤 melanoma of skin	皮肤黑色素瘤 melanoma of skin	C43	皮肤黑色素瘤 melanoma of skin
乳房 breast	乳房 breast	C50	乳腺癌 breast cancer
子宫颈 cervix uteri	子宫颈 cervix uteri	C53	子宫颈癌 cervical cancer
子宫体及子宫部位不明 uterus and unspecified	子宫体 uterus	C54-55	子宫体癌 corpus cancer
卵巢 ovary	卵巢 ovary	C56	卵巢癌 ovarian cancer
前列腺 prostate	前列腺 prostate	C61	前列腺癌 prostate cancer
睾丸 testis	睾丸 testis	C62	睾丸癌 testicular cancer
肾及泌尿系统不明 kidney and unspecified urinary organs	肾 kidney	C64-66，C68	肾癌 renal cancer
膀胱 bladder	膀胱 bladder	C67	膀胱癌 bladder cancer
脑、神经系统 brain，nervous system	脑 brain	C70-72	脑瘤 brain tumor
甲状腺 thyroid	甲状腺 thyroid	C73	甲状腺癌 thyroid cancer
淋巴瘤 lymphoma	淋巴瘤 lymphoma	C81-86，C88，C90，C96	淋巴瘤 lymphoma
白血病 leukemia	白血病 leukemia	C91-95，D45-47	白血病 leukemia
其他及部位不明 other and unspecified	其他 other	other	其他恶性肿瘤 other cancers

1.2　按地区分类

我国共计 34 个省级行政区（简称省份），包括 23 个省、5 个自治区、4 个直辖市、2 个特别行政区。纳入本次年报的监测点所在省份不包含中国香港、中国澳门和中国台湾省。本年报地区分类根据原国家卫生和计划生育委员会印发的《"十三五"国家医学中心及国家区域医疗中心设置规划》，依据覆盖面积和人口分布现状情况，划分为华北地区、东北地区、华东地区、中南地区、西南地区、西北地区 6 个区域（表 4-1-2）。

2　统计分析指标

本年报的统计指标主要包括出院人次、疾病构成比、年龄别构成比、次均住院费用、平均住院日。

2.1　出院人次

【定义】某一时期内某疾病的出院病例报告的总次数。

【单位】人次。

【说明】从入院到出院记为 1 次，同一患儿多次入出院记为多次。本省就医出院人次指户籍地为某省份的肿瘤患儿在该省份诊疗机构就医的出院人次。省外就医出院人次指户籍地为某省份的肿瘤患儿到该省份外的其他省份就医的出院人次。

1.2　Classification by region

There are 34 provincial-level administrative regions (provincial-level regions in short) in China, including 23 provinces, five autonomous regions, four municipalities directly under the central government, and two special administrative regions. In this annual report, the provincial-level regions of surveillance sites do not include Hong Kong, China, Macao, China and Taiwan Province, China. According to the 13th Five-year Plan of National Medical Centers and National Regional Medical Centers issued by the Former National Health and Family Planning Commission, the annual report is classified by six regions according to their coverage of area and population distribution, including North China, Northeast China, East China, Central and Southern China, Southwest China and Northwest China (Table 4-1-2).

2　Statistical analysis indicators

The indicators of annual report mainly includes the number of discharges, disease composition ratio, age composition ratio, expenses per hospitalization, and average length of hospitalization.

2.1　Number of discharges

Definition: The number of cases of a given disease reported to be discharged from hospital during a given period.

Unit: Discharge.

Note: One discharge is counted when a patient is admitted by and then discharged from hospital. Multiple discharges of the same patient will be counted as multiple. The number of discharges from a hospital in the provincial-level region refers to the number of children with cancer in a provincial-level region who have been admitted to and later discharged from medical institutions in the said provincial-level region. The number of discharges from a hospital out of the provincial-level region refers to the number of children with cancer in a provincial-level region who have been admitted to and later discharged from medical institutions out of said provincial-level region.

表 4-1-2　地区分类表

Table 4-1-2　Classification of regions

区域 Regions	省份 Provincial-level regions
华北地区 North China	北京 Beijing
	天津 Tianjin
	河北 Hebei
	山西 Shanxi
	内蒙古 Inner Mongolia
东北地区 Northeast China	辽宁 Liaoning
	吉林 Jilin
	黑龙江 Heilongjiang
华东地区 East China	上海 Shanghai
	江苏 Jiangsu
	浙江 Zhejiang
	安徽 Anhui
	福建 Fujian
	江西 Jiangxi
	山东 Shandong
中南地区 Central and Southern China	河南 Henan
	湖北 Hubei
	湖南 Hunan
	广东 Guangdong
	广西 Guangxi
	海南 Hainan
西南地区 Southwest China	重庆 Chongqing
	四川 Sichuan
	贵州 Guizhou
	云南 Yunnan
	西藏 Xizang
西北地区 Northwest China	陕西 Shaanxi
	甘肃 Gansu
	青海 Qinghai
	宁夏 Ningxia
	新疆 Xinjiang

2.2　疾病构成比

【定义】某一时期内某疾病出院人次占全部疾病出院人次的比例。

$$疾病构成比 = \frac{某疾病出院人次}{全部疾病出院人次} \times 100\%$$

【单位】百分比。

【说明】疾病范围:恶性肿瘤、中枢神经系统良性肿瘤。

2.3　年龄别构成比

【定义】某一时期内某疾病在某年龄段的出院人次占该疾病全部年龄段出院人次的比例。

$$年龄别构成比 = \frac{某年龄段出院人次}{该疾病全部年龄段出院人次} \times 100\%$$

【单位】百分比。

【说明】全部年龄段范围:0~19周岁。

2.4　次均住院费用

【定义】某一时期内某疾病的每一出院人次的平均住院费用。本报告按均数及中位数分别计算。

$$次均住院费用(均数) = \frac{某疾病出院人次的住院费用合计}{该疾病出院人次} \times 100\%$$

次均住院费用(中位数):将某疾病每一出院人次住院费用的金额由小到大排序后取居于中间位置的值(如果样本数是偶数则取两个中间值的平均)。

【单位】元。

2.2　Disease composition ratio

Definition: The proportion of discharges of a given disease to all diseases during a given period.

$$\text{Disease composition ratio} = \frac{\text{discharges of a given disease}}{\text{discharges of all diseases}} \times 100\%$$

Unit: Percentage.

Note: The scope of disease includes cancers, and benign tumors of the central nervous system.

2.3　Age composition ratio

Definition: The proportion of discharges of a given disease within a certain age range to discharges of the full age range of said disease during a given period.

$$\text{Age composition ratio} = \frac{\text{discharges of a given disease within a certain age range}}{\text{discharges of a given disease within the full age range}} \times 100\%$$

Unit: Percentage.

Note: The full age range is 0-19 years old.

2.4　Expenses per hospitalization

Definition: The average hospitalization expenses of discharges of a given disease during a given period, calculated in this report by both the mean and the median.

$$\text{Expenses per hospitalization (by the mean)} = \frac{\text{total hospitalization expenses of all discharges of a given disease}}{\text{number of discharges of a given disease}} \times 100\%$$

Expenses per hospitalization (by the median): the middle number when all the hospitalization expenses of children of a given disease are placed in value order (If there is an even set of samples, the median is determined by adding the middle two numbers and dividing them by two).

Unit: CNY.

2.5　平均住院日

【定义】某一时期某疾病的每一出院人次的平均住院时间,本报告按均数及中位数分别计算。

$$平均住院日(均数)=\frac{某疾病出院人次占用总床日数}{该疾病出院人次}\times 100\%$$

平均住院日(中位数):将某疾病每一出院人次占用床的天数由小到大排序后取居于中间位置的值(如果样本数是偶数则取两个中间值的平均)。

【单位】天。

【说明】入出院为同一天,住院天数按1天计。

2.5　Average length of hospitalization

Definition: The average length of hospitalization of discharges of a given disease during a given period, calculated by both the mean and median.

$$\text{Average length of hospitalization (by the mean)}=\frac{\text{total number of bed days of discharges of a given disease}}{\text{number of discharges of a given disease}}\times 100\%$$

Average length of hospitalization (by the median): the middle number when all the numbers of bed days of discharges of a given disease are placed in value order (If there is an even set of samples, the median is determined by adding the middle two numbers and dividing them by two).

Unit: Day.

Note: If a patient is admitted to and discharged from hospital on the same day, the length of hospitalization is counted as 1 day.

第五章
本年报数据纳入范围与分析内容

Chapter 5
Scope and analysis of data in this annual report

1 数据来源

本年报收录全国 31 个省份 313 家儿童肿瘤监测点的登记资料,包括定点机构 184 家、非定点机构 129 家;按照机构性质包括 236 家综合性医院、49 家儿童专科及妇幼保健院、21 家肿瘤专科医院和 7 家其他专科医院;按照机构级别包括三级医院 301 家、二级医院 11 家、其他 1 家。

1 Data source

This annual report contained the data registered in 313 pediatric cancer surveillance sites in 31 provincial-level regions in China, including 184 designated treatment institutions, and 129 non-designated institutions; according to specialties of the institutions, there were 236 comprehensive medical institutions, 49 children's hospitals and child and maternal healthcare institutions, 21 cancer hospitals, and 7 other specialized hospitals; there were 301 tertiary hospitals, 11 secondary hospitals, and 1 other hospital by institutional level.

2 疾病范围

本年报分析的疾病范围包括恶性肿瘤和中枢神经系统良性肿瘤。

2 Disease scope

The scope of diseases analyzed in this annual report included cancers, and benign tumors of the central nervous system.

3 时间范围

本年报采用出院时间为 2017 年 1 月 1 日至 2018 年 12 月 31 日的报告卡进行汇总、分析。统计截止日期为 2020 年 10 月 20 日。

3 Time range

This annual report collected and analyzed the report cards from January 1, 2017 to December 31, 2018. Data has been collected as of October 20, 2020.

4　分析内容

本年报分析了全部恶性肿瘤、中枢神经系统良性肿瘤的病例信息。描述并对比全国、六大区、31个省份监测点肿瘤患儿的年龄、性别及癌谱分布；分析不同省份来源的肿瘤患儿就医省份分布、医疗付费方式、住院费用及平均住院日等（本年报未包括中国香港、中国澳门及中国台湾省的数据）。

本年报将新疆维吾尔自治区和新疆生产建设兵团的监测点病例信息进行合并分析。分析患儿年龄/性别构成时，出院人次不足100人次的省份不展示年龄/性别构成分布图。分析住院费用医疗付费方式时，以患儿户籍地进行六大区和省份的统计。

4　Analysis content

This annual report analyzed the cases of all cancers and benign tumors of the central nervous system. It described and compared the age, gender, and cancer spectra of children with cancer in the surveillance sites in the 31 provincial-level regions in six regions in China. It analyzed the provincial distribution of medical treatment, medical payment methods, hospitalization expenses, and average lengths of hospitalization of children with cancer in different provincial-level regions (the data of Hong Kong, China, Macao, China and Taiwan Province, China were not included in this annual report).

This annual report had combined the analysis of the case information from surveillance sites in Xinjiang Uygur Autonomous Region and Xinjiang Production and Construction Corps. In the analysis of age/gender composition of patients, the diagrams were not shown for the province-level regions with less than 100 discharges. In the analysis of medical payment methods for hospitalization expenses, the statistics had been collected from the six regions and from provincial-level regions according to patients' registered places of residence.

第六章

本年报数据质量控制结果

Chapter 6

Results after data quality control in this annual report

通过对上报中的报告卡质量控制后，共计有 339 741 张报告卡纳入监测数据库。监测中心根据本中心质控方案（第三章），参考全国三级公立医院绩效考核与医疗质量管理住院病案首页采集系统对接接口标准（2019 年）的标准，以及世界卫生组织国际癌症研究署的肿瘤资料登记质量控制标准；采用 EXCEL、SAS9.4 等软件对报告卡进行整理；最终 329 093 张报告卡纳入年报，纳入率为 96.87%（表 6-0-1，图 6-0-1，表 6-0-2）。

A total of 339, 741 report cards were included in the surveillance database after quality control according to the quality control plan of the NCPCS (Chapter 3), the docking standard for the collection system of first-page information of in-patient medical records in the performance appraisal and medical quality management of national tertiary public hospitals (2019), and the quality control standard for cancer data registration of the International Agency for Research on Cancer (IARC) of the World Health Organization. The report cards were then sorted out via EXCEL, SAS9.4 and other software. Finally, 329, 093 report cards were included in the annual report, with an inclusion rate of 96.87% (Table 6-0-1, Figure 6-0-1, Table 6-0-2).

表 6-0-1　全国六大区及各省份报告卡纳入情况统计表

Table 6-0-1　Statistics on the inclusion of report cards in provincial-level regions and in the six regions

地区 / 省份 Region/provincial-level regions	报告卡数量 Number of report cards	纳入数量 Number of report cards included	纳入率 /% Inclusion rate/%
全国合计 National total	339 741	329 093	96.87
华北地区 North China	91 062	89 507	98.29
北京 Beijing	75 024	74 288	99.02
天津 Tianjin	3 284	3 135	95.46
河北 Hebei	6 932	6 513	93.96
山西 Shanxi	4 097	3 916	95.58
内蒙古 Inner Mongolia	1 725	1 655	95.94
东北地区 Northeast China	19 000	18 664	98.23
辽宁 Liaoning	10 184	10 026	98.45
吉林 Jilin	7 221	7 111	98.48

续表 Table（Continued）

地区 / 省份 Region/provincial-level regions	报告卡数量 Number of report cards	纳入数量 Number of report cards included	纳入率 /% Inclusion rate/%
黑龙江 Heilongjiang	1 595	1 527	95.74
华东地区 East China	99 147	95 874	96.70
上海 Shanghai	9 736	9 370	96.24
江苏 Jiangsu	25 556	25 003	97.84
浙江 Zhejiang	9 347	8 783	93.97
安徽 Anhui	7 159	6 934	96.86
福建 Fujian	13 487	13 091	97.06
江西 Jiangxi	13 557	13 030	96.11
山东 Shandong	20 305	19 663	96.84
中南地区 Central and Southern China	69 760	66 375	95.15
河南 Henan	28 600	27 133	94.87
湖北 Hubei	10 506	10 275	97.80
湖南 Hunan	8 017	7 550	94.17
广东 Guangdong	16 996	16 076	94.59
广西 Guangxi	2 864	2 627	91.72
海南 Hainan	2 777	2 714	97.73
西南地区 Southwest China	37 048	35 767	96.54
重庆 Chongqing	16 461	15 781	95.87
四川 Sichuan	6 632	6 507	98.12
贵州 Guizhou	5 706	5 479	96.02
云南 Yunnan	8 200	7 957	97.04
西藏 Xizang	49	43	87.76
西北地区 Northwest China	23 724	22 906	96.55
陕西 Shaanxi	10 971	10 719	97.70
甘肃 Gansu	3 256	3 060	93.98
青海 Qinghai	335	318	94.93
宁夏 Ningxia	1 307	1 265	96.79
新疆 Xinjiang	7 855	7 544	96.04

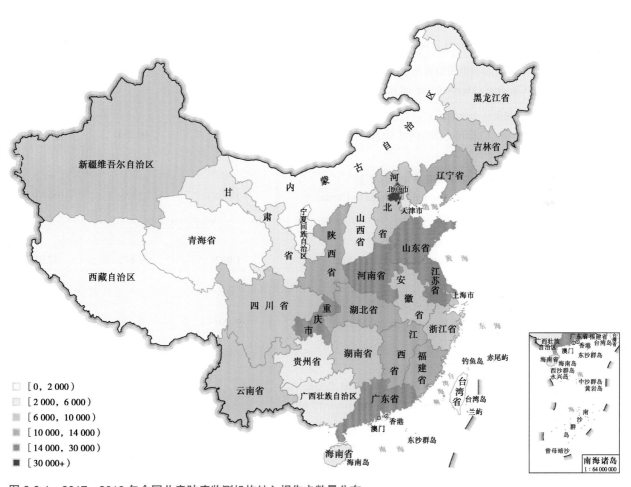

图例
[0, 2 000)
[2 000, 6 000)
[6 000, 10 000)
[10 000, 14 000)
[14 000, 30 000)
[30 000+)

图 6-0-1   2017—2018 年全国儿童肿瘤监测机构纳入报告卡数量分布

Figure 6-0-1   The distribution of the number of case report cards included by the pediatric cancer surveillance sites in 2017-2018

表 6-0-2　儿童肿瘤监测点报告卡纳入情况统计表

Table 6-0-2　Statistics on the inclusion of report cards in pediatric cancer surveillance sites

省份 Provincial- level regions	监测点名称 Name of surveillance sites	报告卡数量 Number of report cards	纳入数量 Number of report cards included	纳入率（%） Inclusion rate（%）
北京 Beijing	北京大学第一医院 Peking University First Hospital	2 623	2 601	99.16
	北京大学人民医院 Peking University People's Hospital	14 956	14 921	99.77
	首都儿科研究所附属儿童医院 Children's Hospital Capital Institute of Pediatrics	2 031	1 974	97.19
	首都医科大学附属北京儿童医院 Beijing Children's Hospital, Capital Medical University	41 081	40 753	99.20
	首都医科大学附属北京世纪坛医院 Beijing Shijitan Hospital Affiliated to Capital Medical University	2 849	2 838	99.61
	首都医科大学附属北京天坛医院 Beijing Tiantan Hospital, Capital Medical University	1 902	1 672	87.91
	首都医科大学附属北京同仁医院 Beijing Tongren Hospital, Capital Medical University	9 550	9 499	99.47
	中国医学科学院北京协和医院 Peking Union Medical College Hospital, Peking Union Medical College and Chinese Academy of Medical Sciences	32	30	93.75
天津 Tianjin	天津市儿童医院 Tianjin Children's Hospital	2 372	2 241	94.48
	天津市肿瘤医院 Tianjin Cancer Hospital	897	880	98.10
	天津中医药大学第一附属医院 First Teaching Hospital of Tianjin University of Traditional Chinese Medicine	15	14	93.33
河北 Hebei	保定市儿童医院 Baoding Children's Hospital	490	402	82.04
	承德市医学院附属医院 Affiliated Hospital of Chengde Medical University	170	154	90.59
	河北省儿童医院 Hebei Children's Hospital	2 880	2 732	94.86
	河北省人民医院 Hebei General Hospital	52	52	100.00

续表 Table（Continued）

省份 Provincial- level regions	监测点名称 Name of surveillance sites	报告卡数量 Number of report cards	纳入数量 Number of report cards included	纳入率（%） Inclusion rate（%）
河北 Hebei	河北省眼科医院 Hebei Eye Hospital	44	40	90.91
	河北省中医院 Traditional Chinese Medicine Hospital of Hebei Province	8	8	100.00
	河北医科大学第二医院 the Second Hospital of Hebei Medical University	1 858	1 800	96.88
	河北医科大学第三医院 the Third Hospital of Hebei Medical University	289	257	88.93
	河北医科大学第四医院 the Fourth Hospital of Hebei Medical Univercity	500	474	94.80
	河北医科大学第一医院 the First Hospital of Hebei Medical University	75	70	93.33
	廊坊市中医医院 Langfang Traditional Chinese Medicine Hospital	133	132	99.25
	邢台市第一医院 the First Hospital of Xingtai	1	1	100.00
	邢台市人民医院 Xingtai People's Hospital	432	391	90.51
山西 Shanxi	国药同煤总医院 Sinopharm Tongmei General Hospital	55	50	90.91
	大同市第三人民医院 the Third People's Hospital of Datong	173	169	97.69
	大同市第一人民医院 the First People's Hospital of Datong	99	99	100.00
	晋城市人民医院 Jincheng People's Hospital	44	41	93.18
	临汾市人民医院 Linfen People's Hospital	98	96	97.96
	吕梁市人民医院 Lvliang People's Hospital	6	5	83.33
	山西白求恩医院 Shanxi Bethune Hospital	161	154	95.65
	晋城大医院 Jincheng General Hospital	3	3	100.00
	大同市第五人民医院 the Fifth People's Hospital of Datong	45	40	88.89

省份 Provincial- level regions	监测点名称 Name of surveillance sites	报告卡数量 Number of report cards	纳入数量 Number of report cards included	纳入率（%） Inclusion rate（%）
山西 Shanxi	山西省儿童医院 Children's Hospital of Shanxi	1 510	1 479	97.95
	临汾市中心医院 Linfen Central Hospital	43	40	93.02
	山西省人民医院 Shanxi Provincial People's Hospital	158	150	94.94
	山西省眼科医院 Shanxi Eye Hospital	3	3	100.00
	山西省运城市中心医院 Yuncheng Central Hospital	134	102	76.12
	山西省肿瘤医院 Shanxi Cancer Hospital	746	714	95.71
	山西医科大学第二医院 the Second Hospital of Shanxi Medical University	643	627	97.51
	山西医科大学第一医院 First Hospital of Shanxi Medical University	158	126	79.75
	长治市人民医院 Changzhi People's Hospital	9	9	100.00
	长治医学院附属和平医院 Heping Hospital Affiliated to Changzhi Medical College	9	9	100.00
内蒙古 Inner Mongolia	包头市第四医院 the Fourth Hospital of Baotou	10	8	80.00
	赤峰市医院 Chifeng Municipal Hospital	393	381	96.95
	赤峰学院附属医院 Affiliated Hospital of Chifeng University	104	89	85.58
	鄂尔多斯市中心医院 Ordos Central Hospital	56	49	87.50
	呼伦贝尔市人民医院 Hulunbeir People's Hospital	30	29	96.67
	内蒙古自治区妇幼保健院 Inner Mongolia Maternity and Child Health Care Hospital	18	15	83.33
	呼和浩特市第一医院 Huhhot First Hospital	9	8	88.89

省份 Provincial- level regions	监测点名称 Name of surveillance sites	报告卡数量 Number of report cards	纳入数量 Number of report cards included	纳入率(%) Inclusion rate(%)
内蒙古 Inner Mongolia	内蒙古科技大学包头医学院第一附属医院 the First Affiliated Hospital of Baotou Medical College，Inner Mongolia University of Science and Technology	157	139	88.54
	内蒙古医科大学附属医院 the Affiliated Hospital of Inner Mongolia Medical University	320	314	98.13
	内蒙古自治区国际蒙医医院 Inner Mongolia International Mongolian Hospital	25	25	100.00
	内蒙古自治区人民医院 Inner Mongolia People's Hospital	468	468	100.00
	通辽市医院 Tongliao City Hospital	14	13	92.86
	兴安盟人民医院 Xing'an League People's Hospital	121	117	96.69
辽宁 Liaoning	本溪市中心医院 Benxi Central Hospital	10	10	100.00
	朝阳市第二医院 the Second Hospital of Chaoyang	92	84	91.30
	大连市儿童医院 Dalian Children's Hospital	102	87	85.29
	大连市妇女儿童医疗中心 Dalian Municipal Women and Children's Medical Center	253	253	100.00
	大连医科大学附属第二医院 the Second Hospital of Dalian Medical University	74	66	89.19
	锦州医科大学附属第一医院 the First Affiliated Hospital of Jinzhou Medical University	39	28	71.79
	辽宁省肿瘤医院 Liaoning Cancer Hospital&Institute	727	714	98.21
	中国医科大学附属第一医院 the First Hospital of China Medical University	1 171	1 166	99.57
	中国医科大学附属盛京医院 Shengjing Hospital of China Medical University	7 716	7 618	98.73

省份 Provincial- level regions	监测点名称 Name of surveillance sites	报告卡数量 Number of report cards	纳入数量 Number of report cards included	纳入率（%） Inclusion rate（%）
吉林 Jilin	吉林大学第二医院 the Second Hospital of Jilin University	215	211	98.14
	吉林大学第一医院 the First Hospital of Jilin University	6 601	6 510	98.62
	吉林大学中日联谊医院 China-Japan Union Hospital of Jilin University	54	44	81.48
	松原市中西医结合医院 Songyuan Integrated Traditional Chinese and Western Medicine Hospital	1	1	100.00
	吉林省一汽总医院 Jilin Province FAW General Hospital	31	30	96.77
	吉林省肿瘤医院 Jilin Cancer Hospital	203	203	100.00
	梅河口市中心医院 Meihekou Central Hospital	4	3	75.00
	松原市中心医院 Songyuan Central Hospital	7	7	100.00
	延边大学附属医院 Yanbian University Hospital	92	90	97.83
	长春市儿童医院 Changchun Children's Hospital	13	12	92.31
黑龙江 Heilongjing	哈尔滨市儿童医院 Harbin Children's Hospital	173	152	87.86
	哈尔滨市第一医院 Harbin First Hospital	33	33	100.00
	哈尔滨医科大学附属第二医院 the 2nd Affiliated Hospital of Harbin Medical University	281	262	93.24
	哈尔滨医科大学附属肿瘤医院 Harbin Medical University Cancer Hospital	1 101	1 074	97.55
	伊春林业管理局中心医院 Central Hospital of Yichun Forestry Administration	7	6	85.71
上海 Shanghai	复旦大学附属儿科医院 the Children's Hospital of Fudan University	9 448	9 098	96.30
	上海市同济医院 Shanghai Tongji Hospital	288	272	94.44

省份 Provincial- level regions	监测点名称 Name of surveillance sites	报告卡数量 Number of report cards	纳入数量 Number of report cards included	纳入率（%） Inclusion rate（%）
江苏 Jiangsu	南京医科大学附属常州第二人民医院 the Affiliated Changzhou No.2 People's Hospital of Nanjing Medical University	18	16	88.89
	常州市第一人民医院 the First People's Hospital of Changzhou	22	22	100.00
	常州市儿童医院 Changzhou Children's Hospital	83	69	83.13
	东南大学附属中大医院 Zhongda Hospital Southeast University	128	120	93.75
	淮安市第二人民医院 Huai'an Second People's Hospital	143	139	97.20
	江苏省妇幼保健院 Jiangsu Women and Children Health Hospital	264	264	100.00
	淮安市第一人民医院 Huai'an First People's Hospital	404	356	88.12
	淮安市妇幼保健院 Huai'an Maternal and Child Health Care Hospital	37	33	89.19
	苏北人民医院 Northern Jiangsu People's Hospital	96	76	79.17
	镇江市第一人民医院 Zhenjiang First People's Hospital	36	33	91.67
	江苏省肿瘤医院 Jiangsu Cancer Hospital	136	121	88.97
	连云港市第一人民医院 the First People's Hospital of Lianyungang	664	621	93.52
	南京医科大学附属儿童医院 Children's Hospital of Nanjing Medical University	9 408	9 211	97.91
	南京医科大学第二附属医院 the Second Affiliated Hospital of Nanjing Medical University	59	55	93.22
	南通大学附属医院 Affiliated Hospital of Nantong University	60	54	90.00
	苏州大学附属第一医院 the First Affiliated Hospital of Soochow University	484	472	97.52

续表 Table（Continued）

省份 Provincial- level regions	监测点名称 Name of surveillance sites	报告卡数量 Number of report cards	纳入数量 Number of report cards included	纳入率（%） Inclusion rate（%）
江苏 Jiangsu	苏州大学附属儿童医院 Children's Hospital of Soochow University	12 946	12 847	99.24
	宿迁市第一人民医院 Suqian First People's Hospital	49	40	81.63
	宿迁市人民医院 Suqian People's Hospital of Nanjing Drum-Tower Hospital Group	50	42	84.00
	徐州医科大学第二附属医院 the Second Affiliated Hospital of Xuzhou Medical Hospital	6	6	100.00
	徐州市儿童医院 Xuzhou Children's Hospital	364	333	91.48
	徐州市肿瘤医院 Xuzhou Cancer Hospital	69	56	81.16
	扬州大学附属医院 Affiliated Hospital of Yangzhou University	30	17	56.67
浙江 Zhejiang	杭州市儿童医院 Hangzhou Children's Hospital	24	18	75.00
	浙江大学医学院附属金华医院 Affiliated Jinhua Hospital, Zhejiang University School of Medicine	297	282	94.95
	温州医科大学附属第二医院 the Second Affiliated Hospital of Wenzhou Medical University	2 542	2 467	97.05
	浙江大学医学院附属第二医院 the Second Affiliated Hospital, Zhejiang University School of Medicine	172	148	86.05
	浙江大学医学院附属第一医院 the First Affiliated Hospital, Zhejiang University School of Medicine	1 879	1 833	97.55
	浙江大学医学院附属儿童医院 the Children's Hospital of Zhejiang University School of Medicine	3 813	3 424	89.80
	中国科学院大学附属肿瘤医院 Cancer Hospital of the University of Chinese Academy of Sciences	620	611	98.55

续表 Table（Continued）

省份 Provincial- level regions	监测点名称 Name of surveillance sites	报告卡数量 Number of report cards	纳入数量 Number of report cards included	纳入率（%） Inclusion rate（%）
安徽 Anhui	安徽省第二人民医院 Anhui No.2 Provincial People's Hospital	15	12	80.00
	安徽省儿童医院 Anhui Children's Hospital	439	377	85.88
	霍邱县第一人民医院 Huoqiu County First People's Hospital	5	2	40.00
	中国科学技术大学附属第一医院 the First Affiliated Hospital of University of Science and Technology of China	930	875	94.09
	芜湖市第一人民医院 Wuhu No.1 People's Hospital	13	8	61.54
	安徽医科大学第二附属医院 the Second Hospital of Anhui Medical University	4 510	4 484	99.42
	安徽医科大学第一附属医院 the First Affiliated Hospital of Anhui Medical University	723	722	99.86
	蚌埠市第三人民医院 the Third People's Hospital of Bengbu	7	7	100.00
	蚌埠医学院第一附属医院 the First Affiliated Hospital of Bengbu Medical College	327	271	82.87
	阜阳市妇女儿童医院 Fuyang Women and Children's Hospital	33	28	84.85
	马鞍山市人民医院 Maanshan People's Hospital	24	23	95.83
	南京鼓楼医院集团安庆市石化医院 Anqing Shihua Hosptial of Nanjing Drum-Tower Hospital Group	1	1	100.00
	太和县中医院 Traditional Chinese Medical Hospital of Taihe County	33	32	96.97
	天长市人民医院 Tianchang City People's Hospital	4	0	0.00
	铜陵市人民医院 Tongling People's Hospital	19	16	84.21
	皖南医学院第一附属医院 the First Affiliated Hospital of Wannan Medical College	76	76	100.00

省份 Provincial- level regions	监测点名称 Name of surveillance sites	报告卡数量 Number of report cards	纳入数量 Number of report cards included	纳入率（%） Inclusion rate（%）
福建 Fujian	福鼎市医院 Fuding Hospital	18	14	77.78
	福建省福州儿童医院 Fuzhou Children's Hospital of Fujian Province	450	428	95.11
	福建省妇幼保健院 Fujian Maternity and Child Health Hospital	84	75	89.29
	福建省立医院 Fujian Provincial Hospital	21	21	100.00
	福建省南平市第一医院 the First Hospital of Fujian Nanping	117	89	76.07
	三明市第一医院 Sanming First Hospital	73	72	98.63
	漳州市医院 Zhangzhou Municipal Hospital	395	361	91.39
	福建医科大学附属第二医院 the Second Affiliated Hospital of Fujian Medical University	68	57	83.82
	福建医科大学附属第一医院 the First Affiliated Hospital of Fujian Medical University	784	729	92.98
	福建医科大学附属协和医院 Fujian Medical University Union Hospital	7 205	7 181	99.67
	福州市第二医院 Fuzhou Second Hospital	97	76	78.35
	福州市第一医院 the First Hospital of Fuzhou	3	1	33.33
	福建省龙岩市第一医院 Longyan First Hospital	81	70	86.42
	宁德市闽东医院 Mindong Hospital of Ningde City	55	40	72.73
	宁德师范学院附属宁德市医院 Ningde Municipal Hospital of Ningde Normal University	24	23	95.83
	莆田市第一医院 the First Hospital of Putian City	172	142	82.56
	莆田学院附属医院 the Affiliated Hospital Putian University	92	90	97.83
	泉州市第一医院 Quanzhou First Hospital，Fujian	1 098	1 068	97.27

续表 Table（Continued）

省份 Provincial- level regions	监测点名称 Name of surveillance sites	报告卡数量 Number of report cards	纳入数量 Number of report cards included	纳入率（%） Inclusion rate（%）
福建 Fujian	泉州市儿童医院 Quan Zhou Women's and Children's Hospital	98	87	88.78
	厦门大学附属第一医院 the First Affiliated Hospital of Xiamen University	2 394	2 356	98.41
	厦门大学附属中山医院 Zhongshan Hospital Affiliated to Xiamen University	85	73	85.88
	厦门市儿童医院 Xiamen Children's Hospital	73	38	52.05
江西 Jiangxi	赣南医学院第一附属医院 First Affiliated Hospital of Gannan Medical University	1 983	1 939	97.78
	江西省赣州市人民医院 Ganzhou People's Hospital	232	227	97.84
	江西省儿童医院 Jiangxi Provincial Children's Hospital	7 763	7 538	97.10
	江西省人民医院 Jiangxi Provincial People's Hospital	230	200	86.96
	江西省肿瘤医院 Jiangxi Cancer Hospital	824	783	95.02
	南昌大学第二附属医院 the Second Affiliated Hospital of Nanchang University	279	279	100.00
	南昌大学第一附属医院 the First Affiliated Hospital of Nanchang University	2 246	2 064	91.90
山东 Shandong	聊城市人民医院 Liaocheng People's Hospital	637	609	95.60
	临沂市人民医院 Linyi People's Hospital	2 074	1 960	94.50
	临沂市中心医院 Linyi Central Hospital	25	25	100.00
	临沂市肿瘤医院 Linyi Cancer Hospital	133	116	87.22
	青岛大学附属医院 the Affiliated Hospital of Qingdao University	606	568	93.73
	青岛市妇女儿童医院 Qingdao Women and Children's Hospital	814	724	88.94
	济南市儿童医院 Jinan Children's Hospital	1 037	962	92.77

省份 Provincial- level regions	监测点名称 Name of surveillance sites	报告卡数量 Number of report cards	纳入数量 Number of report cards included	纳入率（%） Inclusion rate（%）
山东 Shandong	山东大学齐鲁医院 Qilu Hospital of Shandong University	5 450	5 344	98.06
	山东省立医院 Shandong Provincial Hospital	5 029	4 922	97.87
	山东第一医科大学第一附属医院 the First Affiliated Hospital of Shandong First Medical University	1 642	1 599	97.38
	山东省肿瘤医院 Shandong Cancer Hospital and Institute	1 338	1 324	98.95
	烟台毓璜顶医院 Yantai Yuhuangding Hospital	1 520	1 510	99.34
河南 Henan	河南科技大学第一附属医院 the First Affiliated Hospital of Henan University of Science & Technology	1 105	1 062	96.11
	河南省儿童医院 Henan Children's Hospital	2 713	2 300	84.78
	河南省人民医院 Henan Provincial People's Hospital	3 080	3 080	100.00
	河南省肿瘤医院 Henan Cancer Hospital	6 220	6 070	97.59
	河南中医药大学第一附属医院 the First Affiliated Hospital of Henan University of CM	56	42	75.00
	新乡医学院第一附属医院 the First Affiliated Hospital of Xinxiang Medical University	1 057	1 001	94.70
	郑州大学第二附属医院 the Second Affiliated Hospital of Zhengzhou University	115	109	94.78
	郑州大学第三附属医院 the Third Affiliated Hospital of Zhengzhou University	515	492	95.53
	郑州大学第一附属医院 the First Affiliated Hospital of Zhengzhou University	13 739	12 977	94.45
湖北 Hubei	湖北省妇幼保健院 Hubei Maternal and Child Health Hospital	53	42	79.25
	荆门市第一人民医院 Jingmen No.1 People's Hospital	142	135	95.07

省份 Provincial- level regions	监测点名称 Name of surveillance sites	报告卡数量 Number of report cards	纳入数量 Number of report cards included	纳入率（%） Inclusion rate（%）
湖北 Hubei	湖北省肿瘤医院 Hubei Cancer Hospital	332	327	98.49
	华中科技大学同济医学院附属同济医院 Tongji Hospital, Tongji Medical College, Huazhong University of Science and Technology	777	766	98.58
	华中科技大学同济医学院附属协和医院 Union Hospital, Tongji Medical College of Huazhong University of Science and Technology	8 059	7 958	98.75
	荆门市第二人民医院 Jingmen No.2 People's Hospital	45	39	86.67
	荆州市第一人民医院 the First People's Hospital of Jingzhou	243	235	96.71
	武汉大学人民医院 Renmin Hospital of Wuhan University	55	55	100.00
	武汉大学中南医院 Zhongnan Hospital of Wuhan University	625	569	91.04
	武汉儿童医院 Wuhan Children's Hospital	160	138	86.25
	应城市人民医院 Yingcheng People's Hospital	15	11	73.33
湖南 Hunan	湖南省儿童医院 Hunan Children's Hospital	3 932	3 559	90.51
	湖南省人民医院 Hunan Provincial People's Hospital	684	652	95.32
	湖南省肿瘤医院 Hunan Cancer Hospital	253	239	94.47
	南华大学附属第二医院 the Second Hospital, University of South China	90	78	86.67
	南华大学附属第一医院 the First Affiliated Hospital of University of South China	375	359	95.73
	中南大学湘雅二医院 the Second Xiangya Hospital of Central South University	2 116	2 116	100.00
	中南大学湘雅三医院 the Third Xiangya Hospital of Central South University	567	547	96.47

续表 Table（Continued）

省份 Provincial- level regions	监测点名称 Name of surveillance sites	报告卡数量 Number of report cards	纳入数量 Number of report cards included	纳入率（%） Inclusion rate（%）
广东 Guangdong	广东省妇幼保健院 Guangdong Women and Children's Hospital	104	58	55.77
	广州市妇女儿童医疗中心 Guangzhou Women and Children's Medical Center	1 790	1 682	93.97
	南方医科大学第三附属医院 the Third Affiliated Hospital of Southern Medical University	200	187	93.50
	南方医科大学南方医院 Nanfang Hospital, Southern Medical University	2 119	2 013	95.00
	深圳市儿童医院 Shenzhen Children's Hospital	3 605	3 316	91.98
	中山大学附属第一医院 the First Affiliated Hospital of Sun Yat-Sen University	2 035	1 907	93.71
	中山大学孙逸仙纪念医院 Sun Yat-Sen Memorial Hospital, Sun Yat-Sen University	4 552	4 384	96.31
	中山大学中山眼科中心 Zhongshan Ophthalmic Center, Sun Yat-Sen University	683	679	99.41
	中山大学肿瘤防治中心 Sun Yat-Sen University Cancer Center	1 908	1 850	96.96
广西 Guangxi	广西医科大学第一附属医院 the First Affiliated Hospital of Guangxi Medical University	213	94	44.13
	广西壮族自治区妇幼保健院 Maternity and Child Health Care of Guangxi Zhuang Autonomous Region	74	50	67.57
	广西壮族自治区人民医院 the People's Hospital of Guangxi Zhuang Autonomous Region	1 299	1 265	97.38
	梧州市红十字会医院 Wuzhou Red Cross Hospital	133	122	91.73
	柳州市妇幼保健院 Liuzhou Maternity and Child Healthcare Hospital	457	445	97.37
	柳州市人民医院 Liuzhou People's Hospital	565	552	97.70
	钦州市第一人民医院 the First People's Hospital of Qinzhou	123	99	80.49

省份 Provincial- level regions	监测点名称 Name of surveillance sites	报告卡数量 Number of report cards	纳入数量 Number of report cards included	纳入率（%） Inclusion rate（%）
海南 Hainan	海南省妇女儿童医学中心 Hainan Maternal and Children's Medical Center	69	61	88.41
	海南省人民医院 Hainan General Hospital	2 455	2 425	98.78
	海南省眼科医院 Eye Hospital of Hainan Province	13	13	100.00
	海南省肿瘤医院 Hainan Cancer Hospital	116	110	94.83
	解放军总医院海南医院 Hainan Hospital of PLA General Hospital	21	20	95.24
	海南省三亚市人民医院 Sanya People's Hospital	21	12	57.14
	海南省第三人民医院 Hainan Third People's Hospital	82	73	89.02
重庆 Chongning	陆军军医大学第二附属医院 the Second Affiliated Hospital of Army Medical University	2 037	1 985	97.45
	重庆大学附属肿瘤医院 Chongqing University Cancer Hospital	385	361	93.77
	重庆大学附属三峡医院 Chongqing University Three Gorges Hospital	176	152	86.36
	重庆医科大学附属第二医院 the Second Affiliated Hospital of Chongqing Medical University	217	205	94.47
	重庆医科大学附属儿童医院 Children's Hospital of Chongqing Medical University	13 601	13 035	95.84
	重庆医科大学附属永川医院 Yongchuan Hospital of Chongqing Medical University	45	43	95.56
四川 Sichuan	成都市妇女儿童中心医院 Chengdu Women's and Children's Central Hospital	1 288	1 275	98.99
	四川大学华西第二医院 West China Second University Hospital, Sichuan University	1 536	1 507	98.11
	四川省妇幼保健院 Sichuan Provincial Maternity and Child Health Care Hospital	16	13	81.25
	四川省人民医院 Sichuan Provincial People's Hospital	2 876	2 829	98.37

续表 Table（Continued）

省份 Provincial- level regions	监测点名称 Name of surveillance sites	报告卡数量 Number of report cards	纳入数量 Number of report cards included	纳入率（%） Inclusion rate（%）
四川 Sichuan	四川省肿瘤医院 Sichuan Cancer Hospital	764	731	95.68
	西南医科大学附属医院 the Affiliated Hospital of Southwest Medical University	152	152	100.00
贵州 Guizhou	贵阳市妇幼保健院 Guiyang Maternal and Child Health Care Hospital	1 508	1 459	96.75
	贵州省人民医院 Guizhou Provincial People's Hospital	1 683	1 631	96.91
	贵州医科大学附属医院 the Affiliated Hospital of Guizhou Medical University	1 311	1 283	97.86
	遵义医科大学附属医院 Affiliated Hospital of Zunyi Medical University	1 204	1 106	91.86
云南 Yunnan	昆明市儿童医院 Kunming Children's Hospital	5 895	5 803	98.44
	昆明医科大学第二附属医院 the Second Affiliated Hospital of Kunming Medical University	155	150	96.77
	昆明医科大学第一附属医院 First Affiliated Hospital of Kunming Medical University	1 003	957	95.41
	云南省第二人民医院 the Second People's Hospital of Yunnan Province	60	57	95.00
	云南省第一人民医院 the First People's Hospital of Yunnan Province	684	648	94.74
	云南省肿瘤医院 Yunnan Cancer Hospital	403	342	84.86
西藏 Xizang	拉萨市人民医院 Lhasa People's Hospital	11	8	72.73
	林芝市人民医院 Linzhi People's Hospital	1	1	100.00
	日喀则市人民医院 Xigaze People's Hospital	23	22	95.65
	昌都市人民医院 Changdu People's Hospital	2	0	0.00
	西藏自治区人民医院 Tibet Autonomous Region People's Hospital	12	12	100.00

续表 Table（Continued）

省份 Provincial- level regions	监测点名称 Name of surveillance sites	报告卡数量 Number of report cards	纳入数量 Number of report cards included	纳入率（%） Inclusion rate（%）
陕西 Shaanxi	汉中市中心医院 Hanzhong Central Hospital	44	29	65.91
	三二〇一医院 3201 Hospital	166	155	93.37
	陕西省人民医院 Shaanxi Provincial People's Hospital	110	89	80.91
	西乡县中医医院 Xixiang Traditional Chinese Medicine Hospital	3	3	100.00
	石泉县医院 Shiquan County Hospital	2	1	50.00
	铜川市人民医院 People's Hospital of Tongchuan	40	39	97.50
	西安交通大学第二附属医院 the Second Affiliated Hospital of Xi'an Jiaotong University	1 041	928	89.15
	西安交通大学第一附属医院 the First Affiliated Hospital of Xi'an Jiaotong University	462	429	92.86
	西安市儿童医院 Xi'an Children's Hospital	7 735	7 707	99.64
	西北妇女儿童医院 Northwest Women's and Children's Hospital	1 309	1 292	98.70
	咸阳市中心医院 Xian Yang Central Hospital	59	47	79.66
甘肃 Gansu	定西市人民医院 Dingxi People's Hospital	17	13	76.47
	甘肃宝石花医院 Gansu Gem Flower Hospital	6	5	83.33
	甘肃省第二人民医院 Second Provincial People's Hospital of Gansu	12	11	91.67
	甘肃省妇幼保健院 Gansu Provincial Maternity and Child-Care Hospital	377	328	87.00
	嘉峪关市第一人民医院 Jiayuguan First People's Hospital	1	1	100.00
	甘肃省人民医院 Gansu Provincial Hospital	299	286	95.65

续表 Table（Continued）

省份 Provincial- level regions	监测点名称 Name of surveillance sites	报告卡数量 Number of report cards	纳入数量 Number of report cards included	纳入率（%） Inclusion rate（%）
甘肃 Gansu	甘肃省武威肿瘤医院 Gansu Wuwei Tumour Hospital	49	41	83.67
	甘肃省中医院 Gansu Provincial Hospital of Traditional Chinese Medicine	16	11	68.75
	河西学院附属张掖人民医院 Zhang Ye People's Hospital Affiliated to Hexi University	10	10	100.00
	兰州大学第二医院 Lanzhou University Second Hospital	1 923	1 832	95.27
	兰州大学第一医院 the First Hospital of Lanzhou University	516	501	97.09
	甘肃省临夏回族自治州人民医院 the People's Hospital of Linxia Hui Autonomous Prefecture	7	7	100.00
	民勤县人民医院 Minqin County People's Hospital	4	4	100.00
	天水市第一人民医院 First People's Hospital of Tianshui	15	6	40.00
	武威市人民医院 Wuwei People's Hospital	4	4	100.00
青海 Qinghai	青海大学附属医院 Qinghai University Affiliated Hospital	237	221	93.25
	青海省第五人民医院 the Fifth People's Hospital of Qinghai Province	24	24	100.00
	青海省妇女儿童医院 Qinghai Women and Children's Hospital	1	1	100.00
	青海省人民医院 Qinghai Provincial People's Hospital	73	72	98.63
宁夏 Ningxia	宁夏回族自治区人民医院 People's Hospital of Ningxia Hui Autonomous Region	126	113	89.68
	宁夏医科大学总医院 General Hospital of Ningxia Medical University	1 150	1 127	98.00
	银川市第一人民医院 the First People's Hospital of Yinchuan	23	21	91.30
	中卫市人民医院 People's Hospital of Zhongwei	8	4	50.00

省份 Provincial- level regions	监测点名称 Name of surveillance sites	报告卡数量 Number of report cards	纳入数量 Number of report cards included	纳入率（%） Inclusion rate（%）
新疆 Xinjiang	阿克苏地区第一人民医院 the First People's Hospital of Aksu Prefecture	114	87	76.32
	阿勒泰地区人民医院 Altay Region People's Hospital	11	11	100.00
	巴音郭楞蒙古自治州人民医院 Bayingol Mongolian Autonomous Prefecture People's Hospital	35	25	71.43
	博尔塔拉州博州人民医院 Bozhou Peoples Hospital，Boltala Prefecture	3	3	100.00
	昌吉回族自治州人民医院 People's Hospital of Changji Hui Autonomous Prefecture	9	8	88.89
	哈密市第二人民医院 the Second People's Hospital of Hami City	6	6	100.00
	和田地区人民医院 Hetian District People's Hospital	88	88	100.00
	喀什地区第二人民医院 Kashgar Prefecture Second People's Hospital	135	118	87.41
	喀什地区第一人民医院 First People's Hospital of Kashgar	669	639	95.52
	克拉玛依市中心医院 Karamay Central Hospital	11	8	72.73
	克孜勒苏柯尔克孜自治州人民医院 Kizilsu Kirgiz Autonomous Prefecture People's Hospital	30	21	70.00
	伊犁哈萨克自治州塔城地区人民医院 Yili Kazakh Autonomous Prefecture Tacheng District People's Hospital	1	1	100.00
	吐鲁番市人民医院 Turpan People's Hospital	6	4	66.67
	乌鲁木齐市第一人民医院 the First People's Hospital of Urumqi	38	28	73.68
	乌鲁木齐市友谊医院 Urumqi Friendship Hospital	13	13	100.00
	独山子人民医院 Dushanzi People's Hospital	5	5	100.00
	新疆维吾尔自治区人民医院 People's Hospital of Xinjiang Uygur Autonomous Region	2 698	2 616	96.96

续表 Table（Continued）

省份 Provincial- level regions	监测点名称 Name of surveillance sites	报告卡数量 Number of report cards	纳入数量 Number of report cards included	纳入率（%） Inclusion rate（%）
新疆 Xinjiang	新疆维吾尔自治区中医医院 Traditional Chinese Medical Hospital of Xinjiang Uygur Autonomous Region	17	16	94.12
	新疆医科大学第二附属医院 the Sencond Affiliated Hospital of Xinjiang Medical University	13	11	84.62
	新疆医科大学第五附属医院 the Fifth Affiliated Hospital of Xinjiang Medical University	1	1	100.00
	新疆医科大学第一附属医院 the First Affiliated Hospital of Xinjiang Medical University	3 368	3 306	98.16
	伊犁哈萨克自治州奎屯市人民医院 Kuitun People's Hospital of Ili Kazakh Autonomous Prefecture	1	1	100.00
	伊犁哈萨克自治州新华医院 Xinhua Hospital of Ili Kazakh Autonomous Prefecture	62	56	90.32
	伊犁哈萨克自治州友谊医院 Yili Friendship Hospital	95	89	93.68
	新疆医科大学附属肿瘤医院 the Affiliated Cancer Hospital of Xinjiang Medical University	258	253	98.06
兵团 Crops	新疆生产建设兵团第九师医院 the Ninth Division Hospital of Xinjiang Production and Construction Corps	4	3	75.00
	新疆生产建设兵团第七师医院 the Seventh Division Hospital of Xinjiang Production and Construction Corps	4	1	25.00
	新疆生产建设兵团第三师医院 the Third Division Hospital of Xinjiang Production and Construction Corps	7	7	100.00
	新疆生产建设兵团第十三师红星医院 Xinjiang Production and Construction Corps 13 Division Red Star Hospital	4	1	25.00
	新疆生产建设兵团第十师北屯医院 Xpcc Tenth Division Beitun Hospital	4	1	25.00
	新疆生产建设兵团第四师医院 the Fourth Division Hospital of Xinjiang Production and Construction Corps	31	23	74.19

省份 Provincial- level regions	监测点名称 Name of surveillance sites	报告卡数量 Number of report cards	纳入数量 Number of report cards included	纳入率（%） Inclusion rate（%）
兵团 Crops	新疆生产建设兵团第一师医院 the First Division Hospital of Xinjiang Production and Construction Corps	14	10	71.43
	新疆生产建设兵团医院 Hospital of Xinjiang Production and Construction Corps	3	1	33.33
	石河子大学医学院第一附属医院 First Affiliated Hospital，School of Medicine， Shihezi University	92	82	89.13
	石河子市人民医院 Shihezi City People's Hospital	5	1	20.00

第七章

全国儿童肿瘤监测数据分析

通过数据清洗质控,纳入出院时间为2017—2018年的报告卡共计 329 093 张。通过对报告卡主诊断及其他诊断的整理,符合 26 大类癌症的出院人次共计 349 530 人次,将其纳入疾病构成、年龄/性别构成以及就医省份分布的数据分析。剔除费用异常数据后,共计 349 318 人次纳入医疗付费方式、住院费用以及平均住院日的数据分析。本章分别从全国、六大区以及 31 个省份这三个维度对监测数据进行分析。

1 全国儿童肿瘤监测机构肿瘤患儿疾病构成

1.1 全国肿瘤患儿疾病构成情况

在所有肿瘤患儿的出院人次中,前 5 位分别为白血病(57.21%)、不明及其他恶性肿瘤(16.21%)、淋巴瘤(8.15%)、脑瘤(5.63%)和骨肿瘤(3.31%)。后 5 位分别为子宫体癌(0.01%)、食管癌(0.01%)、喉癌(0.01%)、胆囊癌(0.02%)和前列腺癌(0.03%)(图 7-1-1)。

Chapter 7

Analysis of national pediatric cancer surveillance data

Through data cleaning and quality control, a total of 329, 093 report cards with discharge time in 2017-2018 were included. Through sorting out the main and other diagnoses of the report cards, a total of 349, 530 discharges covering 26 categories of cancer were included in the data analysis of disease composition, age/gender composition and the distribution of provinces visited by the patients. After excluding the abnormal expenses data, a total of 349, 318 discharges were included in the data analysis of medical payment methods, hospitalization expenses, and average length of hospitalization. This chapter analyzes the surveillance data from the following three dimensions including the whole country, six regions and 31 provincial-level regions.

1 Disease composition of discharges among children with cancer in pediatric cancer surveillance sites in China

1.1 Disease composition of discharges among children with cancer nationally

Among all discharges of children with cancer, the top five diseases were leukemia (57.21%), unknown and other cancers (16.21%), lymphoma (8.15%), brain tumor (5.63%) and bone cancer (3.31%). The last five were corpus cancer (0.01%), esophageal cancer (0.01%), laryngeal cancer (0.01%), gallbladder cancer (0.02%) and prostate cancer (0.03%) (Figure 7-1-1).

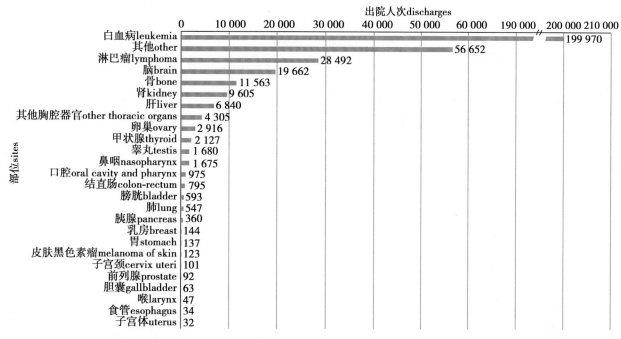

图 7-1-1　2017—2018 年全国儿童肿瘤监测机构肿瘤患儿出院人次疾病构成（按部位计）

Figure 7-1-1　Disease composition of discharges among children with cancer in pediatric cancer surveillance sites nationally in 2017-2018（by the sites）

1.2　六大区肿瘤患儿疾病构成情况

华北地区、东北地区和中南地区的出院人次前 5 位顺位一致，分别为白血病、不明及其他恶性肿瘤、淋巴瘤、脑瘤和骨肿瘤；华东地区和西南地区前 5 位分别为白血病、不明及其他恶性肿瘤、淋巴瘤、脑瘤和肾癌；西北地区前 5 位分别为白血病、不明及其他恶性肿瘤、淋巴瘤、肾癌和脑瘤（图 7-1-2~图 7-1-7）。

1.2　Disease composition of discharges among children with cancer in the six regions

In terms of discharges among children with cancer, in North China, Northeast China, and Central and Southern China, the top five cancers were leukemia, unknown and other cancers, lymphoma, brain tumor and bone cancer. In East China and Southwest China, the top five were leukemia, unknown and other cancers, lymphoma, brain tumor and kidney cancer. The top five in Northwest China were leukemia, unknown and other cancers, lymphoma, kidney cancer and brain tumor (Figure 7-1-2~Figure 7-1-7).

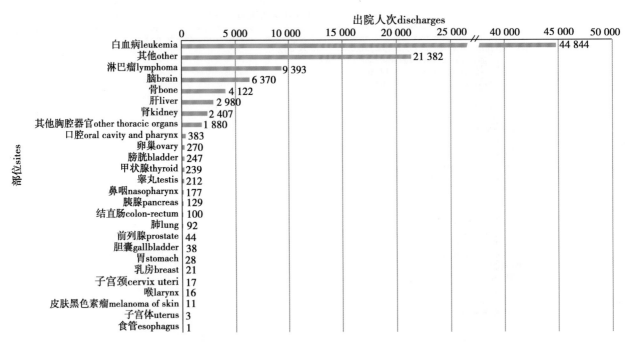

图 7-1-2　2017—2018 年全国华北地区儿童肿瘤监测机构肿瘤患儿出院人次疾病构成（按部位计）

Figure 7-1-2　Disease composition of discharges among children with cancer in pediatric cancer surveillance sites in North China in 2017-2018（by the sites）

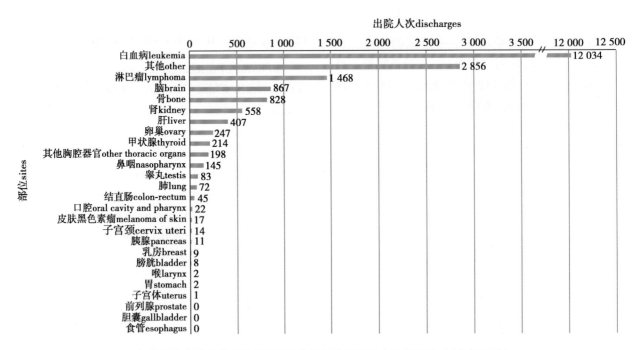

图 7-1-3　2017—2018 年全国东北地区儿童肿瘤监测机构肿瘤患儿出院人次疾病构成（按部位计）

Figure 7-1-3　Disease composition of discharges among children with cancer in pediatric cancer surveillance sites in Northeast China in 2017-2018（by the sites）

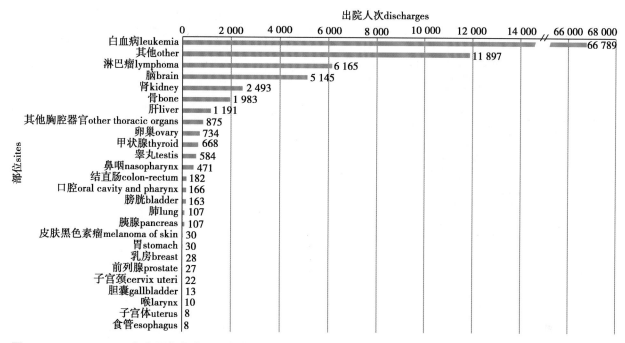

图 7-1-4　2017—2018 年全国华东地区儿童肿瘤监测机构肿瘤患儿出院人次疾病构成（按部位计）

Figure 7-1-4　Disease composition of discharges among children with cancer in pediatric cancer surveillance sites in East China in 2017-2018（by the sites）

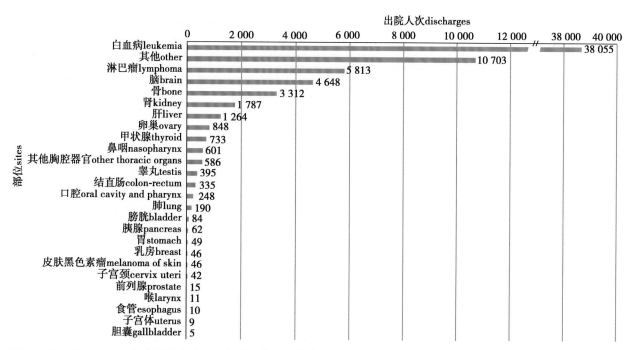

图 7-1-5　2017—2018 年全国中南地区儿童肿瘤监测机构肿瘤患儿出院人次疾病构成（按部位计）

Figure 7-1-5　Disease composition of discharges among children with cancer in pediatric cancer surveillance sites in Central and Southern China in 2017-2018（by the sites）

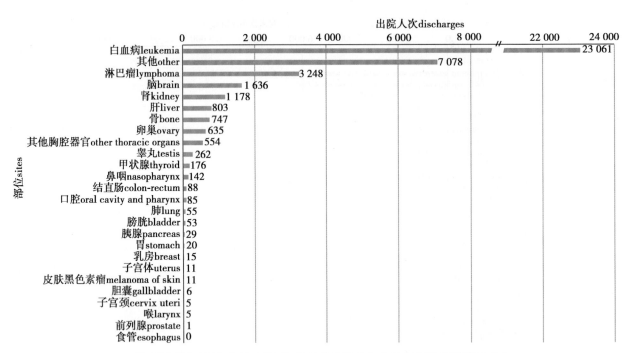

图 7-1-6 2017—2018 年全国西南地区儿童肿瘤监测机构肿瘤患儿出院人次疾病构成（按部位计）

Figure 7-1-6 Disease composition of discharges among children with cancer in pediatric cancer surveillance sites in Southwest China in 2017-2018（by the sites）

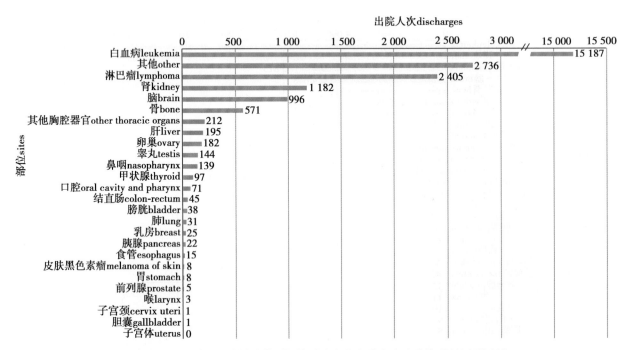

图 7-1-7 2017—2018 年全国西北地区儿童肿瘤监测机构肿瘤患儿出院人次疾病构成（按部位计）

Figure 7-1-7 Disease composition of discharges among children with cancer in pediatric cancer surveillance sites in Northwest China in 2017-2018（by the sites）

1.3　各省份肿瘤患儿疾病构成情况

总体而言,各省份癌谱分布略有差异,但主要癌种构成基本相同,包括白血病、不明及其他恶性肿瘤、淋巴瘤、脑瘤、骨肿瘤、肾癌和肝癌。以浙江省为例,出院人次前6位分别为白血病(58.04%)、不明及其他恶性肿瘤(15.01%)、淋巴瘤(10.02%)、脑瘤(5.47%)、肾癌(2.79%)和肝癌(1.71%)(图7-1-8~图7-1-38)。

1.3　Disease composition of discharges among children with cancer in each provincial-level region

In general, despite a slight difference in the cancer spectra in different provincial-level regions, the compositions of main cancers were basically the same, including leukemia, unknown and other cancers, lymphoma, brain tumor, bone cancer, kidney cancer and liver cancer. Taking Zhejiang as an example, the 6 diseases with the most discharges were leukemia (58.04%), unknown and other cancers (15.01%), lymphoma (10.02%), brain tumor (5.47%), kidney cancer (2.79%) and liver cancer (1.71%) (Figure 7-1-8~Figure 7-1-38).

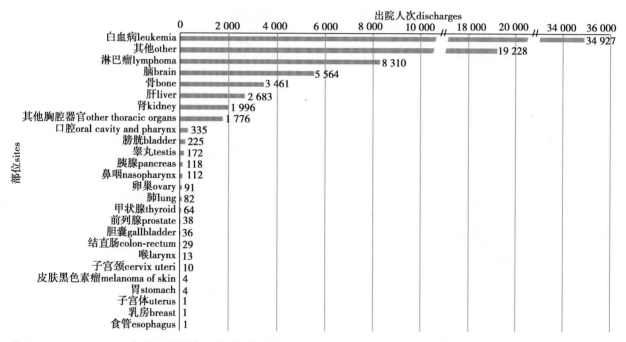

图 7-1-8　2017—2018 年北京儿童肿瘤监测机构肿瘤患儿出院人次疾病构成(按部位计)

Figure 7-1-8　Disease composition of discharges among children with cancer in pediatric cancer surveillance sites in Beijing in 2017-2018 (by the sites)

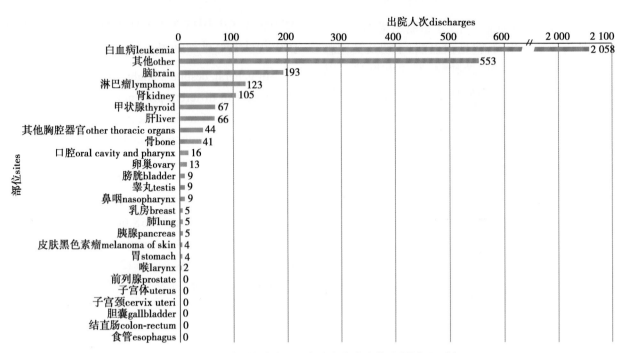

图 7-1-9　2017—2018 年天津儿童肿瘤监测机构肿瘤患儿出院人次疾病构成（按部位计）

Figure 7-1-9　Disease composition of discharges among children with cancer in pediatric cancer surveillance sites in Tianjin in 2017-2018（by the sites）

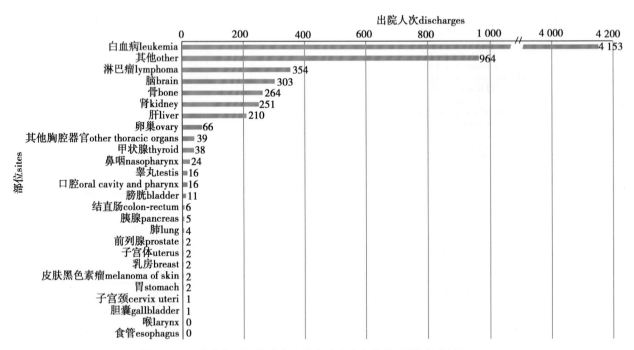

图 7-1-10　2017—2018 年河北儿童肿瘤监测机构肿瘤患儿出院人次疾病构成（按部位计）

Figure 7-1-10　Disease composition of discharges among children with cancer in pediatric cancer surveillance sites in Hebei in 2017-2018（by the sites）

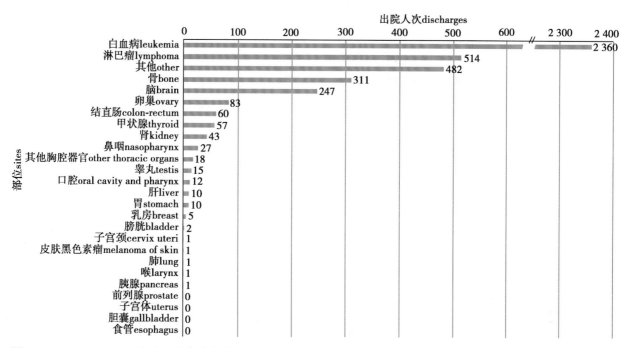

图 7-1-11　2017—2018 年山西儿童肿瘤监测机构肿瘤患儿出院人次疾病构成（按部位计）

Figure 7-1-11　Disease composition of discharges among children with cancer in pediatric cancer surveillance sites in Shanxi in 2017-2018（by the sites）

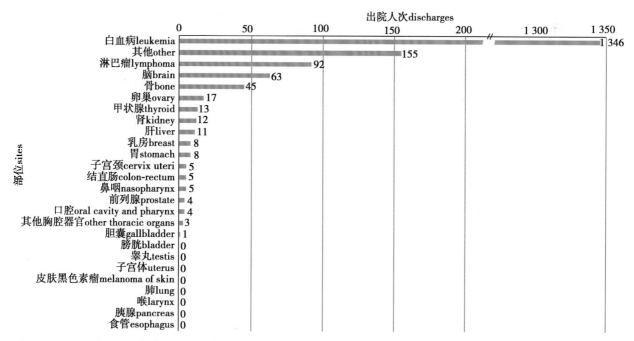

图 7-1-12　2017—2018 年内蒙古儿童肿瘤监测机构肿瘤患儿出院人次疾病构成（按部位计）

Figure 7-1-12　Disease composition of discharges among children with cancer in pediatric cancer surveillance sites in Inner Mongolia in 2017-2018（by the sites）

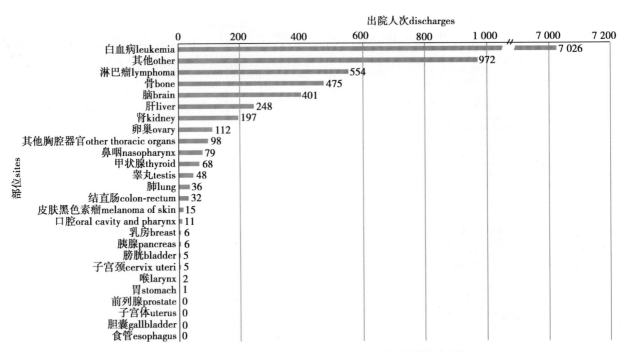

图 7-1-13　2017—2018 年辽宁儿童肿瘤监测机构肿瘤患儿出院人次疾病构成（按部位计）

Figure 7-1-13　Disease composition of discharges among children with cancer in pediatric cancer surveillance sites in Liaoning in 2017-2018（by the sites）

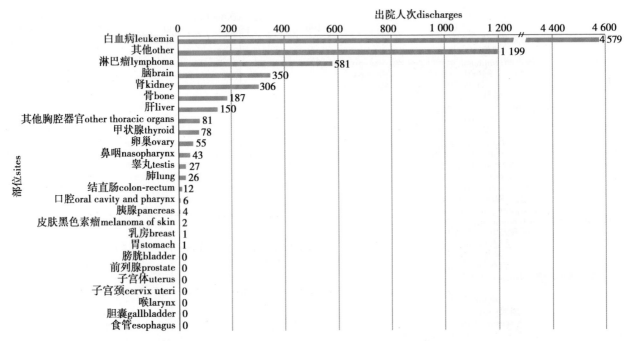

图 7-1-14　2017—2018 年吉林儿童肿瘤监测机构肿瘤患儿出院人次疾病构成（按部位计）

Figure 7-1-14　Disease composition of discharges among children with cancer in pediatric cancer surveillance sites in Jilin in 2017-2018（by the sites）

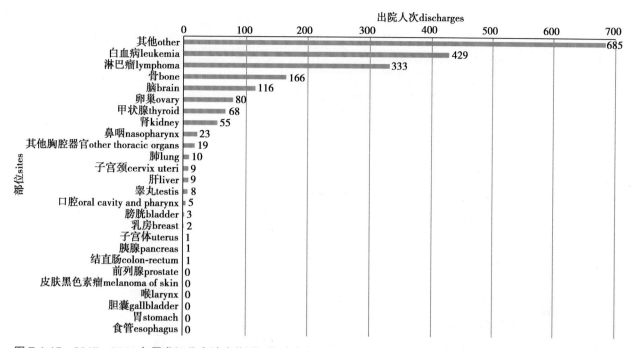

图 7-1-15　2017—2018 年黑龙江儿童肿瘤监测机构肿瘤患儿出院人次疾病构成（按部位计）

Figure 7-1-15　Disease composition of discharges among children with cancer in pediatric cancer surveillance sites in Heilongjiang in 2017-2018（by the sites）

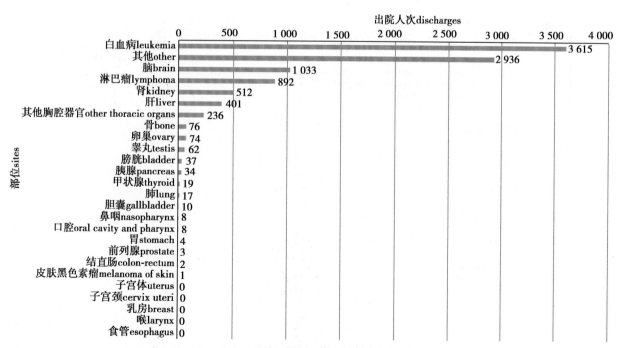

图 7-1-16　2017—2018 年上海儿童肿瘤监测机构肿瘤患儿出院人次疾病构成（按部位计）

Figure 7-1-16　Disease composition of discharges among children with cancer in pediatric cancer surveillance sites in Shanghai in 2017-2018（by the sites）

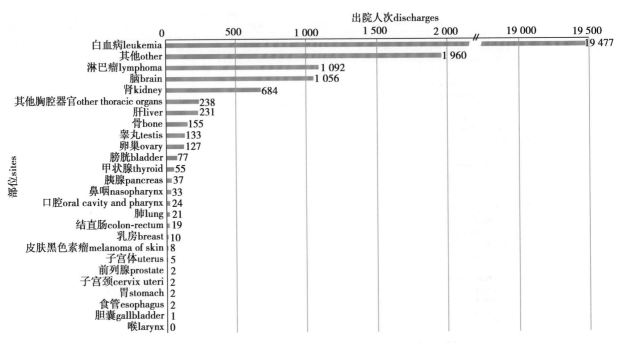

图 7-1-17　2017—2018 年江苏儿童肿瘤监测机构肿瘤患儿出院人次疾病构成（按部位计）

Figure 7-1-17　Disease composition of discharges among children with cancer in pediatric cancer surveillance sites in Jiangsu in 2017-2018（by the sites）

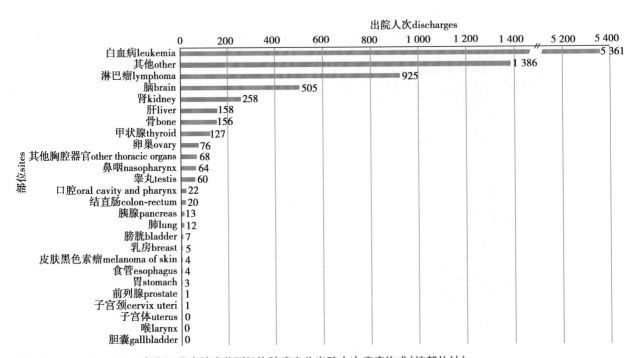

图 7-1-18　2017—2018 年浙江儿童肿瘤监测机构肿瘤患儿出院人次疾病构成（按部位计）

Figure 7-1-18　Disease composition of discharges among children with cancer in pediatric cancer surveillance sites in Zhejiang in 2017-2018（by the sites）

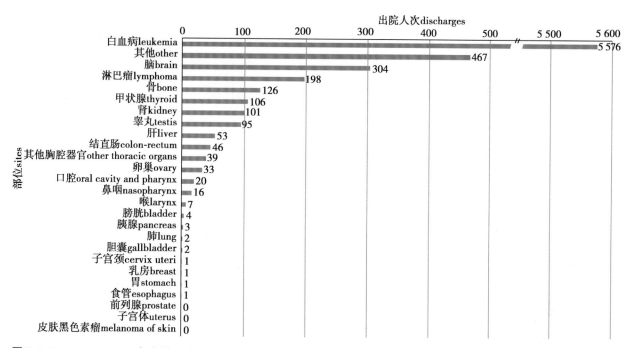

图 7-1-19　2017—2018 年安徽儿童肿瘤监测机构肿瘤患儿出院人次疾病构成（按部位统计）

Figure 7-1-19　Disease composition of discharges among children with cancer in pediatric cancer surveillance sites in Anhui in 2017-2018（by the sites）

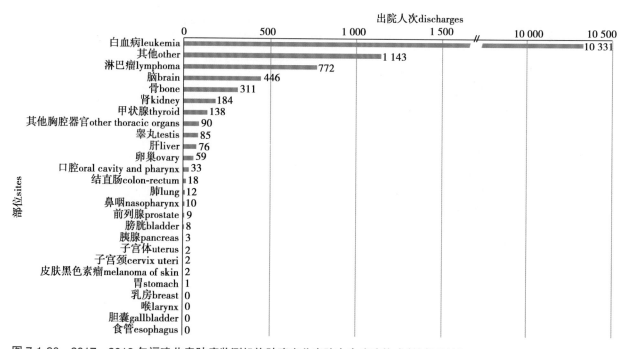

图 7-1-20　2017—2018 年福建儿童肿瘤监测机构肿瘤患儿出院人次疾病构成（按部位计）

Figure 7-1-20　Disease composition of discharges among children with cancer in pediatric cancer surveillance sites in Fujian in 2017-2018（by the sites）

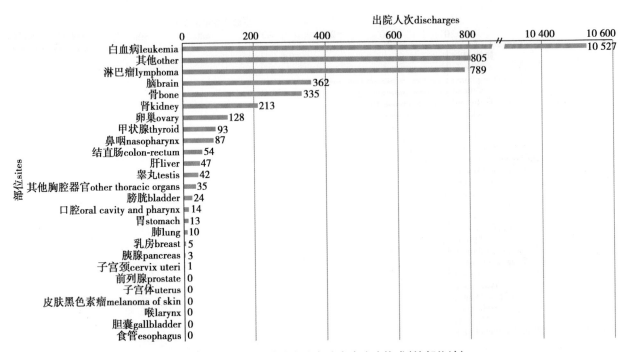

图 7-1-21　2017—2018 年江西儿童肿瘤监测机构肿瘤患儿出院人次疾病构成（按部位计）

Figure 7-1-21　Disease composition of discharges among children with cancer in pediatric cancer surveillance sites in Jiangxi in 2017-2018（by the sites）

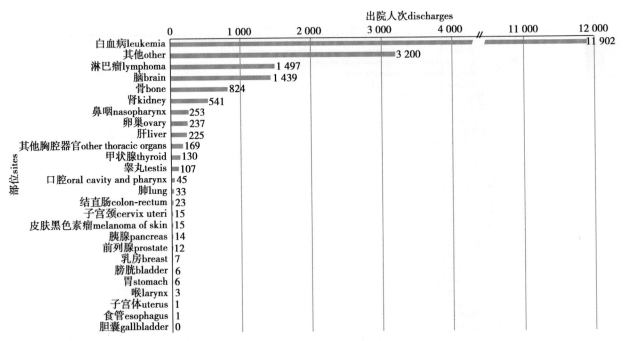

图 7-1-22　2017—2018 年山东儿童肿瘤监测机构肿瘤患儿出院人次疾病构成（按部位计）

Figure 7-1-22　Disease composition of discharges among children with cancer in pediatric cancer surveillance sites in Shandong in 2017-2018（by the sites）

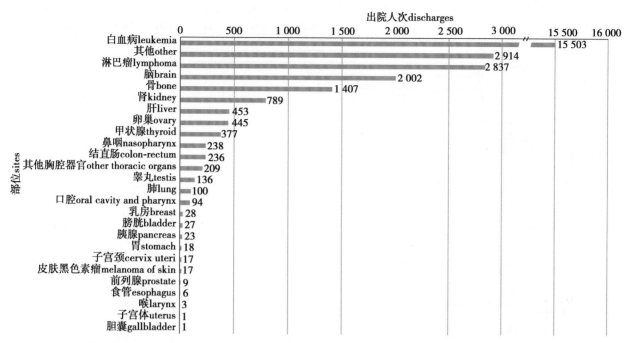

图 7-1-23　2017—2018 年河南儿童肿瘤监测机构肿瘤患儿出院人次疾病构成（按部位计）

Figure 7-1-23　Disease composition of discharges among children with cancer in pediatric cancer surveillance sites in Henan in 2017-2018（by the sites）

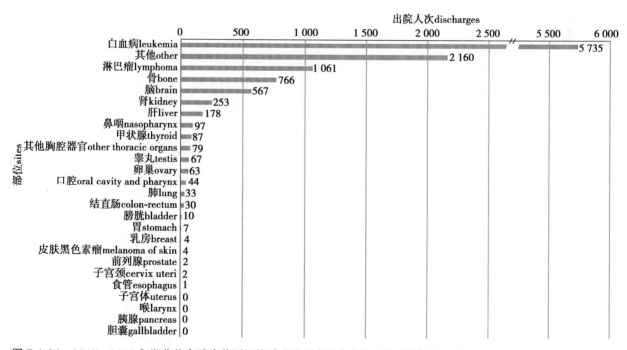

图 7-1-24　2017—2018 年湖北儿童肿瘤监测机构肿瘤患儿出院人次疾病构成（按部位计）

Figure 7-1-24　Disease composition of discharges among children with cancer in pediatric cancer surveillance sites in Hubei in 2017-2018（by the sites）

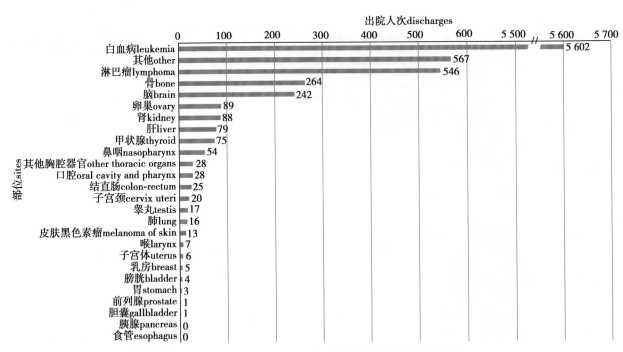

图 7-1-25　2017—2018 年湖南儿童肿瘤监测机构肿瘤患儿出院人次疾病构成（按部位计）

Figure 7-1-25　Disease composition of discharges among children with cancer in pediatric cancer surveillance sites in Hunan in 2017-2018（by the sites）

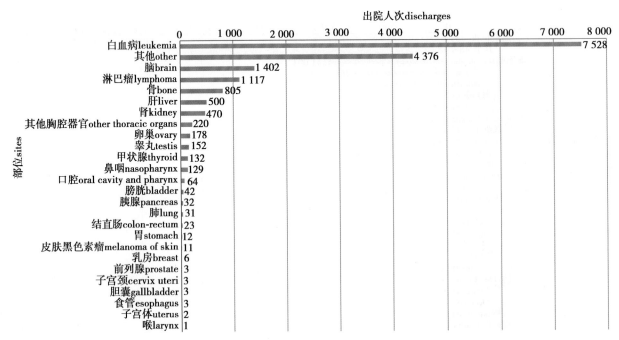

图 7-1-26　2017—2018 年广东儿童肿瘤监测机构肿瘤患儿出院人次疾病构成（按部位计）

Figure 7-1-26　Disease composition of discharges among children with cancer in pediatric cancer surveillance sites in Guangdong in 2017-2018（by the sites）

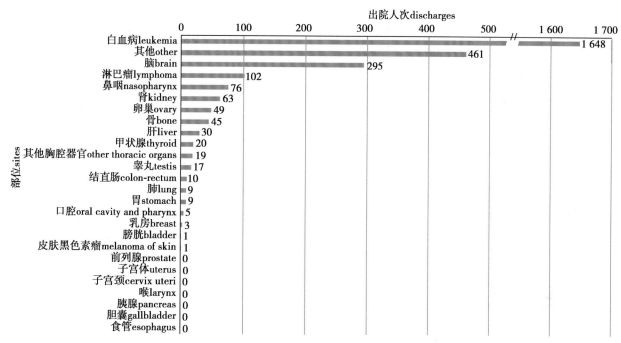

图 7-1-27　2017—2018 年广西儿童肿瘤监测机构肿瘤患儿出院人次疾病构成（按部位计）

Figure 7-1-27　Disease composition of discharges among children with cancer in pediatric cancer surveillance sites in Guangxi in 2017-2018（by the sites）

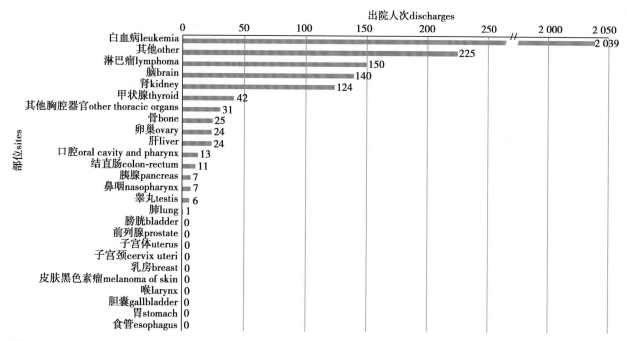

图 7-1-28　2017—2018 年海南儿童肿瘤监测机构肿瘤患儿出院人次疾病构成（按部位计）

Figure 7-1-28　Disease composition of discharges among children with cancer in pediatric cancer surveillance sites in Hainan in 2017-2018（by the sites）

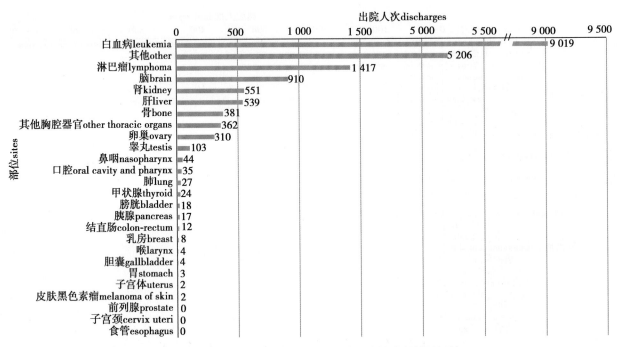

图 7-1-29　2017—2018 年重庆儿童肿瘤监测机构肿瘤患儿出院人次疾病构成（按部位计）

Figure 7-1-29　Disease composition of discharges among children with cancer in pediatric cancer surveillance sites in Chongqing in 2017-2018（by the sites）

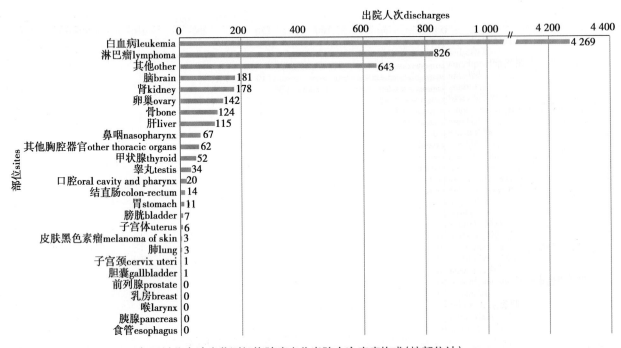

图 7-1-30　2017—2018 年四川儿童肿瘤监测机构肿瘤患儿出院人次疾病构成（按部位计）

Figure 7-1-30　Disease composition of discharges among children with cancer in pediatric cancer surveillance sites in Sichuan in 2017-2018（by the sites）

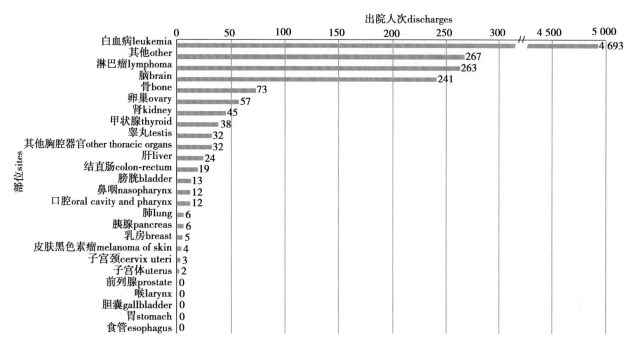

图 7-1-31　2017—2018 年贵州儿童肿瘤监测机构肿瘤患儿出院人次疾病构成（按部位计）

Figure 7-1-31　Disease composition of discharges among children with cancer in pediatric cancer surveillance sites in Guizhou in 2017-2018（by the sites）

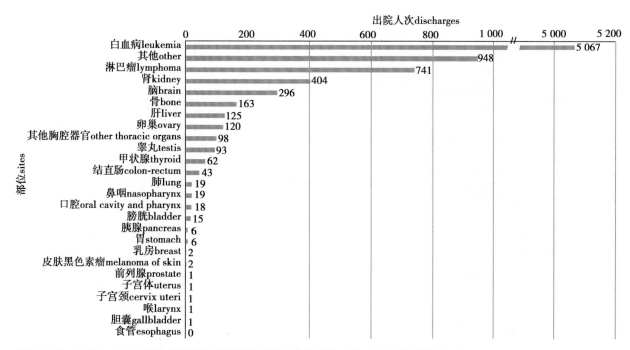

图 7-1-32　2017—2018 年云南儿童肿瘤监测机构肿瘤患儿出院人次疾病构成（按部位计）

Figure 7-1-32　Disease composition of discharges among children with cancer in pediatric cancer surveillance sites in Yunnan in 2017-2018（by the sites）

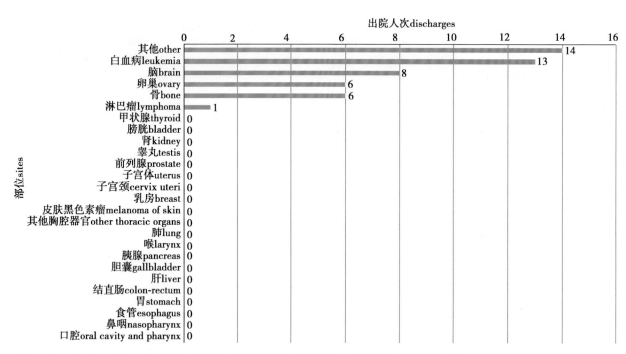

图 7-1-33　2017—2018 年西藏儿童肿瘤监测机构肿瘤患儿出院人次疾病构成（按部位计）

Figure 7-1-33　Disease composition of discharges among children with cancer in pediatric cancer surveillance sites in Xizang in 2017-2018（by the sites）

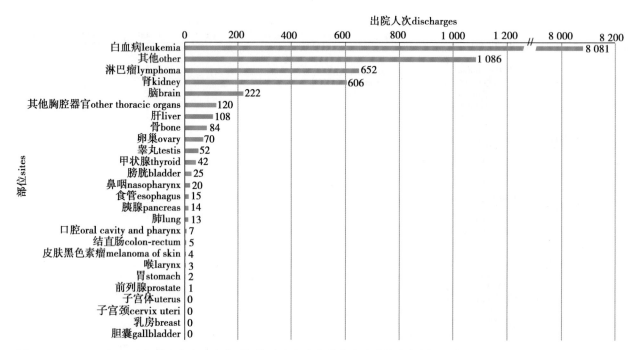

图 7-1-34　2017—2018 年陕西儿童肿瘤监测机构肿瘤患儿出院人次疾病构成（按部位计）

Figure 7-1-34　Disease composition of discharges among children with cancer in pediatric cancer surveillance sites in Shaanxi in 2017-2018（by the sites）

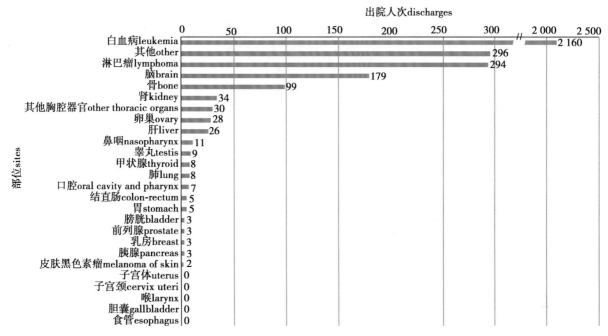

图 7-1-35　2017—2018 年甘肃儿童肿瘤监测机构肿瘤患儿出院人次疾病构成（按部位计）

Figure 7-1-35　Disease composition of discharges among children with cancer in pediatric cancer surveillance sites in Gansu in 2017-2018（by the sites）

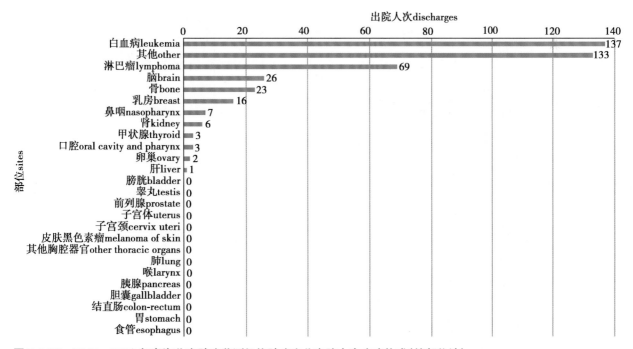

图 7-1-36　2017—2018 年青海儿童肿瘤监测机构肿瘤患儿出院人次疾病构成（按部位计）

Figure 7-1-36　Disease composition of discharges among children with cancer in pediatric cancer surveillance sites in Qinghai in 2017-2018（by the sites）

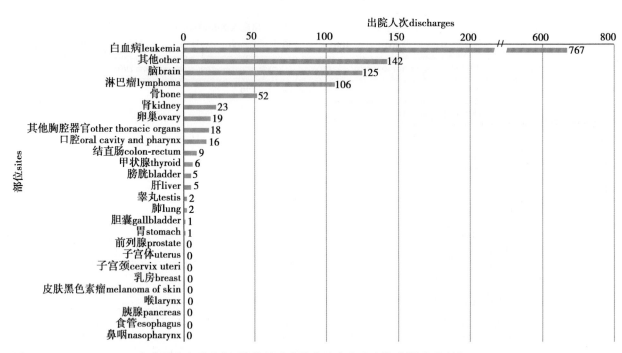

图 7-1-37 2017—2018 年宁夏儿童肿瘤监测机构肿瘤患儿出院人次疾病构成（按部位计）

Figure 7-1-37 Disease composition of discharges among children with cancer in pediatric cancer surveillance sites in Ningxia in 2017-2018（by the sites）

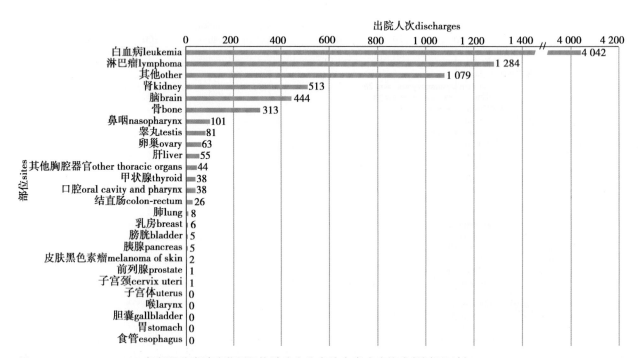

图 7-1-38 2017—2018 年新疆儿童肿瘤监测机构肿瘤患儿出院人次疾病构成（按部位计）

Figure 7-1-38 Disease composition of discharges among children with cancer in pediatric cancer surveillance sites in Xinjiang in 2017-2018（by the sites）

2 全国儿童肿瘤监测机构肿瘤患儿年龄 / 性别构成

2.1 全国肿瘤患儿年龄 / 性别构成情况

从性别分布来看,男性患儿占全部出院人次比例为 59.52%,女性患儿为 40.48%;男性患儿各年龄段的出院人次比例均高于女性患儿。从年龄分布来看,3 岁年龄组所占比例最高(10.04%),其次为 4 岁(9.66%)和 5 岁(8.43%)年龄组(图 7-2-1)。

2 Age/gender composition of children with cancer in pediatric cancer surveillance sites in China

2.1 Age/gender composition of children with cancer nationally

In terms of gender distribution, male children accounted for 59.52% of all discharges, and female for 40.48%. The discharge proportions of male children at all ages were higher than those of female. In terms of age distribution, the 3-year age group accounted for the highest proportion (10.04%), followed by the 4-year age group (9.66%) and the 5-year age group (8.43%) (Figure 7-2-1).

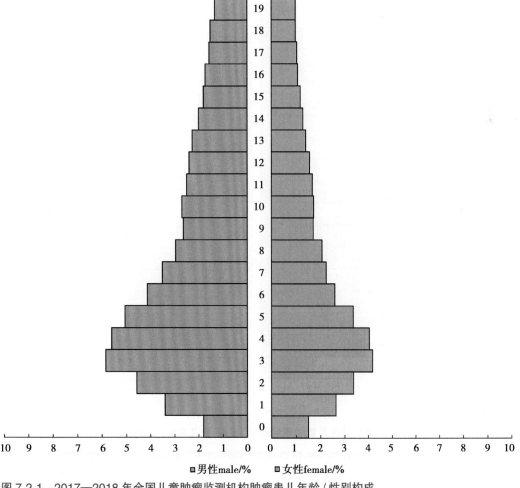

图 7-2-1　2017—2018 年全国儿童肿瘤监测机构肿瘤患儿年龄 / 性别构成

Figure 7-2-1　Age/gender composition of children with cancer in pediatric cancer surveillance sites nationally in 2017-2018

2.2 六大区肿瘤患儿年龄/性别构成情况

从性别分布来看,六大区均显示男性患儿占全部出院人次比例高于女性患儿。从年龄分布来看,六大区的比例各有不同,其中华北地区、华东地区和西南地区的3岁年龄组所占比例最高;东北地区、中南地区和西北地区的4岁年龄组所占比例最高(图7-2-2~图7-2-7)。

2.2 Age/gender composition of children with cancer in the six regions

In terms of gender distribution, male children accounted for a higher proportion of all dischargs than female in the six regions. In terms of age distribution, the proportions of the six regions were different, and the proportions of the 3-year age group in North China, East China and Southwest China were the highest. The proportions of the 4-year age group in Northeast China, Central and Southern China and Northwest China were the highest (Figure 7-2-2~ Figure 7-2-7).

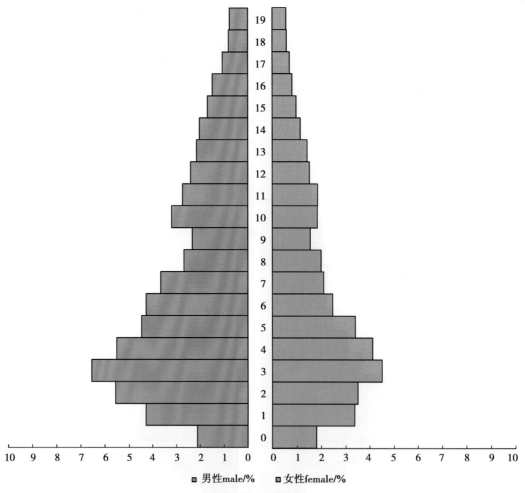

图 7-2-2 2017—2018 年华北地区儿童肿瘤监测机构肿瘤患儿年龄/性别构成

Figure 7-2-2 Age/gender composition of children with cancer in pediatric cancer surveillance sites in North China in 2017-2018

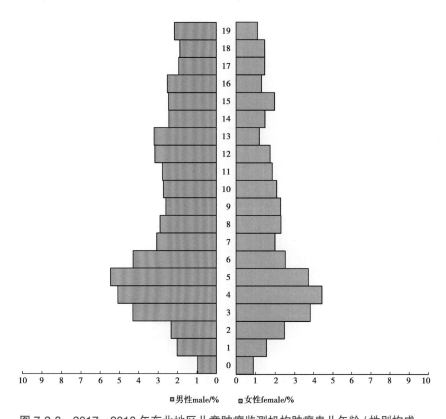

图 7-2-3 2017—2018 年东北地区儿童肿瘤监测机构肿瘤患儿年龄 / 性别构成

Figure 7-2-3 Age/gender composition of children with cancer in pediatric cancer surveillance sites in Northeast China in 2017-2018

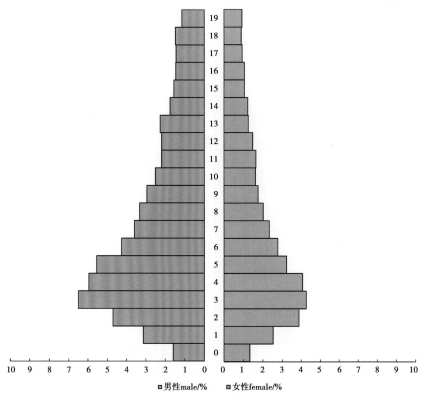

图 7-2-4 2017—2018 年华东地区儿童肿瘤监测机构肿瘤患儿年龄 / 性别构成

Figure 7-2-4 Age/gender composition of children with cancer in pediatric cancer surveillance sites in East China in 2017-2018

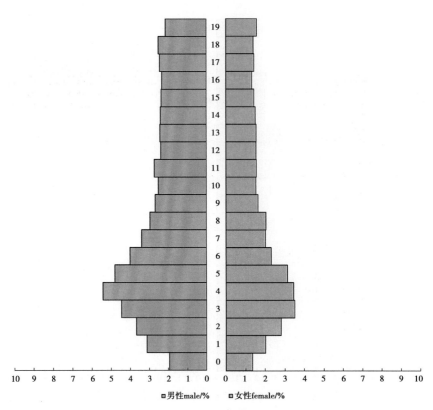

图 7-2-5 2017—2018 年中南地区儿童肿瘤监测机构肿瘤患儿年龄／性别构成

Figure 7-2-5 Age/gender composition of children with cancer in pediatric cancer surveillance sites in Central and Southern China in 2017-2018

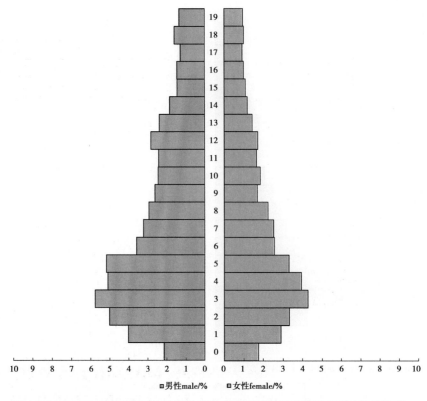

图 7-2-6 2017—2018 年西南地区儿童肿瘤监测机构肿瘤患儿年龄／性别构成

Figure 7-2-6 Age/gender composition of children with cancer in pediatric cancer surveillance sites in Southwest China in 2017-2018

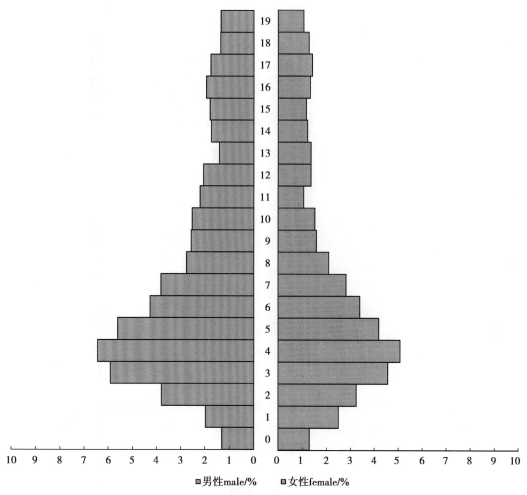

图 7-2-7　2017—2018 年西北地区儿童肿瘤监测机构肿瘤患儿年龄／性别构成

Figure 7-2-7　Age/gender composition of children with cancer in pediatric cancer surveillance sites in Northwest China in 2017-2018

2.3 各省份肿瘤患儿年龄／性别构成情况

各省份出院患儿的性别分布均呈现男性比例高于女性,年龄集中分布在 2~8 岁年龄组。以福建省为例,从性别分布来看,男性患儿占全部出院人次比例为 62.20%,女性患儿为 37.80%。从年龄分布来看,4 岁年龄组所占比例最高(11.59%),其次为 3 岁(11.28%)和 5 岁(10.61%)年龄组(图 7-2-8~图 7-2-38)。

2.3 Age/gender composition of children with cancer in each provincial-level region

The proportions of discharged male children in all provincial-level regions were higher than those of female, concentrated in the age group of 2-8. Taking Fujian as an example, in terms of gender distribution, male children accounted for 62.20% of the total discharges, and female for 37.80% of the total discharges. In terms of age distribution, the 4-year age group accounted for the highest proportion (11.59%), followed by the 3-year age group (11.28%) and the 5-year age group (10.61%) (Figure 7-2-8~Figure 7-2-38).

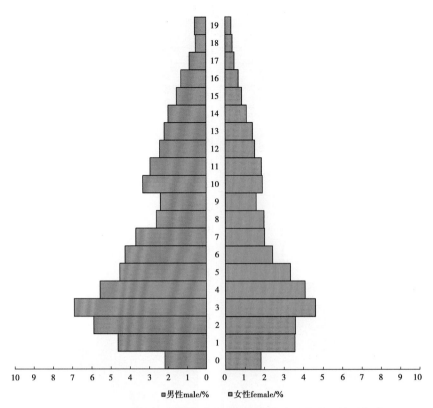

图 7-2-8 2017—2018 年北京儿童肿瘤监测机构肿瘤患儿年龄／性别构成

Figure 7-2-8 Age/gender composition of children with cancer in pediatric cancer surveillance sites in Beijing in 2017-2018

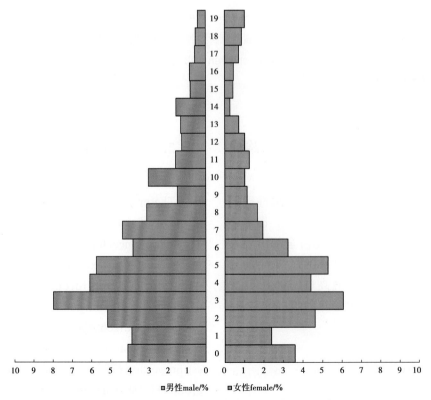

图 7-2-9 2017—2018 年天津儿童肿瘤监测机构肿瘤患儿年龄／性别构成

Figure 7-2-9 Age/gender composition of children with cancer in pediatric cancer surveillance sites in Tianjin in 2017-2018

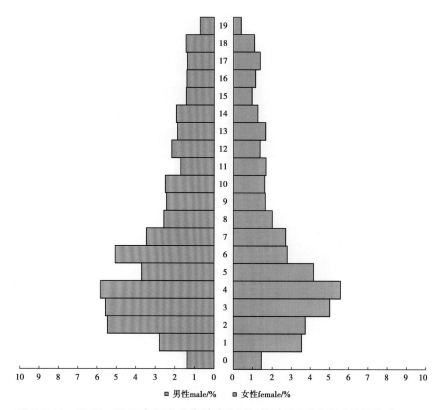

图 7-2-10　2017—2018 年河北儿童肿瘤监测机构肿瘤患儿年龄 / 性别构成

Figure 7-2-10　Age/gender composition of children with cancer in pediatric cancer surveillance sites in Hebei in 2017-2018

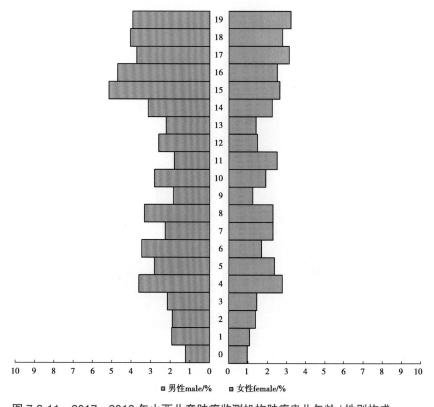

图 7-2-11　2017—2018 年山西儿童肿瘤监测机构肿瘤患儿年龄 / 性别构成

Figure 7-2-11　Age/gender composition of children with cancer in pediatric cancer surveillance sites in Shanxi in 2017-2018

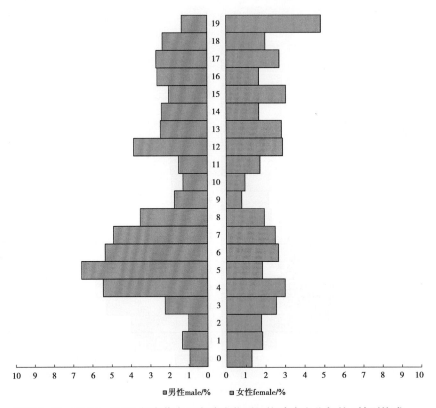

图 7-2-12　2017—2018 年内蒙古儿童肿瘤监测机构肿瘤患儿年龄／性别构成

Figure 7-2-12　Age/gender composition of children with cancer in pediatric cancer surveillance sites in Inner Mongolia in 2017-2018

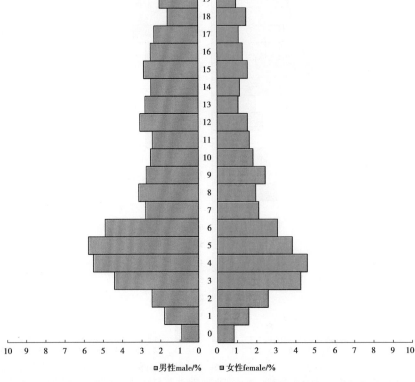

图 7-2-13　2017—2018 年辽宁儿童肿瘤监测机构肿瘤患儿年龄／性别构成

Figure 7-2-13　Age/gender composition of children with cancer in pediatric cancer surveillance sites in Liaoning in 2017-2018

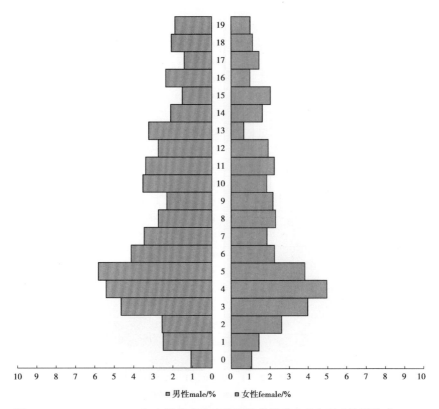

图 7-2-14　2017—2018 年吉林儿童肿瘤监测机构肿瘤患儿年龄／性别构成

Figure 7-2-14　Age/gender composition of children with cancer in pediatric cancer surveillance sites in Jilin in 2017-2018

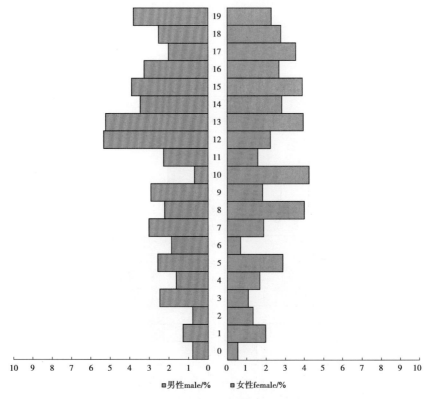

图 7-2-15　2017—2018 年黑龙江儿童肿瘤监测机构肿瘤患儿年龄／性别构成

Figure 7-2-15　Age/gender composition of children with cancer in pediatric cancer surveillance sites in Heilongjiang in 2017-2018

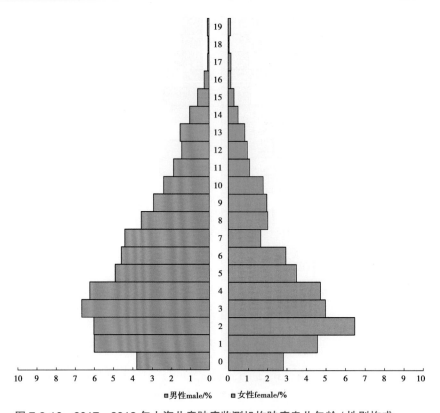

图 7-2-16 2017—2018 年上海儿童肿瘤监测机构肿瘤患儿年龄 / 性别构成

Figure 7-2-16 Age/gender composition of children with cancer in pediatric cancer surveillance sites in Shanghai in 2017-2018

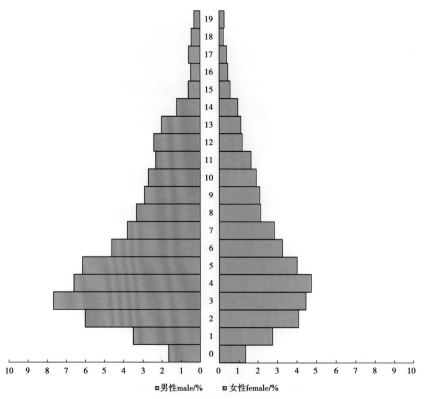

图 7-2-17 2017—2018 年江苏儿童肿瘤监测机构肿瘤患儿年龄 / 性别构成

Figure 7-2-17 Age/gender composition of children with cancer in pediatric cancer surveillance sites in Jiangsu in 2017-2018

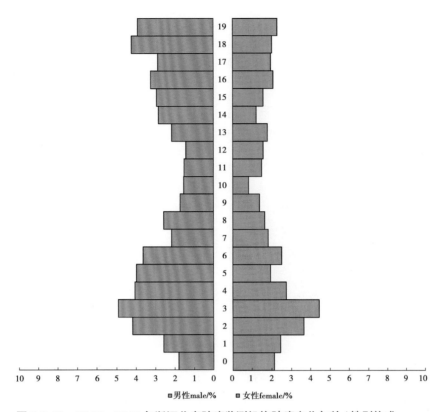

图 7-2-18　2017—2018 年浙江儿童肿瘤监测机构肿瘤患儿年龄／性别构成

Figure 7-2-18　Age/gender composition of children with cancer in pediatric cancer surveillance sites in Zhejiang in 2017-2018

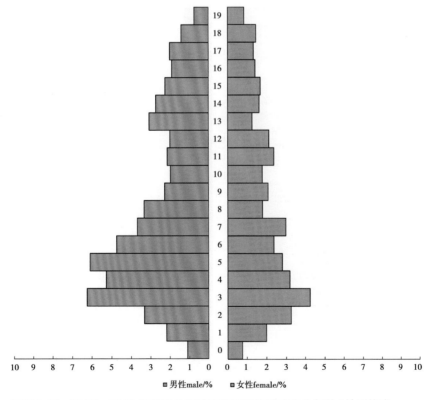

图 7-2-19　2017—2018 年安徽儿童肿瘤监测机构肿瘤患儿年龄／性别构成

Figure 7-2-19　Age/gender composition of children with cancer in pediatric cancer surveillance sites in Anhui in 2017-2018

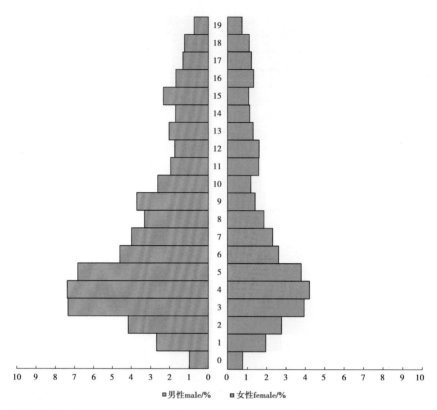

图 7-2-20　2017—2018 年福建儿童肿瘤监测机构肿瘤患儿年龄／性别构成

Figure 7-2-20　Age/gender composition of children with cancer in pediatric cancer surveillance sites in Fujian in 2017-2018

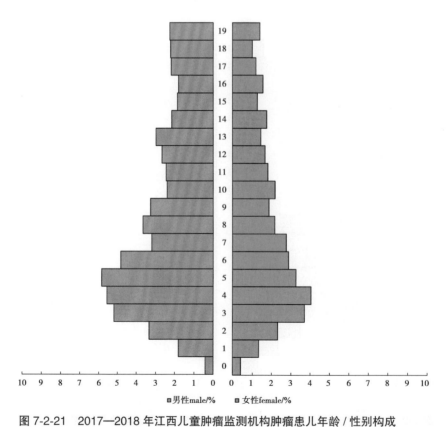

图 7-2-21　2017—2018 年江西儿童肿瘤监测机构肿瘤患儿年龄／性别构成

Figure 7-2-21　Age/gender composition of children with cancer in pediatric cancer surveillance sites in Jiangxi in 2017-2018

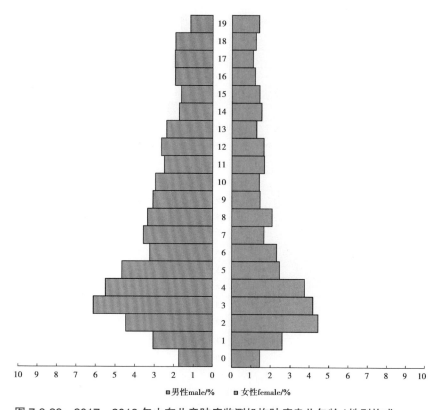

图 7-2-22　2017—2018 年山东儿童肿瘤监测机构肿瘤患儿年龄 / 性别构成

Figure 7-2-22　Age/gender composition of children with cancer in pediatric cancer surveillance sites in Shandong in 2017-2018

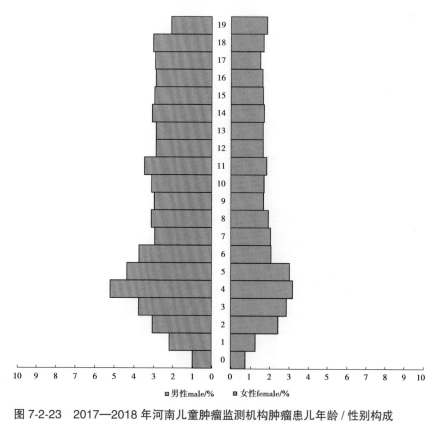

图 7-2-23　2017—2018 年河南儿童肿瘤监测机构肿瘤患儿年龄 / 性别构成

Figure 7-2-23　Age/gender composition of children with cancer in pediatric cancer surveillance sites in Henan in 2017-2018

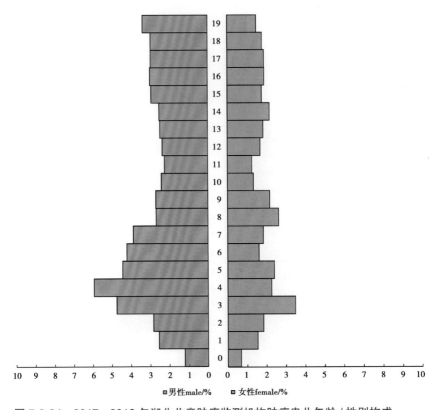

图 7-2-24　2017—2018 年湖北儿童肿瘤监测机构肿瘤患儿年龄 / 性别构成

Figure 7-2-24　Age/gender composition of children with cancer in pediatric cancer surveillance sites in Hubei in 2017-2018

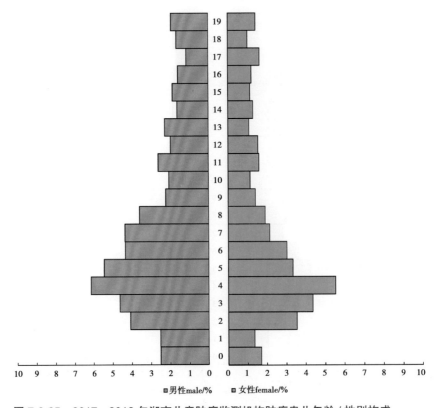

图 7-2-25　2017—2018 年湖南儿童肿瘤监测机构肿瘤患儿年龄 / 性别构成

Figure 7-2-25　Age/gender composition of children with cancer in pediatric cancer surveillance sites in Hunan in 2017-2018

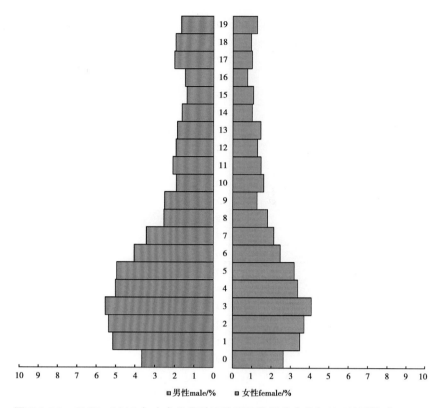

图 7-2-26   2017—2018 年广东儿童肿瘤监测机构肿瘤患儿年龄 / 性别构成

Figure 7-2-26   Age/gender composition of children with cancer in pediatric cancer surveillance sites in Guangdong in 2017-2018

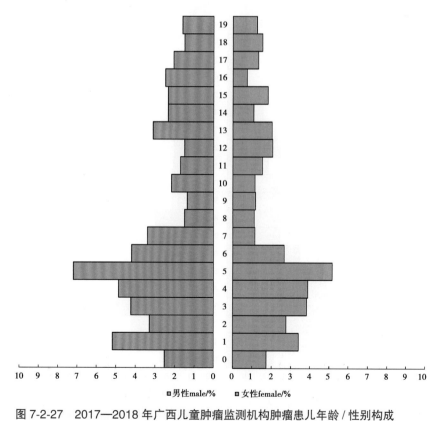

图 7-2-27   2017—2018 年广西儿童肿瘤监测机构肿瘤患儿年龄 / 性别构成

Figure 7-2-27   Age/gender composition of children with cancer in pediatric cancer surveillance sites in Guangxi in 2017-2018

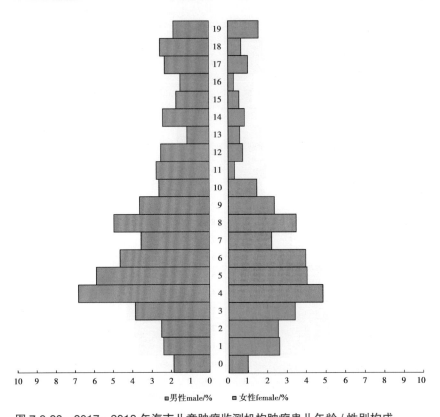

图 7-2-28　2017—2018 年海南儿童肿瘤监测机构肿瘤患儿年龄／性别构成

Figure 7-2-28　Age/gender composition of children with cancer in pediatric cancer surveillance sites in Hainan in 2017-2018

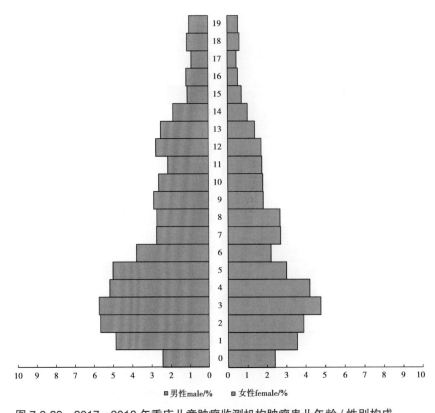

图 7-2-29　2017—2018 年重庆儿童肿瘤监测机构肿瘤患儿年龄／性别构成

Figure 7-2-29　Age/gender composition of children with cancer in pediatric cancer surveillance sites in Chongqing in 2017-2018

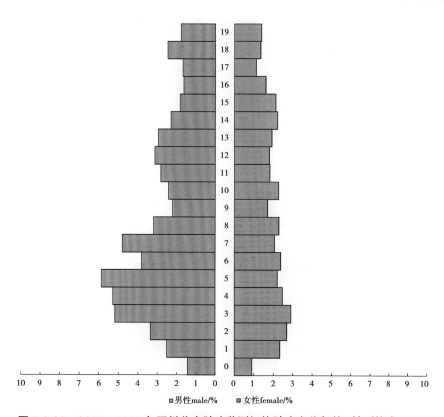

图 7-2-30　2017—2018 年四川儿童肿瘤监测机构肿瘤患儿年龄 / 性别构成

Figure 7-2-30　Age/gender composition of children with cancer in pediatric cancer surveillance sites in Sichuan in 2017-2018

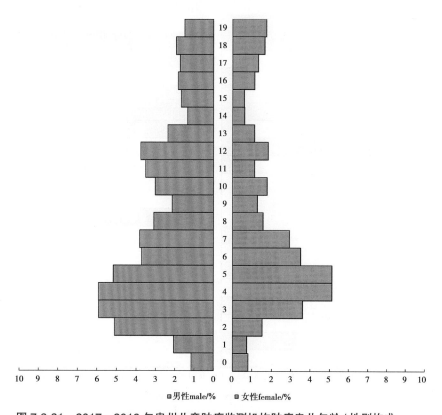

图 7-2-31　2017—2018 年贵州儿童肿瘤监测机构肿瘤患儿年龄 / 性别构成

Figure 7-2-31　Age/gender composition of children with cancer in pediatric cancer surveillance sites in Guizhou in 2017-2018

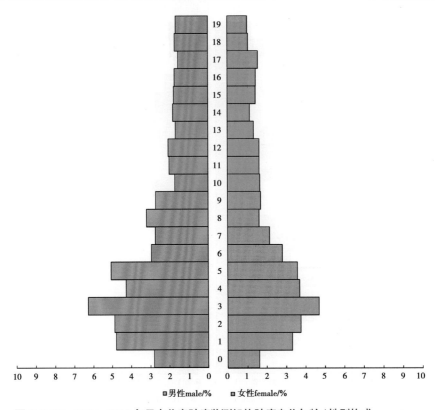

图 7-2-32 2017—2018 年云南儿童肿瘤监测机构肿瘤患儿年龄／性别构成

Figure 7-2-32 Age/gender composition of children with cancer in pediatric cancer surveillance sites in Yunnan in 2017-2018

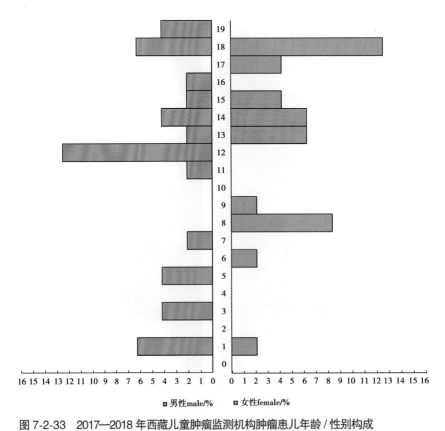

图 7-2-33 2017—2018 年西藏儿童肿瘤监测机构肿瘤患儿年龄／性别构成

Figure 7-2-33 Age/gender composition of children with cancer in pediatric cancer surveillance sites in Xizang in 2017-2018

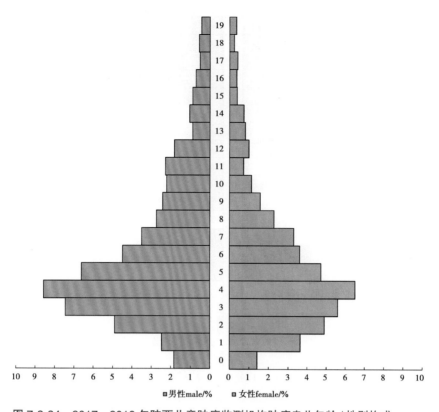

图 7-2-34 2017—2018 年陕西儿童肿瘤监测机构肿瘤患儿年龄 / 性别构成

Figure 7-2-34 Age/gender composition of children with cancer in pediatric cancer surveillance sites in Shaanxi in 2017-2018

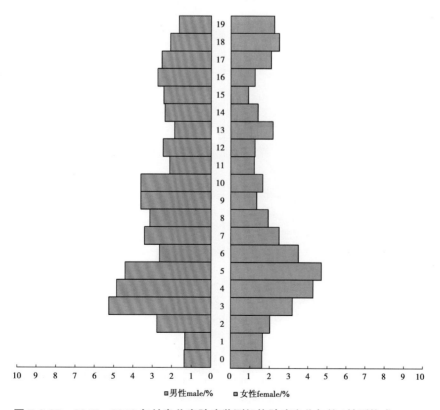

图 7-2-35 2017—2018 年甘肃儿童肿瘤监测机构肿瘤患儿年龄 / 性别构成

Figure 7-2-35 Age/gender composition of children with cancer in pediatric cancer surveillance sites in Gansu in 2017-2018

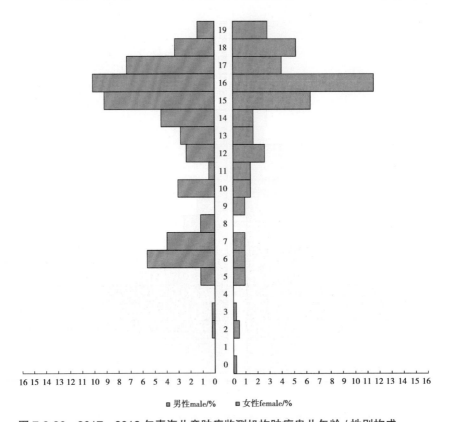

图 7-2-36　2017—2018 年青海儿童肿瘤监测机构肿瘤患儿年龄／性别构成

Figure 7-2-36　Age/gender composition of children with cancer in pediatric cancer surveillance sites in Qinghai in 2017-2018

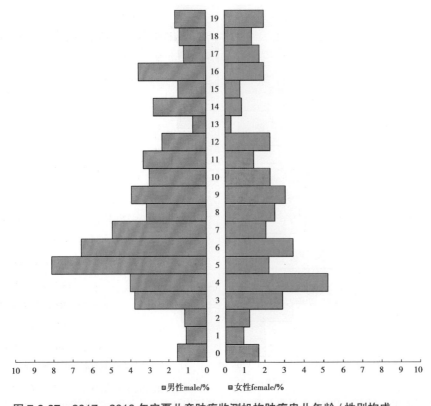

图 7-2-37　2017—2018 年宁夏儿童肿瘤监测机构肿瘤患儿年龄／性别构成

Figure 7-2-37　Age/gender composition of children with cancer in pediatric cancer surveillance sites in Ningxia in 2017-2018

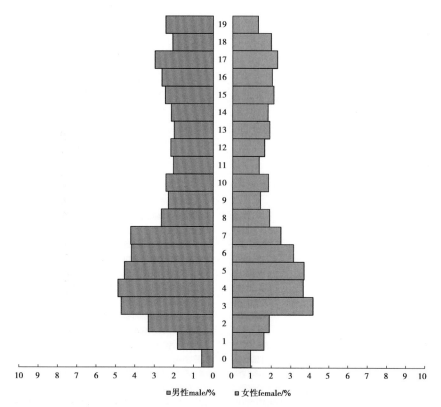

图 7-2-38　2017—2018 年新疆儿童肿瘤监测机构肿瘤患儿年龄 / 性别构成

Figure 7-2-38　Age/gender composition of children with cancer in pediatric cancer surveillance sites in Xinjiang in 2017-2018

3　全国儿童肿瘤监测机构肿瘤患儿就医省份分布

3.1　全国各省份肿瘤患儿本省就医与省外就医的分布情况

总体而言,全国肿瘤患儿本省就医的比例为 66.22%。在所有省份中,本省就医比例前 3 位的省份分别为北京(98.61%)、重庆(90.76%)和广东(90.32%)。省外就医比例前 3 位分别为西藏(78.48%)、内蒙古(77.60%)和河北(71.48%)(图7-3-1)。

3　Distribution of provincial-level regions visited by children with cancer in pediatric cancer surveillance sites in China

3.1　Distribution of children with cancer receiving medical treatment in and out of their own provincial-level regions

In general, 66.22% of all children with cancer sought medical treatment in their own provincial-level regions. Beijing (98.61%), Chongqing (90.76%) and Guangdong (90.32%) were the top three recipients of patients from other provincial-level regions. Xizang (78.48%), Inner Mongolia (77.60%) and Hebei (71.48%) were the top three provincial-level regions in terms of the proportion of patients going to other provincial-level regions for medical treatment (Figure 7-3-1).

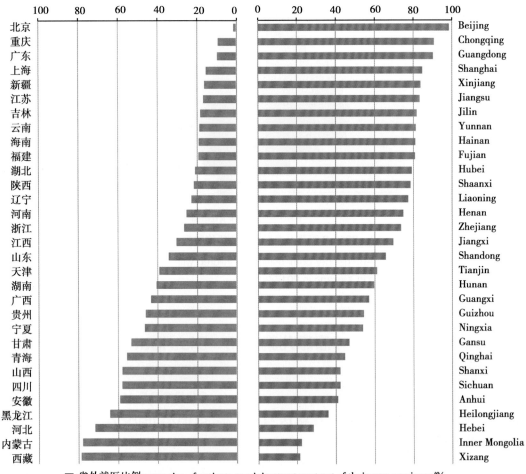

省外就医比例proportion of patients receiving treatment out of their own provinces/%

本省就医比例proportion of patients receiving treatment in their own provinces/%

图 7-3-1　2017—2018 年全国各省份肿瘤患儿本省就医与省外就医比例 /%

Figure 7-3-1　Proportion of children with cancer receiving medical treatment in and out of their own provincial-level regions in 2017-2018/%

3.2　全国各省份肿瘤患儿省外就医的去向省份分布情况

各省份肿瘤患儿选择省外就医的去向分布呈现明显的规律,主要的去向省份为北京、广东、上海、重庆和江苏。如户籍地为江西的肿瘤患儿,选择省外就医的主要去向为北京、上海和广东,分别占户籍地为江西的肿瘤患儿选择省外就医总数的43.5%、21.7%和16.4%。再如户籍地为安徽的肿瘤患儿,选择省外就医的主要去向为江苏、北京和上海,分别占户籍地为安徽的肿瘤患儿选择省外就医总数的46.0%、26.3%和18.2%(图7-3-2,按行方向查看)。

3.3　全国各省份收治肿瘤患儿来源的省份分布情况

各省份儿童肿瘤监测机构收治的省外就医肿瘤患儿来源分布略有差异,多数省份收治的肿瘤患儿来源以其相邻省份为主。如北京,其收治的省外就医患儿主要来源于河北、山东和河南,分别占北京收治的省外就医肿瘤患儿总数的20.0%、12.6%和9.4%。再如湖南,其收治的省外就医患儿主要来源于江西、湖北和广西,分别占湖南收治的省外就医肿瘤患儿总数的31.1%、14.5%和13.2%(图7-3-3,按列方向查看)。

3.2　Distribution of provincial-level regions receiving children with cancer from outside the provincial-level regions

The distribution of provincial-level regions receiving children with cancer from outside the provincial-level regions showed obvious regularity. The main destinations were Beijing, Guangdong, Shanghai, Chongqing and Jiangsu. For Jiangxi children with cancer, the main destinations were Beijing, Shanghai and Guangdong, accounting for 43.5%, 21.7% and 16.4%, respectively, of the total number of Jiangxi children with cancer going outside Jiangxi. For Anhui children with cancer, Jiangsu, Beijing and Shanghai were the main destinations, accounting for 46.0%, 26.3% and 18.2%, respectively, of the total number of Anhui children with cancer going outside Anhui (Figure 7-3-2, view in rows).

3.3　Distribution of the provincial-level regions of origin of children receiving treatment out of their own provincial-level regions

There was a slight difference in the distribution of the provincial-level regions of origin of children with cancer admitted to surveillance sites in different provincial-level regions, and most of the children were mainly from their neighboring provincial-level regions. For example, in Beijing, cancer patients from other provincial-level regions were mainly from Hebei, Shandong and Henan, accounting respectively for 20.0%, 12.6% and 9.4% of the total number of children hospitalized from other provincial-level regions in Beijing. In Hunan, children hospitalized from other provincial-level regions were mainly from Jiangxi, Hubei and Guangxi, accounting for 31.1%, 14.5% and 13.2% of the total number of children hospitalized from other provincial-level regions in Hunan, respectively (Figure 7-3-3, view in lines).

收治省外就医肿瘤患儿的医院省份分布
provincial distribution of hospitals receiving children with cancer from outside the province

户籍地 / 就医省份	北京 Beijing	天津 Tianjin	河北 Hebei	山西 Shanxi	内蒙古 Inner Mongolia	辽宁 Liaoning	吉林 Jilin	黑龙江 Heilongjiang	上海 Shanghai	江苏 Jiangsu	浙江 Zhejiang	安徽 Anhui	福建 Fujian	江西 Jiangxi	山东 Shandong	河南 Henan	湖北 Hubei	湖南 Hunan	广东 Guangdong	广西 Guangxi	海南 Hainan	重庆 Chongqing	四川 Sichuan	贵州 Guizhou	云南 Yunnan	西藏 Xizang	陕西 Shaanxi	甘肃 Gansu	青海 Qinghai	宁夏 Ningxia	新疆 Xinjiang	合计 total
北京 Beijing	95.0	26.0	5.0	0	0	4.0	4.0	0	1.0	9.0	0	0	1.0	0	13.0	1.5	0	1.0	2.0	4.0	1.0	1.0	0	8.0	0	0	8.0	0	0	0	12.0	100
天津 Tianjin	89.9	7.9	0.4	0	0	0.1	0.1	0	1.0	0.3	0	0.3	0.3	0	1.6	0.2	0	0.1	0.1	0.4	0.1	0.1	0.0	0.1	0.1	0	0.2	0	0	0	0	100
河北 Hebei	86.0	0.5	1.0	0.1	0.1	0.1	0.1	0.1	0.2	0.5	0.1	0.0	0.1	0.0	0.5	2.1	0.0	0.0	0.1	0.0	0.0	0.1	0.2	0.2	0.0	0	5.9	0.0	0	0.0	0.4	100
山西 Shanxi	82.9	0.8	0.3		1.0	0.7	0.3	0.4	0.2	0.1	0.1	0.1	0.0	0.1	0.4	2.1	0.0	0.0	0.1	0.1	0.2	0.1	0.1	0.0	0.0	0	0.6	0.0	0	0.0	0.4	100
内蒙古 Inner Mongolia	88.4	1.8	0.1	0.0	1.0	7.0	6.0	0.4	0.0	1.2	0.1	0.0	0.2	0.0	1.6	0.2	0	0.1	0.1	0.1	0.5	0.1	0.1	0.8	0.0	0	0.1	0.1	0	0	1.6	100
辽宁 Liaoning	82.7	1.2	0.3	0.1	0.1	4.3	3.6	1.0	2.1	0.5	0.0	0.1	1.1	0	2.9	0.2	0	0.1	1.6	0.1	0.1	0	0.2	0	0	0	0.1	0.1	0	0.1	0	100
吉林 Jilin	84.7	4.1	0.2	0.1	0.1	2.8	2.3		1.1	0.4	0.1	0.1	0.1	0	2.4	0.1	1.3	0.4	0.5	0.0	0.1	0.1	0.5	0	0	0	0.2	0	0	0.1	4.4	100
黑龙江 Heilongjiang	48.8	0.4	0.1	0.2	0	0.3	0	0.2	47.8	36.8	1.6	0.1	0.1	1.3	1.5	0	1.3	0.4	0.7	0.1	0.4	1.5	0.0	1.8	0	0	0.2	0	0	0.1	0.1	100
上海 Shanghai	44.0	1.1	0.4	0	0	0.1	0	0	47.4	5.3	3.7	0.1	0.1	0.0	0.6	0.5	0.0	0.1	1.1	0.1	0.1	0.3	0.5	0.1	0.0	0	0.3	0.0	0.0	0.1	0.1	100
江苏 Jiangsu	42.1	0.6	0.2	0	0	0.1	0	0	18.2	46.0	5.0	0.1	0.1	0.1	0.6	0.1	0.6	0.2	1.0	0.1	0.1	0.7	0.1	0.0	0.1	0	0.8	0	0	0.0	0.1	100
浙江 Zhejiang	26.3	0.5	0.2	0.1	0.2	0.3	0.1	0.0	23.8	1.8	5.0		4.2	0.0	0.2	0.5	0.8	0.1	10.5	0.3	0.1	0.3	0.1	0.0	0.1	0	0.3	0	0	0.1	0.2	100
安徽 Anhui	54.1	0.3	0	0.0	0	0.4	0.7	0	21.7	2.9	6.1	0.5	4.2		0.2	0.1	0.7	0.2	16.4	0.3	0.0	0.7	0.1	0	0.1	0	0.8	0	0	0.1	0.2	100
福建 Fujian	43.5	0.1	0	0.0	0.1	0.4	0.2	0	2.9	1.5	0.3	0.4		0.0	0.2	0.5	0.1	1.2	0.8	0.1	0.3	0.3	0.0	0	0.1	0	0.1	0.0	0	0.1	0.0	100
江西 Jiangxi	89.0	1.9	0.4	0.0	0.1	1.0	0.2	0.0	3.8	3.1	1.8	0.8	0.6	0.0	1.0	0.1	8.1	0.0	2.3	0.1	0.1	0.2	0.1	0	0.1	0	1.4	0.0	0.1	0	0.6	100
山东 Shandong	73.2	0.6	0.5	0.2	0.0	0.4	1.0	0.1	4.3	2.6	5.4	0.8	3.5	0.4	0.8	0.8	2.3	1.2	14.4	0.4	0.9	3.1	0.2	0.1	0.1	0	0.6	0.0	0	0.0	0.0	100
河南 Henan	58.3	1.5	0.3	0.0	0	0.1	0.2	0	3.5	3.5	2.2	0.8	0.2	1.4	5.7	0.6	2.3	1.2	23.2	0	0.6	0.7	0.1	0.6	0	0	0.6	0.0	0	0.2	0.2	100
湖北 Hubei	54.2	0.4	0.1	0	0	0.0	0.2	0.1	1.2	20.8	2.1	0.3	4.3	1.3	0.2	0.1	2.6	0.9	50.6	2.4	2.3	2.7	1.1	0.6	0	0	0.6	0	0	0.2	1.3	100
湖南 Hunan	51.9	0.9	2.2	0	0	0.6	0.2	0.6	1.3	1.2	0.3	0.3	1.1	0.3	0.4	0.3	0.3	1.5	53.5	1.1	0.9	0.2	0.6	0.1	0.1	0	0	0	0	0.2	1.3	100
广东 Guangdong	37.4	0.4	0.3	0.1	0	0.1	0.1	0	0.3	2.7	0.2	0.1	1.1	0.3	0.5	0.3	5.0	0.3	12.0	0.4		0.2	4.7	0.9	0.3	0	1.2	0	0.0	1.1	0.2	100
广西 Guangxi	37.0	0.6	1.6	0.1	0.4	0.2	0	0.1	5.2	1.4	1.2	0.1	2.6	0.4	4.9	0.4	0.3	0.1	53.5	0.4	0.9	0.2	0.9	0.2	0.3	0	1.2	0	0	1.1	0.1	100
海南 Hainan	57.8	0.9	0.1	0.2	0.4	0.2	0.1	0.0	2.6	0.9	0.7	0.1	1.6	0.2	2.1	0.2	0.7	0.4	2.5	0.6	0.9	73.4	1.1	0.6	0.3	0	0.1	0.0	0	0.1	0.7	100
重庆 Chongqing	12.3	0.2	0	0	0.0	0	0.2	0	3.2	0.4	2.4	0.1	2.9	0	0.6	0.6	0.8	0.5	3.8	0.6	0.1	57.4	1.1	0.6	9.7	0	0.0	0.0	0	0	0	100
四川 Sichuan	16.2	0.5	0.5	0	0	0.3	0.6	0.1	7.7	9.6	5.5	0.2	0.2	1.1	0.6	0.6	0.8	0.6	4.5	0.9	0	18.8	2.4	0.6	0	0	1.4	0	0.1	0	0	100
贵州 Guizhou	45.4	0.1	0	0.2	0	0.1	0	0	0	0.4	2.3	0.2	0.6	1.1	1.1	0.8	0.1	0.6	1.7	0.1	0.5	28.0	26.9	0.6	0	0	1.1	0.0	0	1.3	1.1	100
云南 Yunnan	14.9	0	0.5	0.1	0	0.1	0	0	2.1	0	2.3	0.1	0.3	0	1.1	1.4	0.1	0.6	1.1	0.1	0	0.2	2.4	0.6	0	0	1.1	8.6	0	0.4	0.6	100
西藏 Xizang	85.3	1.3	0.6	0.1	0.9	0.1	0.2	0	1.4	3.8	0.2	0	0	0	1.7	0.8	0.1	0.2	0.5	0.1	0	0.2	1.7	0.3	0.1	0	1.1	0	0	0.4	1.6	100
陕西 Shaanxi	41.1	0.8	0.1	0.0	0	0.2	0.2	0.0	0	2.1	1.5	0.2	0.1	0	0.3	1.4	0.1	0.2	1.1	0.1	0	1.2	1.7	0.3	0.0	0	42.8	0	0.1	1.3	1.6	100
甘肃 Gansu	69.1	0.8	0.4	0	0	0.1	0.2	0.2	0	2.1	2.3	0.2	0	0	0.6	4.6	0.2	0.3	0.5	0	0	0.8	0.8	0.3	0	0	11.6	4.6	0.1	0.4	0.2	100
青海 Qinghai	77.0	0.7	0	0.1	0	0.1	0	0.2	0.5	0.2	0.1	0	0.1	0	0.6	1.8	0.1	0.2	2.5	0	0	0.1	0.1	0	0.1	0	18.2	0.8	0		0.2	100
宁夏 Ningxia	86.3	0.1	0	0	0	0.1	0.1	0	4.3	0.5	0.1	0.2	0	0	0.5	1.9	0.0	0.3	1.1	0	0	0.8	1.0	0	0	0	1.6	1.1	0	0	0	100
新疆 Xinjiang																																100

各省户籍地肿瘤患儿外就医省份分布
distribution of the provinces of origin of children with cancer receiving treatment out of their own provinces

图 7-3-2 2017—2018 年全国各省省份户籍地肿瘤患儿选择省外就医的省份分布 /%

Figure 7-3-2 Distribution of provincial-level regions receiving children with cancer from other provincial-level regions in 2017-2018/%

收治省外级医院肿瘤患儿的医院省份分布

provincial distribution of hospitals receiving children with cancer from outside the province

就诊省份儿童肿瘤监测机构省外就医省份分布 distribution of the provinces of origin of children with cancer receiving treatment out of their own provinces	北京 Beijing	天津 Tianjin	河北 Hebei	山西 Shanxi	内蒙古 Inner Mongolia	辽宁 Liaoning	吉林 Jilin	黑龙江 Heilongjiang	上海 Shanghai	江苏 Jiangsu	浙江 Zhejiang	安徽 Anhui	福建 Fujian	江西 Jiangxi	山东 Shandong	河南 Henan	湖北 Hubei	湖南 Hunan	广东 Guangdong	广西 Guangxi	海南 Hainan	重庆 Chongqing	四川 Sichuan	贵州 Guizhou	云南 Yunnan	西藏 Xizang	陕西 Shaanxi	甘肃 Gansu	青海 Qinghai	宁夏 Ningxia	新疆 Xinjiang
北京 Beijing	1.0	1.2	1.6	0	0	0.6	0.6	0	0.0	0.2	0	0.9	0.1	0	1.1	1.9	0	0.4	0.0	1.9	0.5	0.0	0	5.9	0	0	0.3	0	0	0	3.8
天津 Tianjin	20.0	59.0	0.9	0	0	1.0	0.7	6.9	0.2	0	0	0.4	0.2	0	1.0	1.9	0.3	0.4	0.2	1.4	0	0.2	1.1	0.7	0.2	0	1.3	0	0	2.0	0.3
河北 Hebei	6.8	1.4	17.7	24.3	9.4	4.6	2.4	0	0.1	0.8	0.4	0.9	1.7	1.9	7.2	6.2	0.1	0	0.1	3.8	0.9	0	2.2	8.9	0	0	13.4	1.3	37.5	0.7	7.3
山西 Shanxi	6.7	2.2	5.9	7.0	49.6	47.0	45.2	0	0.1	0.4	0.1	1.3	0.1	1.3	1.8	20.3	0	0.4	0.1	0.9	0	0.4	0.4	0	0.2	0	1.3	2.5	46.7	0.7	0
内蒙古 Inner Mongolia	3.4	2.3	1.2	1.2	0.8	—	13.2	2.8	0.0	0.1	0.2	0.4	0.7	1.3	3.9	1.0	0	0.4	0.4	1.4	6.9	0.5	0.9	15.6	0	0	0.1	2.5	12.5	0	0
辽宁 Liaoning	1.8	0.9	1.5	1.2	0.8	7.6	10.2	20.8	0.4	0.1	0	0.4	1.9	0	3.8	0.7	0	0	0.5	0.5	0.5	0.8	3.8	0	0	0	0.2	0	0	1.3	7.7
吉林 Jilin	4.1	6.7	1.9	5.8	3.3	11.5	—	0	0.4	0.2	0.1	0	0.2	0	7.2	0.7	0.3	0.4	0.3	0.5	0.9	0	0	3.0	0	0	0.2	0	0	1.3	3.2
黑龙江 Heilongjiang	0.2	0.1	0	0	0	0	0.6	—	0.4	1.3	0.1	0	0.2	0	0	0	0.3	0	0.2	0	0.9	0	0	0	0	0	0.4	0	0	0	0.6
上海 Shanghai	2.3	2.0	1.2	7.0	0	1.3	0.1	9.7	20.7	2.1	3.3	1.7	0.2	7.1	4.9	0	0.1	0	0.5	0.9	0	0.6	0.2	3.7	0.2	0	0.4	2.5	0	2.0	0.6
江苏 Jiangsu	1.6	0.7	3.1	0	0	0.2	0	1.4	14.5	68.8	3.1	0.2	0.2	0.6	0.2	2.9	1.3	0.9	0.5	0.5	1.4	0	2.2	2.2	0.2	0	0.4	1.3	0	4.0	0.6
浙江 Zhejiang	3.6	2.1	6.2	16.3	2.6	3.9	1.7	0	20.8	0.8	20.4	1.6	1.6	3.2	5.0	7.8	5.1	7.0	1.9	4.7	0	0.3	11.2	1.5	0.6	0	2.0	2.5	37.5	0.7	1.3
安徽 Anhui	2.3	0.4	1.9	1.2	5.1	3.0	2.8	0	8.3	2.5	8.4	13.1	27.6	1.3	0.2	0.5	2.1	1.3	5.9	3.8	0	0.2	0.9	0.7	0.4	0	0.9	0	0	0.7	3.8
福建 Fujian	3.5	0.4	3.1	0	0	0.1	0.1	0	14.6	2.5	19.9	13.1	27.6	0.9	0	5.4	3.4	1.3	17.8	8.0	0.9	0.1	1.8	3.7	0.4	0	0.6	0	25.0	0.7	1.6
江西 Jiangxi	12.6	8.9	13.6	3.5	1.7	11.6	2.3	6.9	3.4	2.3	1.8	19.7	1.7	0.6	0.9	9.2	0.2	31.1	1.5	2.8	0.5	0.2	5.2	0	0.4	0	0.6	3.8	25.0	5.3	16.9
山东 Shandong	9.4	2.4	13.6	23.3	2.6	3.9	11.8	2.8	4.1	4.2	9.1	31.4	6.2	1.9	7.8	9.2	62.9	0.9	3.9	4.2	2.3	0.2	1.3	0	1.7	0	5.1	1.3	0.7	0.7	0.3
河南 Henan	2.1	1.8	2.5	0	0	0.1	0.6	0	1.3	1.0	7.9	9.2	10.4	7.1	1.9	3.8	—	14.5	7.1	4.7	11.0	0.8	1.1	0.7	0.2	0	0.6	0	12.5	0	0.3
湖北 Hubei	3.8	0.8	0.9	1.2	0	0.2	1.0	5.6	2.1	2.6	6.3	7.9	2.2	0.6	24.8	5.7	9.9	—	21.9	8.9	3.7	0.4	1.6	3.7	0.6	0	0.4	2.5	0	2.0	3.5
湖南 Hunan	0.9	0.5	8.7	1.2	0	0.9	0.4	9.7	0.2	3.9	1.5	1.7	6.0	10.3	0.2	2.6	2.8	4.8	3.4	14.6	13.3	0.6	3.1	5.2	0.2	0	0.3	0	0	0	5.1
广东 Guangdong	1.0	0.4	1.9	1.2	0	0.3	0.1	0	1.8	2.6	5.4	1.7	2.5	4.5	0.9	0.2	0.6	13.2	1.5	7.5	8.3	0.6	2.7	0.7	0.2	0	0.3	0	0	0	0
海南 Hainan	0.3	0.2	3.1	0	0	0.1	0.1	0	0.0	0.3	0.1	0.4	0.1	1.3	0.2	0.3	3.9	0.9	6.1	3.3	0	0.0	10.6	0.7	0	0	0.1	0	0	4.7	0.3
重庆 Chongqing	0.7	0.4	0.3	3.4	0	0.2	0.1	0	0.6	0.2	0.6	2.7	0.9	0.6	3.9	0.7	3.9	0.9	2.0	1.9	0.5	64.0	9.9	5.9	0	0	0.4	2.5	0	0	0.3
四川 Sichuan	1.5	0.7	2.2	7.0	1.7	0.2	1.7	0	2.5	1.2	3.5	1.7	15.5	10.3	15.6	2.9	2.2	4.4	4.0	7.0	36.2	27.9	11.9	9.6	5.7	0	0.4	2.5	12.5	21.3	19.2
贵州 Guizhou	1.1	1.1	1.5	0	0	0.9	1.3	0	1.8	0.3	6.4	1.7	15.5	1.3	0.4	1.9	2.9	9.2	3.4	13.1	1.4	3.4	13.5	—	0	0	0.1	0	0	10.0	18.5
云南 Yunnan	1.1	0.1	2.8	1.2	0	0.6	1.3	1.4	1.6	2.6	5.4	0.4	0.4	2.6	0.9	1.7	1.3	3.9	1.5	7.5	0	3.4	9.7	8.1	88.1	0	0.1	10.1	0	0	0.3
西藏 Xizang	0.0	0	0	0	0	0.1	0.1	1.4	0.0	0.3	0.2	1.3	0.1	1.3	0.2	0.3	0.2	0.4	0.1	0	0	0.5	10.6	0.7	0	—	0.1	10.1	0	4.7	0
陕西 Shaanxi	2.8	1.4	4.3	1.2	18.8	0.3	2.1	0	0.6	0.4	0.2	0.9	0.9	0	3.5	3.5	0.2	2.6	0.5	1.4	5.0	0.1	0	11.1	0.2	0	60.9	2.5	0	21.3	4.5
甘肃 Gansu	2.0	1.4	0.6	0	1.7	0.7	1.0	0	0.6	2.1	3.0	0.9	0.4	1.3	0.8	8.3	0.3	0	0.4	1.4	0	0.4	13.5	7.4	0.2	0	2.4	30.4	25.0	10.0	18.5
青海 Qinghai	0.5	0.3	0.6	0	0	0.1	0	0	0.1	0.4	0.7	0	0.1	0	0.3	4.2	0.1	0	0.2	0	0	0	0.9	0	0	0	7.2	10.1	—	0	0.3
宁夏 Ningxia	1.1	0.0	0.3	0	0	0.1	0.1	1.4	0.8	0.1	0.1	0.9	0.1	0	0.6	3.1	0.2	2.2	0.2	2.2	0	0.0	0.2	0	0.2	0	1.0	20.3	0	—	0
新疆 Xinjiang	1.8	0.3	0	0	0	0.1	0.1	0	0.8	0.1	0.1	0.9	0.3	0	0.6	5.0	0.2	0	0.3	0	0	0.1	3.4	0	0.2	0	1.8	0	0	0	—
合计 Total	100	100	100	100	100	100	100	100	100	100	100	100	100	100	100	100	100	100	100	100	100	100	100	100	100	100	100	100	100	100	100

图 7-3-3　2017—2018 年全国各省份儿童肿瘤监测机构省外就医肿瘤患儿来源分布 /%

Figure 7-3-3　Distribution of provincial-level regions of origin of children with cancer going outside their provincial-level regions for medical treatment in 2017-2018/%

4 全国儿童肿瘤监测机构肿瘤患儿住院费用医疗付费方式构成

4.1 全国肿瘤患儿住院费用医疗付费方式构成情况

全国肿瘤患儿住院费用的医疗付费方式中,占比最高的前 3 种类型分别为全自费(33.56%)、新型农村合作医疗(22.93%)和城镇居民基本医疗保险(19.38%)(图 7-4-1)。

4 Composition of medical payment methods for hospitalization expenses of children with cancer in pediatric cancer surveillance sites in China

4.1 Composition of medical payment methods for hospitalization expenses of children with cancer nationally

Among the medical payment methods of children with cancer nationally, the top three methods were 100% self-pay (33.56%), new rural cooperative medical system (22.93%) and basic medical insurance for urban residents (19.38%)(Figure 7-4-1).

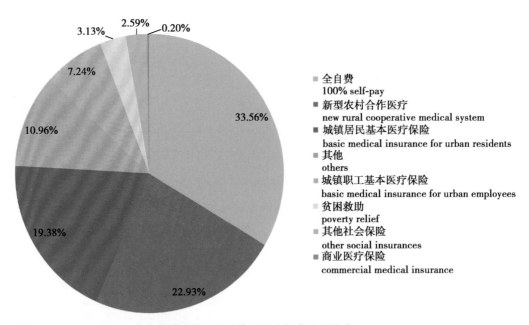

- 全自费
  100% self-pay
- 新型农村合作医疗
  new rural cooperative medical system
- 城镇居民基本医疗保险
  basic medical insurance for urban residents
- 其他
  others
- 城镇职工基本医疗保险
  basic medical insurance for urban employees
- 贫困救助
  poverty relief
- 其他社会保险
  other social insurances
- 商业医疗保险
  commercial medical insurance

图 7-4-1 2017—2018 年全国肿瘤患儿住院费用医疗付费方式构成

Figure 7-4-1 Composition of medical payment methods for hospitalization expenses of children with cancer nationally in 2017-2018

4.2　六大区肿瘤患儿住院费用医疗付费方式构成情况

六大区的医疗付费方式所占比例各不相同，西南地区、华北地区和华东地区均以全自费占比最高，分别为46.04%、41.59% 和35.59%。而中南地区、西北地区和东北地区则以新型农村合作医疗占比最高，分别为37.33%、32.55% 和25.17%（图7-4-2~图7-4-7）。

4.2　Composition of medical payment methods for hospitalization expenses of children with cancer in the six regions

The proportions of medical payment methods in the six regions were different, and the proportion of 100% self-pay was the highest in Southwest China, North China and East China, which was 46.04%, 41.59% and 35.59%, respectively. In Central and Southern China, Northwest China and Northeast China, the proportion of new rural cooperative medical system was the highest, accounting for 37.33%, 32.55% and 25.17%, respectively (Figure 7-4-2~Figure 7-4-7).

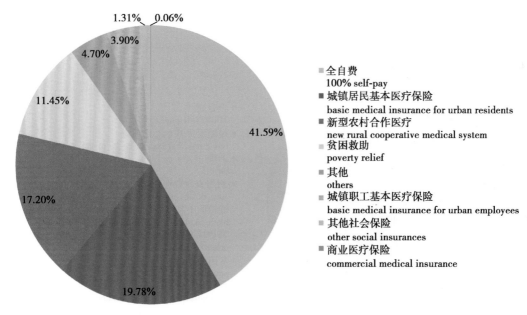

图 7-4-2　2017—2018 年华北地区肿瘤患儿住院费用医疗付费方式构成

Figure 7-4-2　Composition of medical payment methods for hospitalization expenses of children with cancer in North China in 2017-2018

93

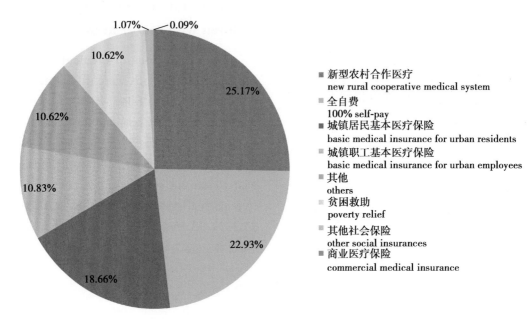

图 7-4-3 2017—2018 年东北地区肿瘤患儿住院费用医疗付费方式构成

Figure 7-4-3 Composition of medical payment methods for hospitalization expenses of children with cancer in Northeast China in 2017-2018

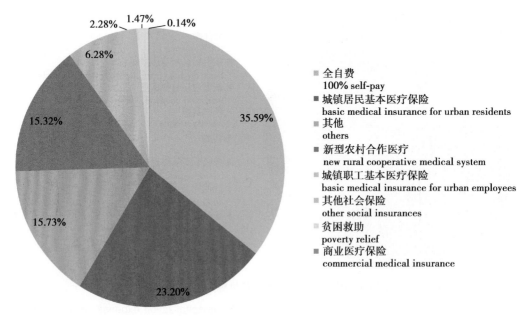

图 7-4-4 2017—2018 年华东地区肿瘤患儿住院费用医疗付费方式构成

Figure 7-4-4 Composition of medical payment methods for hospitalization expenses of children with cancer in East China in 2017-2018

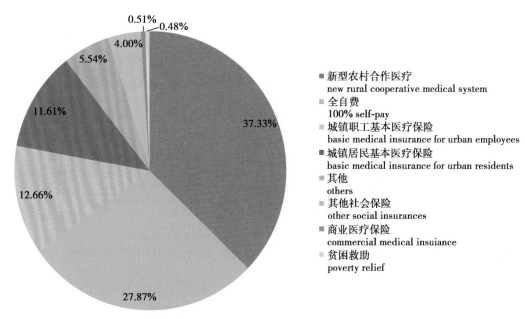

图 7-4-5 2017—2018 年中南地区肿瘤患儿住院费用医疗付费方式构成

Figure 7-4-5 Composition of medical payment methods for hospitalization expenses of children with cancer in Central and Southern China in 2017-2018

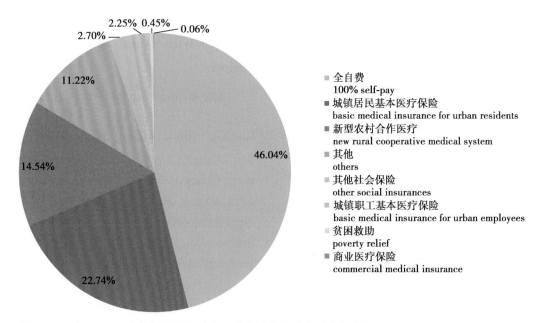

图 7-4-6 2017—2018 年西南地区肿瘤患儿住院费用医疗付费方式构成

Figure 7-4-6 Composition of medical payment methods for hospitalization expenses of children with cancer in Southwest China in 2017-2018

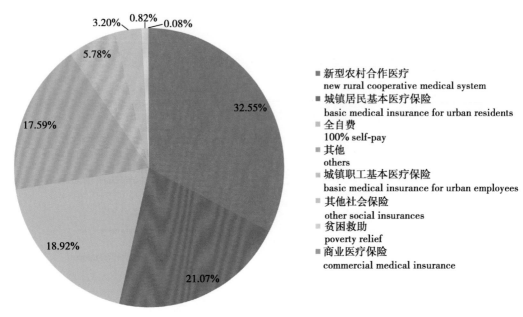

图 7-4-7 2017—2018 年西北地区肿瘤患儿住院费用医疗付费方式构成

Figure 7-4-7 Composition of medical payment methods for hospitalization expenses of children with cancer in Northwest China in 2017-2018

4.3 各省份肿瘤患儿住院费用医疗付费方式构成情况

河北、山西、内蒙古、黑龙江、江苏、安徽、福建、江西、湖南、广东、广西、四川、贵州、云南和西藏 15 个省份均以全自费所占比例最高。吉林、河南、海南、陕西和甘肃 5 个省份的新型农村合作医疗占比最高。天津、上海、山东、重庆和宁夏 5 个省份的城镇居民基本医疗保险占比最高（图 7-4-8～图 7-4-38）。

4.3 Composition of medical payment methods for hospitalization expenses of children with cancer in each provincial-level region

The proportion of 100% self-pay was the highest in the following 15 provincial-level regions: Hebei, Shanxi, Inner Mongolia, Heilongjiang, Jiangsu, Anhui, Fujian, Jiangxi, Hunan, Guangdong, Guangxi, Sichuan, Guizhou, Yunnan and Xizang. Jilin, Henan, Hainan, Shaanxi and Gansu had the highest proportion of payment through new rural cooperative medical system. The following five provincial-level regions—Tianjin, Shanghai, Shandong, Chongqing and Ningxia—had the highest proportion of payment through basic medical insurance for urban residents (Figure 7-4-8~Figure 7-4-38).

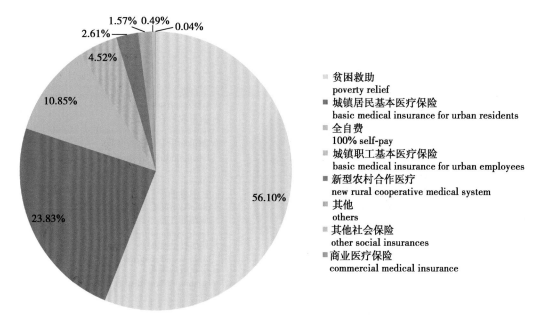

图 7-4-8　2017—2018 年北京肿瘤患儿住院费用医疗付费方式构成

Figure 7-4-8　Composition of medical payment methods for hospitalization expenses of children with cancer in Beijing in 2017-2018

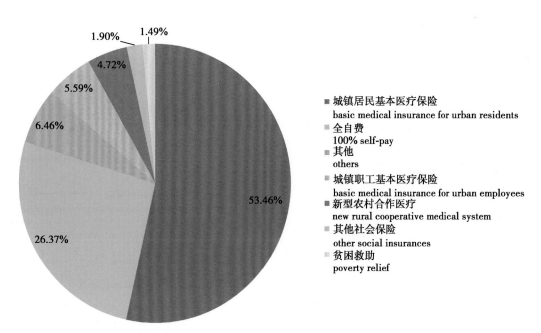

图 7-4-9　2017—2018 年天津肿瘤患儿住院费用医疗付费方式构成

Figure 7-4-9　Composition of medical payment methods for hospitalization expenses of children with cancer in Tianjin in 2017-2018

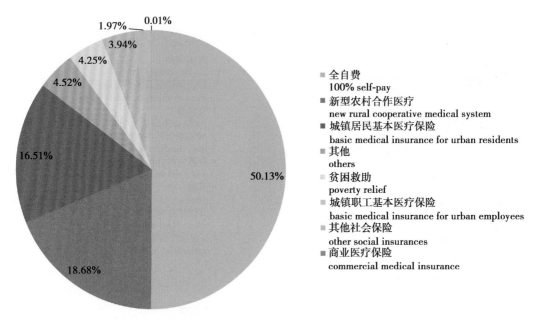

图 7-4-10　2017—2018 年河北肿瘤患儿住院费用医疗付费方式构成

Figure 7-4-10　Composition of medical payment methods for hospitalization expenses of children with cancer in Hebei in 2017-2018

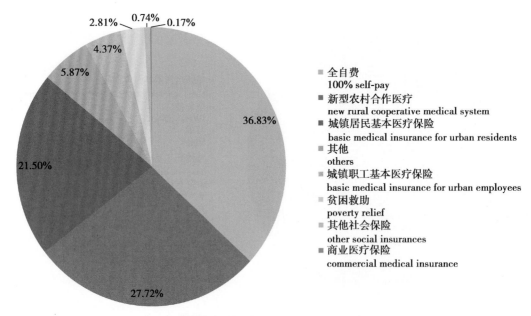

图 7-4-11　2017—2018 年山西肿瘤患儿住院费用医疗付费方式构成

Figure 7-4-11　Composition of medical payment methods for hospitalization expenses of children with cancer in Shanxi in 2017-2018

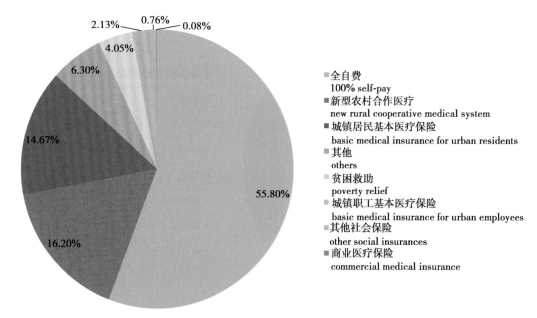

图 7-4-12　2017—2018 年内蒙古肿瘤患儿住院费用医疗付费方式构成

Figure 7-4-12　Composition of medical payment methods for hospitalization expenses of children with cancer in Inner Mongolia in 2017-2018

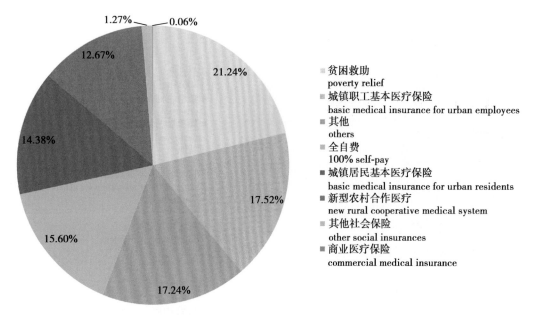

图 7-4-13　2017—2018 年辽宁肿瘤患儿住院费用医疗付费方式构成

Figure 7-4-13　Composition of medical payment methods for hospitalization expenses of children with cancer in Liaoning in 2017-2018

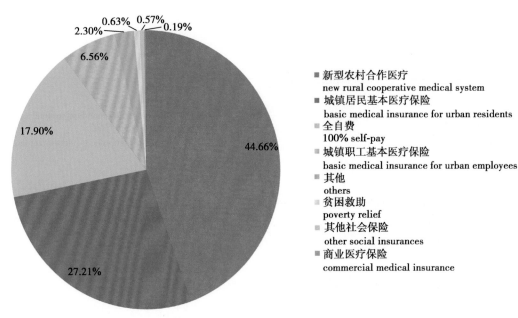

新型农村合作医疗
new rural cooperative medical system

城镇居民基本医疗保险
basic medical insurance for urban residents

全自费
100% self-pay

城镇职工基本医疗保险
basic medical insurance for urban employees

其他
others

贫困救助
poverty relief

其他社会保险
other social insurances

商业医疗保险
commercial medical insurance

图 7-4-14　2017—2018 年吉林肿瘤患儿住院费用医疗付费方式构成

Figure 7-4-14　Composition of medical payment methods for hospitalization expenses of children with cancer in Jilin in 2017-2018

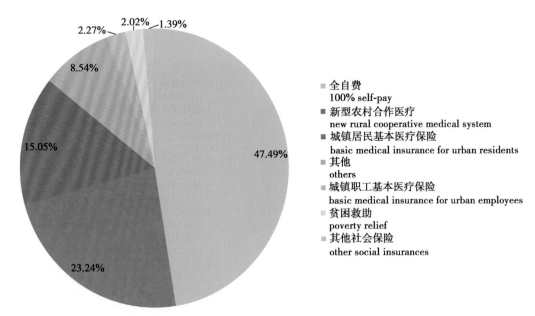

全自费
100% self-pay

新型农村合作医疗
new rural cooperative medical system

城镇居民基本医疗保险
basic medical insurance for urban residents

其他
others

城镇职工基本医疗保险
basic medical insurance for urban employees

贫困救助
poverty relief

其他社会保险
other social insurances

图 7-4-15　2017—2018 年黑龙江肿瘤患儿住院费用医疗付费方式构成

Figure 7-4-15　Composition of medical payment methods for hospitalization expenses of children with cancer in Heilongjiang in 2017-2018

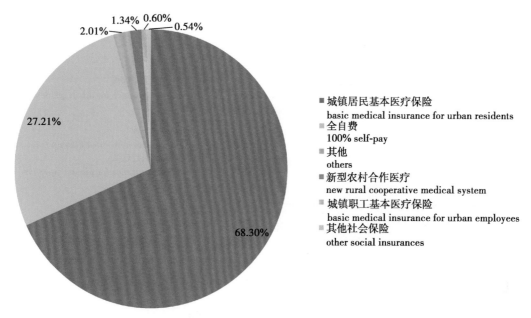

图 7-4-16   2017—2018 年上海肿瘤患儿住院费用医疗付费方式构成

Figure 7-4-16   Composition of medical payment methods for hospitalization expenses of children with cancer in Shanghai in 2017-2018

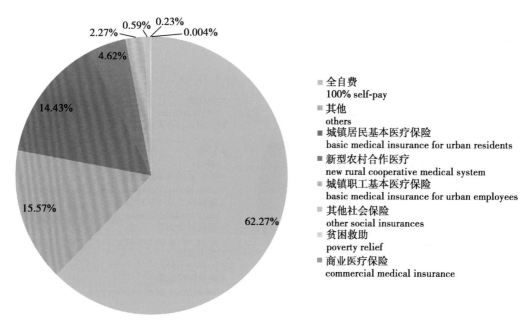

图 7-4-17   2017—2018 年江苏肿瘤患儿住院费用医疗付费方式构成

Figure 7-4-17   Composition of medical payment methods for hospitalization expenses of children with cancer in Jiangsu in 2017-2018

101

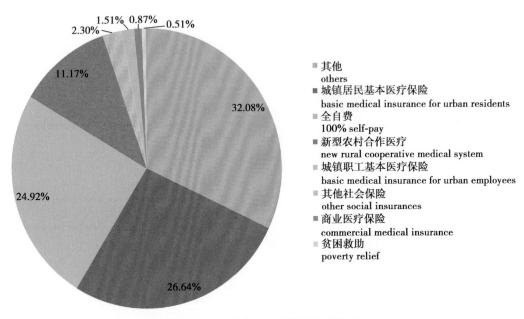

图 7-4-18 2017—2018 年浙江肿瘤患儿住院费用医疗付费方式构成

Figure 7-4-18 Composition of medical payment methods for hospitalization expenses of children with cancer in Zhejiang in 2017-2018

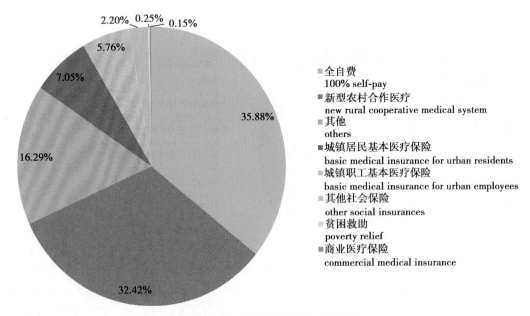

图 7-4-19 2017—2018 年安徽肿瘤患儿住院费用医疗付费方式构成

Figure 7-4-19 Composition of medical payment methods for hospitalization expenses of children with cancer in Anhui in 2017-2018

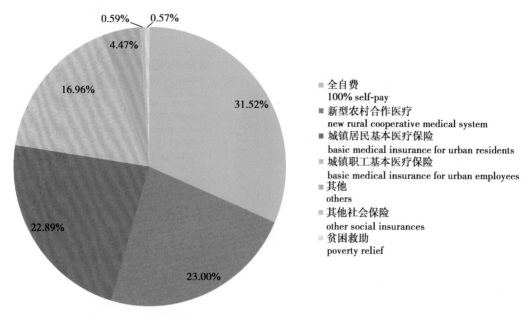

图 7-4-20　2017—2018 年福建肿瘤患儿住院费用医疗付费方式构成

Figure 7-4-20　Composition of medical payment methods for hospitalization expenses of children with cancer in Fujian in 2017-2018

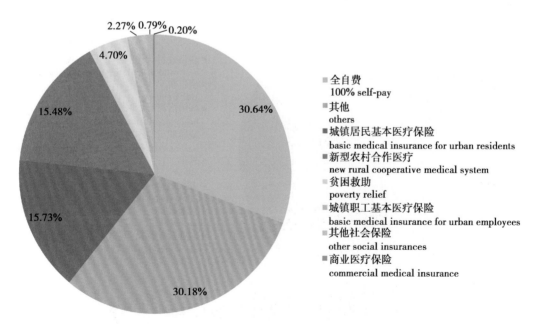

图 7-4-21　2017—2018 年江西肿瘤患儿住院费用医疗付费方式构成

Figure 7-4-21　Composition of medical payment methods for hospitalization expenses of children with cancer in Jiangxi in 2017-2018

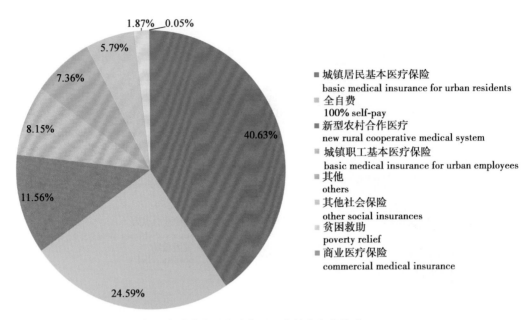

图 7-4-22　2017—2018 年山东肿瘤患儿住院费用医疗付费方式构成

Figure 7-4-22　Composition of medical payment methods for hospitalization expenses of children with cancer in Shandong in 2017-2018

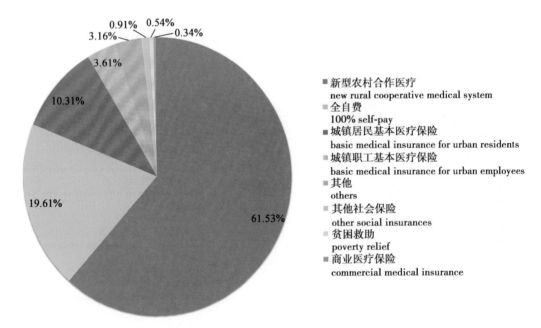

图 7-4-23　2017—2018 年河南肿瘤患儿住院费用医疗付费方式构成

Figure 7-4-23　Composition of medical payment methods for hospitalization expenses of children with cancer in Henan in 2017-2018

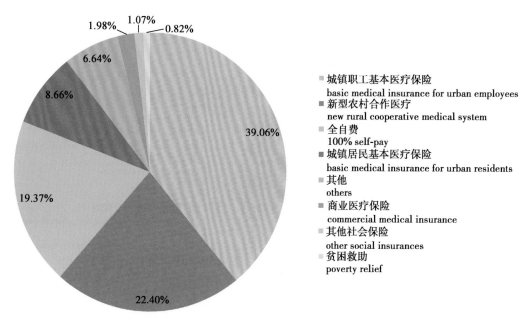

图 7-4-24　2017—2018 年湖北肿瘤患儿住院费用医疗付费方式构成

Figure 7-4-24　Composition of medical payment methods for hospitalization expenses of children with cancer in Hubei in 2017-2018

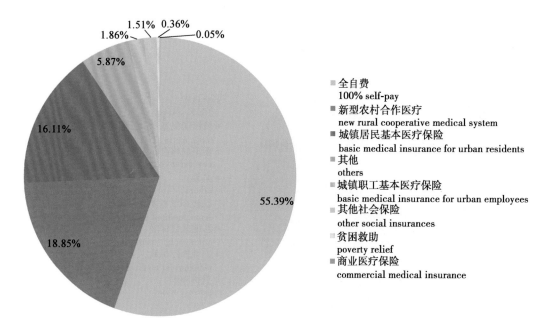

图 7-4-25　2017—2018 年湖南肿瘤患儿住院费用医疗付费方式构成

Figure 7-4-25　Composition of medical payment methods for hospitalization expenses of children with cancer in Hunan in 2017-2018

105

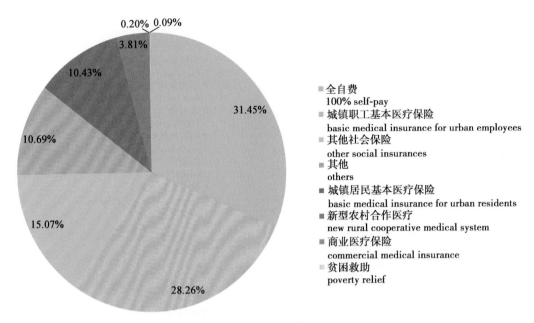

图 7-4-26　2017—2018 年广东肿瘤患儿住院费用医疗付费方式构成

Figure 7-4-26　Composition of medical payment methods for hospitalization expenses of children with cancer in Guangdong in 2017-2018

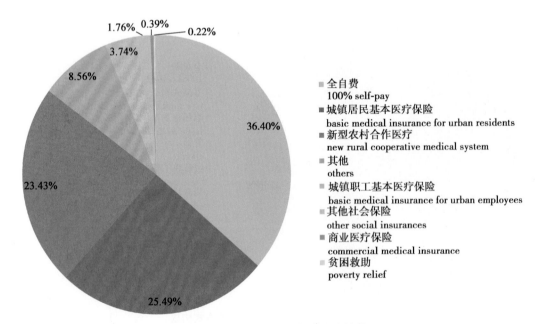

图 7-4-27　2017—2018 年广西肿瘤患儿住院费用医疗付费方式构成

Figure 7-4-27　Composition of medical payment methods for hospitalization expenses of children with cancer in Guangxi in 2017-2018

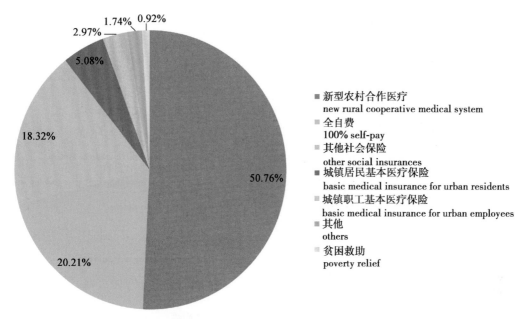

图 7-4-28　2017—2018 年海南肿瘤患儿住院费用医疗付费方式构成

Figure 7-4-28　Composition of medical payment methods for hospitalization expenses of children with cancer in Hainan in 2017-2018

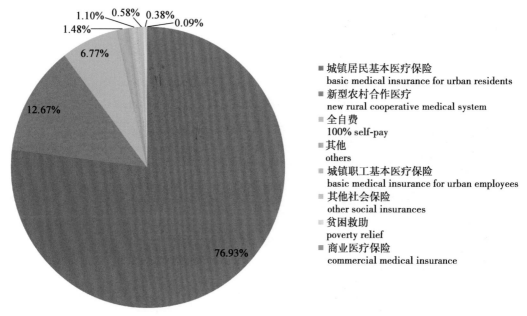

图 7-4-29　2017—2018 年重庆肿瘤患儿住院费用医疗付费方式构成

Figure 7-4-29　Composition of medical payment methods for hospitalization expenses of children with cancer in Chongqing in 2017-2018

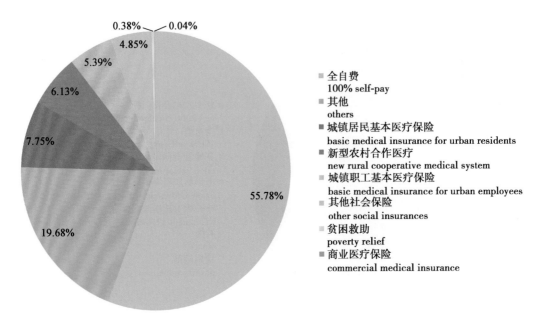

图 7-4-30 2017—2018 年四川肿瘤患儿住院费用医疗付费方式构成

Figure 7-4-30 Composition of medical payment methods for hospitalization expenses of children with cancer in Sichuan in 2017-2018

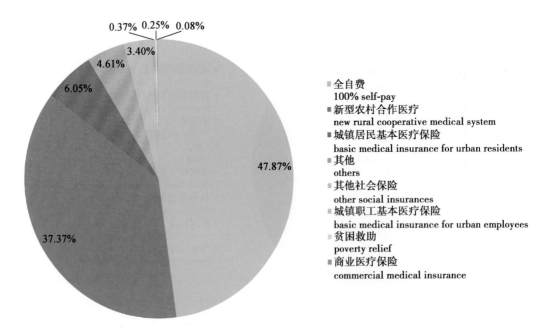

图 7-4-31 2017—2018 年贵州肿瘤患儿住院费用医疗付费方式构成

Figure 7-4-31 Composition of medical payment methods for hospitalization expenses of children with cancer in Guizhou in 2017-2018

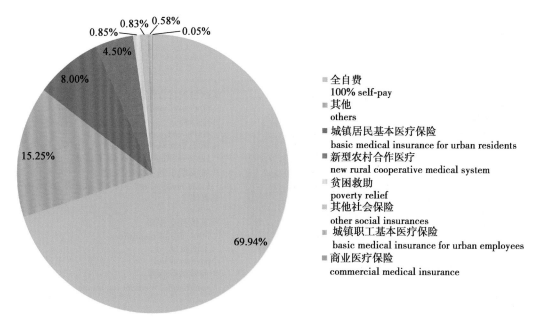

图 7-4-32　2017—2018 年云南肿瘤患儿住院费用医疗付费方式构成

Figure 7-4-32　Composition of medical payment methods for hospitalization expenses of children with cancer in Yunnan in 2017-2018

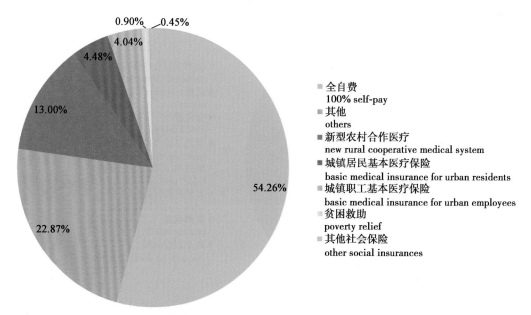

图 7-4-33　2017—2018 年西藏肿瘤患儿住院费用医疗付费方式构成

Figure 7-4-33　Composition of medical payment methods for hospitalization expenses of children with cancer in Xizang in 2017-2018

109

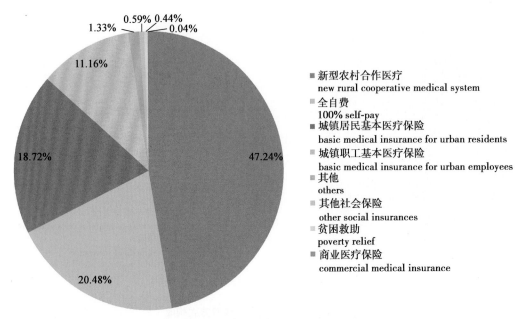

图 7-4-34　2017—2018 年陕西肿瘤患儿住院费用医疗付费方式构成

Figure 7-4-34　Composition of medical payment methods for hospitalization expenses of children with cancer in Shaanxi in 2017-2018

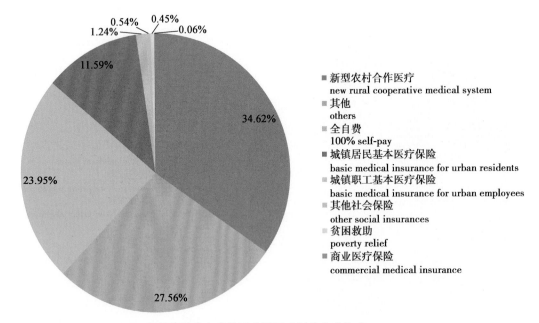

图 7-4-35　2017—2018 年甘肃肿瘤患儿住院费用医疗付费方式构成

Figure 7-4-35　Composition of medical payment methods for hospitalization expenses of children with cancer in Gansu in 2017-2018

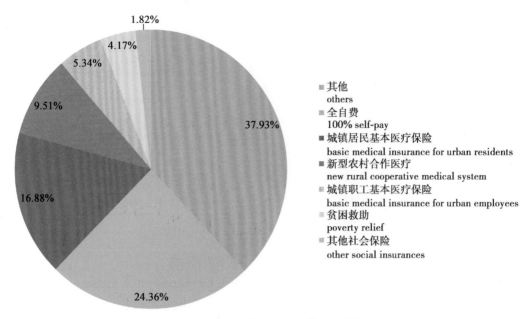

图 7-4-36　2017—2018 年青海肿瘤患儿住院费用医疗付费方式构成

Figure 7-4-36　Composition of medical payment methods for hospitalization expenses of children with cancer in Qinghai in 2017-2018

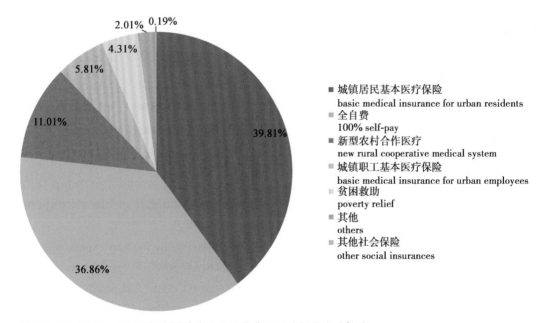

图 7-4-37　2017—2018 年宁夏肿瘤患儿住院费用医疗付费方式构成

Figure 7-4-37　Composition of medical payment methods for hospitalization expenses of children with cancer in Ningxia in 2017-2018

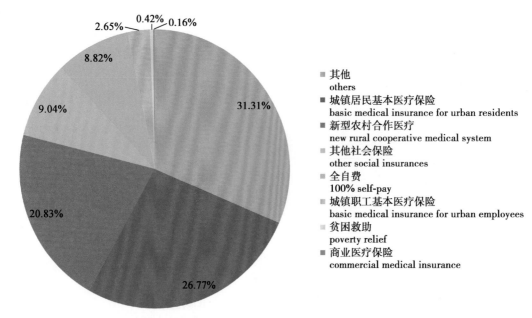

图 7-4-38　2017—2018 年新疆肿瘤患儿住院费用医疗付费方式构成

Figure 7-4-38　Composition of medical payment methods for hospitalization expenses of children with cancer in Xinjiang in 2017-2018

图例：
- 其他 others
- 城镇居民基本医疗保险 basic medical insurance for urban residents
- 新型农村合作医疗 new rural cooperative medical system
- 其他社会保险 other social insurances
- 全自费 100% self-pay
- 城镇职工基本医疗保险 basic medical insurance for urban employees
- 贫困救助 poverty relief
- 商业医疗保险 commercial medical insurance

5　全国儿童肿瘤监测机构肿瘤患儿住院费用分析

5.1　全国儿童肿瘤监测机构肿瘤患儿次均住院费用情况

5.1.1　全国及六大区肿瘤患儿次均住院费用情况

全国肿瘤患儿次均住院费用（中位数）为 6 647.30 元。高于全国中位数水平的地区分别为中南地区（10 078.23 元）、东北地区（7 741.24 元）和西南地区（6 759.76 元），低于全国中位数水平的地区分别为西北地区（4 980.13 元）、华东地区（5 642.47元）和华北地区（6 164.30 元）（图 7-5-1）。

5　Analysis of hospitalization expenses of children with cancer in pediatric cancer surveillance sites in China

5.1　Expenses per hospitalization of children with cancer in pediatric cancer surveillance sites in China

5.1.1　Expenses per hospitalization of children with cancer in the six regions and the whole country

Nationally, the median expenses per hospitalization was 6, 647.30 CNY. The regions above the national median were Central and Southern China (10, 078.23 CNY), Northeast China (7, 741.24 CNY) and Southwest China (6, 759.76 CNY), while those below the national median were Northwest China (4, 980.13 CNY), East China (5, 642.47 CNY) and North China (6, 164.30 CNY) (Figure 7-5-1).

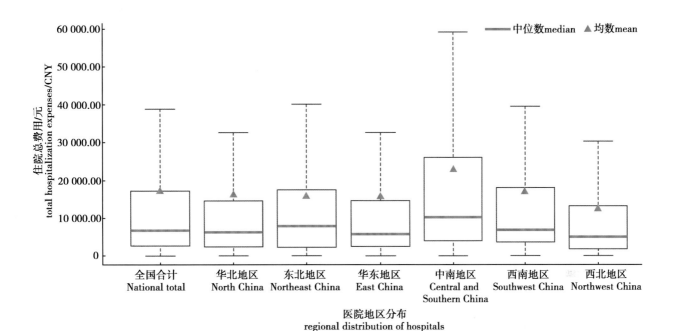

图 7-5-1　2017—2018 年全国及六大区肿瘤患儿次均住院费用

Figure 7-5-1　Expenses per hospitalization of children with cancer in the six regions and the whole country in 2017-2018

5.1.2　各省份肿瘤患儿次均住院费用情况

根据肿瘤患儿次均住院费用(中位数),前 3 位的省份分别为广东(13 873.30 元)、河南(10 599.00 元)和青海(10 559.94 元),后 3 位分别为陕西(2 693.52 元)、福建(4 025.47 元)和上海(4 203.03 元)(图 7-5-2)。

5.1.2　Expenses per hospitalization of children with cancer in each provincial-level region

In terms of the median expenses of each child with cancer per hospitalization, the top three provincial-level regions were Guangdong (13, 873.30 CNY), Henan (10, 599.00 CNY) and Qinghai (10, 559.94 CNY), while the last three were Shaanxi (2, 693.52 CNY), Fujian (4, 025.47 CNY) and Shanghai (4, 203.03 CNY) (Figure 7-5-2).

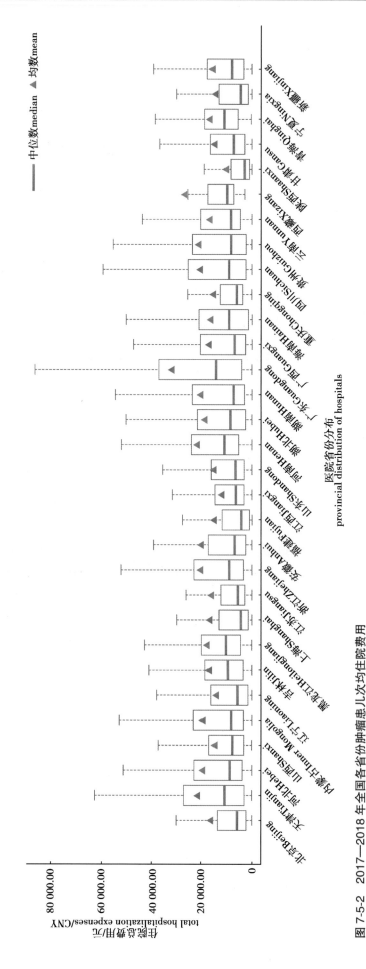

图 7-5-2　2017—2018 年全国各省份肿瘤患儿次均住院费用

Figure 7-5-2　Expenses per hospitalization of children with cancer in each provincial-level region in 2017-2018

5.2　全国儿童肿瘤监测机构肿瘤患儿次均住院分项费用情况

5.2.1　全国及六大区肿瘤患儿次均住院分项费用情况

根据全国肿瘤患儿次均住院分项费用(中位数),前3位分别为诊断类费用(1 449.00元)、西药类费用(1 383.51元)和综合医疗服务类费用(950.60元)。六大区分项费用中位数的顺位与全国相比略有不同,如西南地区,次均住院分项费用(中位数)前3位分别为西药类费用(2 010.45元)、诊断类费用(1 843.00元)和综合医疗服务类费用(1 268.80元)(图7-5-3)。按均数统计的结果详见图7-5-4。

5.2.2　各省份肿瘤患儿次均住院分项费用情况

根据各省份肿瘤患儿次均住院分项费用(中位数),以综合医疗服务类费用为例,前3位的省份依次为西藏(2 341.00元)、天津(2 046.50元)和吉林(1 714.50元),后3位依次为陕西(527.00元)、宁夏(651.72元)和江苏(658.55元)(图7-5-5)。按均数统计的结果详见图7-5-6。

5.2　Expenses of each item per hospitalization of children with cancer in pediatric cancer surveillance sites in China

5.2.1　Expenses of each item per hospitalization of children with cancer in the six regions and the whole country

In terms of the median expenses of each item per hospitalization of children with cancer, the top three items were diagnostic expenses (1, 449.00 CNY), western medication expenses (1, 383.51 CNY) and comprehensive medical service expenses (950.60 CNY). The rank of the median expenses of each item in the six regions was slightly different from the national median. For example, in Southwest China, the top three median expenses of each item per hospitalization were western medication expenses (2, 010.45 CNY), diagnostic expenses (1, 843.00 CNY) and comprehensive medical service expenses (1, 268.80 CNY)(Figure 7-5-3). Data by the mean expenses in Figure 7-5-4.

5.2.2　Expenses of each item per hospitalization of children with cancer in each provincial-level region

In terms of the median expenses of each item per hospitalization of children with cancer in each provincial-level region, taking comprehensive medical services expenses as an example, the top three provincial-level regions were Xizang (2, 341.00 CNY), Tianjin (2, 046.50 CNY) and Jilin (1, 714.50 CNY). The last three were Shaanxi (527.00 CNY), Ningxia (651.72 CNY) and Jiangsu (658.55 CNY)(Figure 7-5-5). Data by the mean expenses in Figure 7-5-6.

行政区分布 regional distribution of hospitals	综合医疗服务类费用 comprehensive medical service expenses	诊断类费用 diagnostic expenses	治疗类费用 treatment expenses	康复类费用 rehabilitation expenses	分项费用/元 expenses of each item/CNY					
					中医类费用 traditional chinese medicine service expenses	西药类费用 western medication expenses	中药类费用 traditional chinese medication expenses	血液和血液制品类费用 blood and blood product expenses	耗材类费用 medical consumable expenses	其他类费用 others
全国合计 National total	950.60	1 449.00	30.00	0	0	1 383.51	0	0	330.10	0.03
华北地区 North China	841.65	1 236.00	0	0	0	1 204.05	0	0	505.88	0
东北地区 Northeast China	1 091.00	1 570.00	77.16	0	0	1 380.25	0	0	466.80	36.00
华东地区 East China	842.10	1 370.00	65.00	0	0	1 214.17	0	0	273.87	30.00
中南地区 Central and Southern China	1 096.00	1 827.00	130.00	0	0	2 072.30	0	0	363.87	8.00
西南地区 Southwest China	1 268.80	1 843.00	52.00	0	0	2 010.45	0	0	252.59	2.97
西北地区 Northwest China	742.00	1 254.00	102.00	0	0	1 018.49	0	0	74.80	0

图 7-5-3　2017—2018 年全国及六大区肿瘤患儿次均住院分项费用（按中位数计）

Figure 7-5-3　Expenses of each item per hospitalization of children with cancer in the six regions and the whole country in 2017-2018 (by the median)

行政区分布 regional distribution of hospitals	综合医疗服务类费用 comprehensive medical service expenses	诊断类费用 diagnostic expenses	治疗类费用 treatment expenses	康复类费用 rehabilitation expenses	分项费用/元 expenses of each item/CNY					
					中医类费用 traditional chinese medicine service expenses	西药类费用 western medication expenses	中药类费用 traditional chinese medication expenses	血液和血液制品类费用 blood and blood product expenses	耗材类费用 medical consumable expenses	其他类费用 others
全国合计 National total	2 236.20	3 360.37	1 103.81	14.93	19.36	4 967.65	137.85	1 246.57	1 994.82	819.64
华北地区 North China	2 038.42	3 173.66	652.44	2.18	4.08	4 641.85	96.64	1 433.74	2 631.57	501.50
东北地区 Northeast China	2 119.19	3 035.21	1 397.43	11.41	10.13	4 325.81	351.74	1 428.41	1 762.10	1 311.86
华东地区 East China	2 185.69	3 046.22	1 084.52	30.23	8.77	4 955.53	111.31	1 105.06	1 659.99	775.30
中南地区 Central and Southern China	2 560.09	4 302.00	2 098.17	11.13	66.34	6 097.89	222.54	1 123.60	2 550.78	1 933.54
西南地区 Southwest China	2 770.07	3 804.11	927.02	27.24	21.28	5 160.76	140.59	1 417.22	1 273.53	219.49
西北地区 Northwest China	1 722.01	2 693.00	979.04	5.75	18.15	4 139.85	84.13	844.34	958.21	376.60

图 7-5-4　2017—2018 年全国及六大区肿瘤患儿次均住院分项费用（按均数计）

Figure 7-5-4　Expenses of each item per hospitalization of children with cancer in the six regions and the whole country in 2017-2018 (by the mean)

医院省份分布 provincial distribution of hospitals	分项费用/元 expenses of each item/CNY									
	综合医疗服务类费用 comprehensive medical service expenses	诊断类费用 diagnostic expenses	治疗类费用 treatment expenses	康复类费用 rehabilitation expenses	中医类费用 traditional chinese medicine service expenses	西药类费用 western medication expenses	中药类费用 traditional chinese medication expenses	血液和血液制品类费用 blood and blood product expenses	耗材类费用 medical consumable expenses	其他类费用 others
北京Beijing	741.70	1 123.50	0	0	0	1 040.02	0	0	525.94	0
天津Tianjin	2 046.50	3 030.00	30.00	0	0	1 612.23	0	0	582.04	10.00
河北Hebei	912.00	1 673.50	118.00	0	0	2 303.14	0	162.00	412.87	0
山西Shanxi	1 129.10	1 741.30	40.00	0	0	1 771.69	0	0	369.70	2.00
内蒙古Inner Mongolia	692.29	1 480.50	400.00	0	0	2 598.37	0	0	152.72	40.00
辽宁Liaoning	786.00	1 072.24	83.49	0	0	901.33	44.40	297.93	275.22	819.11
吉林Jilin	1 714.50	2 560.00	43.00	0	0	1 822.73	0	0	896.00	0
黑龙江Heilongjiang	1 040.00	1 485.10	0	0	0	3 127.49	0	0	862.50	84.00
上海Shanghai	923.00	970.50	40.00	0	0	856.14	0	0	374.48	0
江苏Jiangsu	658.55	1 398.50	36.00	9.00	0	1 218.83	40.00	0	327.62	340.40
浙江Zhejiang	872.00	1 880.00	170.00	0	0	2 573.08	0	0	327.70	5.00
安徽Anhui	1 215.00	1 418.50	90.00	60.00	0	1 133.76	39.80	516.00	177.28	60.00
福建Fujian	686.98	418.00	0	0	0	691.26	0	0	0	4.80
江西Jiangxi	818.00	1 802.00	72.00	30.00	0	1 795.20	123.25	80.75	244.71	30.00
山东Shandong	1 048.00	1 398.00	130.00	0	0	977.16	0	0	402.23	2.30
河南Henan	1 239.00	1 049.60	192.10	0	0	3 523.04	0	0	125.22	0
湖北Hubei	940.25	1 985.00	50.00	0	0	2 270.93	0	0	369.73	6.00
湖南Hunan	967.00	1 706.50	92.00	0	0	1 414.35	0	0	528.32	92.00
广东Guangdong	1 151.76	2 890.64	251.50	0	0	1 787.33	0	0	722.20	2.28
广西Guangxi	884.10	1 745.95	272.80	0	0	873.14	0	0	221.34	0
海南Hainan	1 073.35	1 438.76	195.00	0	0	1 005.97	79.64	0	395.86	0
重庆Chongqing	1 158.72	1 750.33	0	0	0	1 639.93	0	0	312.50	5.00
四川Sichuan	1 620.00	1 604.00	184.00	0	0	1 953.38	4.60	0	548.63	0
贵州Guizhou	1 214.95	2 105.75	120.00	0	0	1 666.51	0	0	0	49.00
云南Yunnan	1 545.00	2 050.00	190.00	0	0	3 119.09	69.00	1 400.00	115.13	0.04
西藏Xizang	2 341.00	2 107.75	15.00	100.00	0	2 305.56	0	0	129.86	157.15
陕西Shaanxi	527.00	687.00	50.00	0	0	627.11	0	0	74.58	0
甘肃Gansu	1 265.00	1 622.50	57.50	6.00	0	1 551.84	0	0	0	0
青海Qinghai	896.00	3 151.00	40.00	0	0	3 254.00	0	0	240.87	0
宁夏Ningxia	651.72	922.85	190.10	0	0	821.50	115.45	820.20	265.16	12.00
新疆Xinjiang	816.00	2 276.00	190.00	0	0	1 902.35	0	0	74.67	32.00

图 7-5-5 2017—2018 年全国各省份肿瘤患儿次均住院分项费用(按中位数计)

Figure 7-5-5 Expenses of each item per hospitalization of children with cancer in each provincial-level region in 2017-2018(by the median)

分项费用/元
expenses of each item/CNY

图表省份分布 provincial distribution of hospitals	综合医疗服务类费用 comprehensive medical service expenses	诊断类费用 diagnostic expenses	治疗类费用 treatment expenses	康复类费用 rehabilitation expenses	中医类费用 traditional chinese medicine service expenses	西药类费用 western medication expenses	中药类费用 traditional chinese medication expenses	血液和血液制品类费用 blood and blood product expenses	耗材类费用 medical consumable expenses	其他类费用 others
北京Beijing	1 905.29	3 069.42	534.13	1.69	2.77	4 409.85	92.35	1 443.47	2 816.31	491.17
天津Tianjin	4 334.40	4 857.76	1 420.45	0.21	0.55	5 361.31	47.64	1 049.04	1 975.87	184.47
河北Hebei	2 217.57	3 577.14	972.36	3.64	18.07	6 430.38	132.18	1 952.02	1 979.82	1 047.69
山西Shanxi	2 357.13	3 222.62	1 234.47	10.95	8.01	4 374.06	160.35	828.96	1 511.90	192.01
内蒙古Inner Mongolia	2 228.06	3 023.39	1 924.08	5.64	34.08	7 509.29	134.64	1 599.62	767.28	439.98
辽宁Liaoning	1 678.47	2 225.77	1 530.95	30.54	0.36	3 923.69	363.09	2 241.50	1 284.93	2 332.97
吉林Jilin	2 786.09	4 134.53	1 119.28	6.74	16.02	4 475.94	334.10	1 121.10	2 213.26	147.32
黑龙江Heilongjiang	1 845.63	2 610.21	1 978.32	0	22.67	5 722.52	394.93	810.25	2 481.18	1 319.28
上海Shanghai	2 482.14	3 675.23	1 161.26	32.69	1.62	4 097.37	25.07	345.52	3 375.34	259.69
江苏Jiangsu	1 786.00	3 425.28	799.67	32.17	29.84	5 244.14	116.56	1 537.63	1 715.17	1 073.16
浙江Zhejiang	2 296.89	3 398.04	1 882.68	30.91	24.50	7 453.62	67.99	1 280.35	1 963.82	411.26
安徽Anhui	3 269.79	3 419.32	864.74	162.79	1.31	6 334.46	171.42	2 663.47	1 216.87	313.03
福建Fujian	2 620.75	1 852.19	758.94	1.83	4.01	5 085.18	14.37	562.16	625.78	433.02
江西Jiangxi	1 680.55	2 676.21	881.75	24.69	1.98	4 024.39	349.85	1 464.97	908.69	166.92
山东Shandong	2 189.37	2 914.27	1 432.81	3.35	57.78	3 970.31	91.75	949.91	1 828.76	1 551.79
河南Henan	2 381.89	2 331.82	1 383.10	7.63	3.21	7 431.43	127.81	1 018.44	819.43	677.34
湖北Hubei	2 151.21	4 478.80	1 333.64	6.43	3.21	6 001.33	174.06	666.16	1 621.67	602.49
湖南Hunan	2 716.27	4 087.61	827.68	12.48	305.97	5 404.74	798.12	1 483.64	2 260.13	907.99
广东Guangdong	3 068.60	6 407.81	3 539.18	17.78	6.93	6 421.20	55.63	1 371.99	4 365.05	4 449.34
广西Guangxi	2 217.19	3 654.13	2 568.20	7.87	9.18	4 118.66	34.36	1 054.59	1 980.79	123.99
海南Hainan	1 924.13	2 158.49	1 491.09	0.03	45.34	4 478.20	223.87	771.89	1 513.21	160.01
重庆Chongqing	2 416.60	3 864.07	689.71	24.96	27.63	3 392.06	40.01	971.25	1 220.31	20.33
四川Sichuan	3 757.73	3 605.56	1 629.55	40.00	23.62	5 456.70	111.73	1 718.83	1 716.61	276.86
贵州Guizhou	2 796.47	4 568.03	1 037.38	2.95	3.36	6 983.69	320.64	1 776.69	1 236.56	810.12
云南Yunnan	2 648.18	3 282.99	769.74	91.18	11.02	7 263.76	320.02	2 471.92	1 047.35	127.52
西藏Xizang	6 731.58	6 243.77	1 013.10	187.66	0	8 007.43	148.02	161.48	479.99	1 934.66
陕西Shaanxi	1 479.23	1 729.61	537.94	0.70	16.47	3 115.15	16.02	650.55	682.41	302.53
甘肃Gansu	2 276.22	2 912.77	910.80	25.44	55.40	4 470.35	168.89	1 274.37	1 489.28	346.11
青海Qinghai	1 434.66	4 042.47	1 493.88	13.31	0	5 428.62	123.34	1 138.00	1 156.83	482.12
宁夏Ningxia	1 687.00	2 681.79	1 343.71	96.75	22.71	3 052.65	350.38	3 475.56	1 843.47	27.39
新疆Xinjiang	1 861.43	3 776.94	1 547.83	2.11	9.67	5 413.18	124.86	715.53	1 009.41	487.44

图 7-5-6 2017—2018 年全国各省份肿瘤患儿次均住院分项费用（按均数计）

Figure 7-5-6 Expenses of each item per hospitalization of children with cancer in each provincial-level region in 2017-2018 (by the mean)

6 全国儿童肿瘤监测机构肿瘤患儿平均住院日分析

6.1 全国及六大区肿瘤患儿平均住院日情况

全国肿瘤患儿平均住院日的中位数为 5 天。高于全国中位数水平的地区分别为东北地区(7 天)、中南地区(7 天)、西南地区(7 天)和西北地区(6 天),与全国中位数水平相同的地区分别为华东地区(5 天),低于全国中位数水平的地区为华北地区(4 天)(图 7-6-1)。

6.2 各省份肿瘤患儿平均住院日情况

根据各省份肿瘤患儿平均住院日的中位数,肿瘤患儿平均住院日最长的省份是西藏(11 天),其次是青海(10 天)、内蒙古(9 天)和河南(9 天),最短的是北京(3 天)(图 7-6-2)。

6 Analysis of the average length of hospitalization of children with cancer in pediatric cancer surveillance sites in China

6.1 Average length of hospitalization of children with cancer in the six regions and the whole country

Nationally, the median of average length of hospitalization was five days. Northeast China (7 days), Central and Southern China (7 days), Southwest China (7 days) and Northwest China (6 days) were above the national median. East China (5 days) was the same with the national median. North China (4 days) was below the national median (Figure 7-6-1).

6.2 Average length of hospitalization of children with cancer in each provincial-level region

In terms of the median of average length of hospitalization of children with cancer in each provincial-level region, the provincial-level region with the longest average hospital stay was Xizang (11 days), followed by Qinghai (10 days), Inner Mongolia (9 days) and Henan (9 days), and the shortest was Beijing (3 days) (Figure 7-6-2).

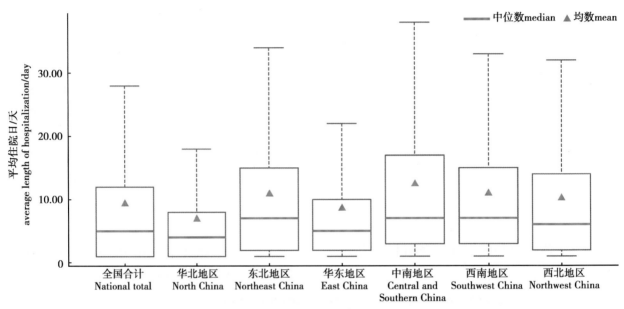

图 7-6-1　2017—2018 年全国及六大区肿瘤患儿平均住院日

Figure 7-6-1　Average length of hospitalization of children with cancer in the six regions and the whole country in 2017-2018

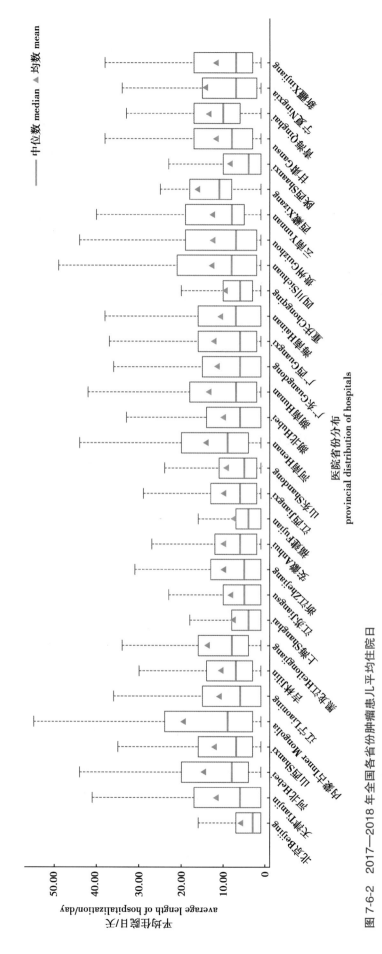

图 7-6-2 2017—2018 年全国各省份肿瘤患儿平均住院日

Figure 7-6-2 Average length of hospitalization of children with cancer in each provincial-level region in 2017-2018

第八章

主要癌种监测数据分析结果

---

1 白血病

1.1 全国儿童肿瘤监测机构白血病患儿出院人次分析

1.1.1 六大区白血病患儿出院人次构成情况

在白血病患儿出院人次中,各大区出院人次占全部出院人次的比例由高到低依次为华东地区(33.40%)、华北地区(22.43%)、中南地区(19.03%)、西南地区(11.53%)、西北地区(7.59%)和东北地区(6.02%)(图 8-1-1)。

1.1.2 各省份白血病患儿出院人次构成情况

在所有省份中,白血病患儿出院人次占全部出院人次比例前 3 位的省份分别为北京(17.47%)、江苏(9.74%)和河南(7.75%),后 3 位分别为西藏(0.01%)、青海(0.07%)和黑龙江(0.21%)(图 8-1-2,图 8-1-3)。

Chapter 8

Analysis results of surveillance data of main cancers

---

1 Leukemia

1.1 Analysis of discharges among children with leukemia in pediatric cancer surveillance sites in China

1.1.1 Composition of discharges among children with leukemia in the six regions

In terms of the discharges among children with leukemia, the regions with the highest to the lowest proportions of discharges among children with leukemia in all discharges were East China (33.40%), North China (22.43%), Central and Southern China (19.03%), Southwest China (11.53%), Northwest China (7.59%) and Northeast China (6.02%) (Figure 8-1-1).

1.1.2 Composition of discharges among children with leukemia in each provincial-level region

Among all provincial-level regions, Beijing (17.47%), Jiangsu (9.74%) and Henan (7.75%) were the three provincial-level regions with the highest proportions of discharges among children with leukemia in all discharges, and Xizang (0.01%), Qinghai (0.07%) and Heilongjiang (0.21%) had the lowest proportions of discharges among children with leukemia (Figure 8-1-2, Figure 8-1-3).

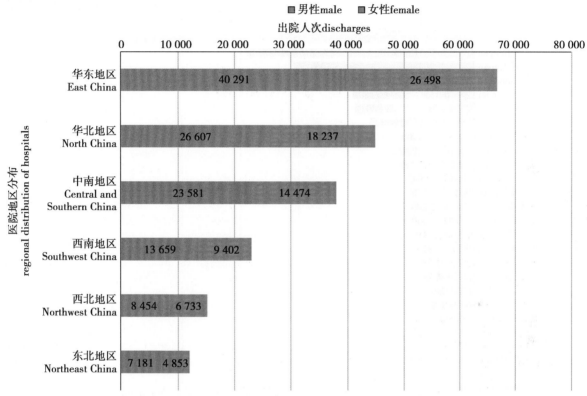

图 8-1-1　2017—2018 年全国六大区儿童肿瘤监测机构白血病出院人次构成

Figure 8-1-1　Composition of discharges among children with leukemia in pediatric cancer surveillance sites in the six regions in 2017-2018

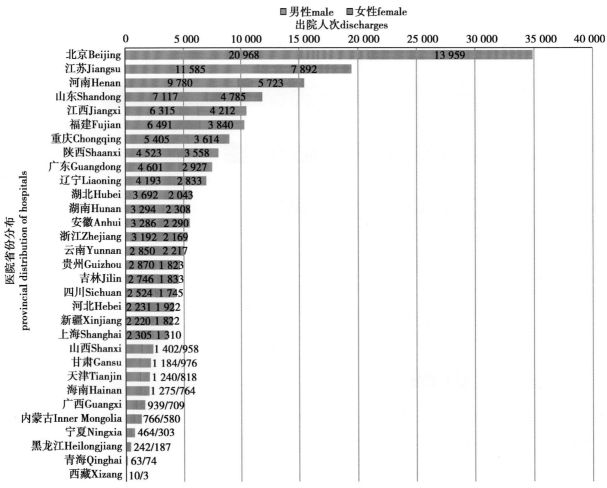

图 8-1-2　2017—2018 年全国各省份儿童肿瘤监测机构白血病出院人次构成

Figure 8-1-2　Composition of discharges among children with leukemia in pediatric cancer surveillance sites in each provincial-level region in 2017-2018

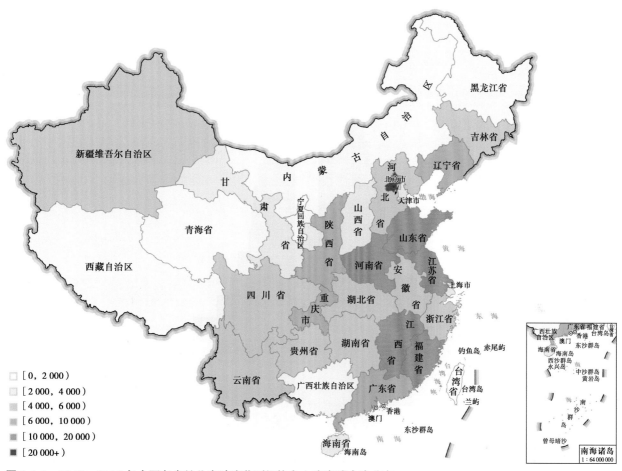

图 8-1-3　2017—2018 年全国各省份儿童肿瘤监测机构白血病出院人次分布

Figure 8-1-3　Distribution of discharges among children with leukemia in pediatric cancer surveillance sites in each provincial-level region in 2017-2018

1.2　全国儿童肿瘤监测机构白血病患儿年龄 / 性别构成

1.2.1　全国白血病患儿年龄 / 性别构成情况

从性别分布来看,男性患儿占全部出院人次比例为 59.90%,女性患儿为 40.10%,男性患儿各年龄段的出院人次比例均高于女性患儿。从年龄分布来看,4 岁年龄组所占比例最高(11.90%),其次为 3 岁(11.62%)和 5 岁(10.43%)年龄组(图 8-1-4)。

1.2　Age/gender composition of children with leukemia in pediatric cancer surveillance sites in China

1.2.1　Age/gender composition of children with leukemia nationally

In terms of gender distribution, male children accounted for 59.90% of all discharges, and female for 40.10%.The discharge proportions of male children at all ages were higher than those of female. In terms of age distribution, the 4-year age group accounted for the highest proportion (11.90%), followed by the 3-year age group (11.62%) and the 5-year age group (10.43%) (Figure 8-1-4).

125

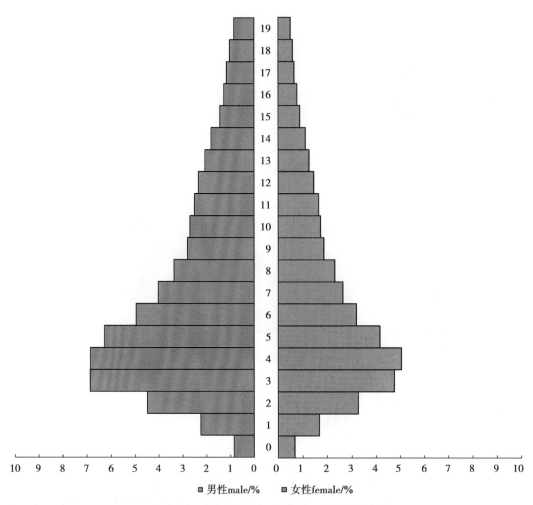

图 8-1-4　2017—2018 年全国儿童肿瘤监测机构白血病患儿年龄／性别构成

Figure 8-1-4　Age/gender composition of children with leukemia in pediatric cancer surveillance sites in China in 2017-2018

1.2.2　六大区白血病患儿年龄／性别构成情况

从性别分布来看，六大区均显示男性患儿占全部出院人次比例高于女性患儿。从年龄分布来看，六大区的比例各有不同，其中华北地区、华东地区和西南地区的 3 岁年龄组所占比例最高；东北地区、中南地区和西北地区的 4 岁年龄组所占比例最高（图 8-1-5～图 8-1-10）。

1.2.2　Age/gender composition of children with leukemia in the six regions

In terms of gender distribution, male children accounted for a higher proportion of all discharges than female in all the six regions. In terms of age distribution, the proportions of the six regions were different, among which the proportions of the 3-year age group in North China, East China and Southwest China were the highest. The proportions of the 4-year age group in Northeast China, Central and Southern China and Northwest China were the highest (Figure 8-1-5~Figure 8-1-10).

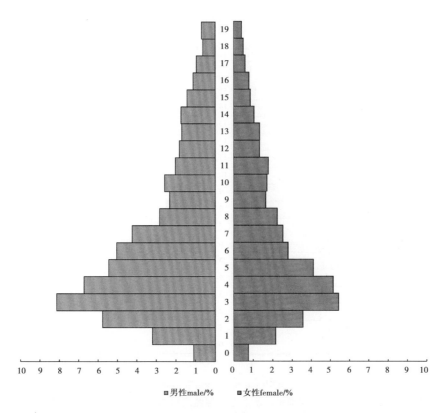

图 8-1-5　2017—2018 年华北地区儿童肿瘤监测机构白血病患儿年龄／性别构成

Figure 8-1-5　Age/gender composition of children with leukemia in pediatric cancer surveillance sites in North China in 2017-2018

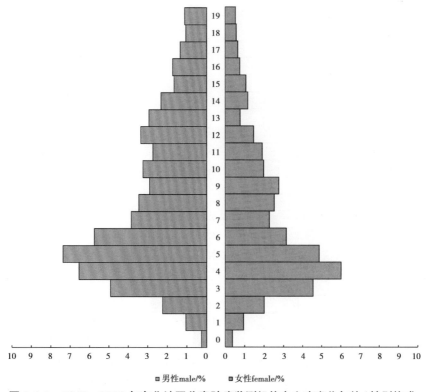

图 8-1-6　2017—2018 年东北地区儿童肿瘤监测机构白血病患儿年龄／性别构成

Figure 8-1-6　Age/gender composition of children with leukemia in pediatric cancer surveillance sites in Northeast China in 2017-2018

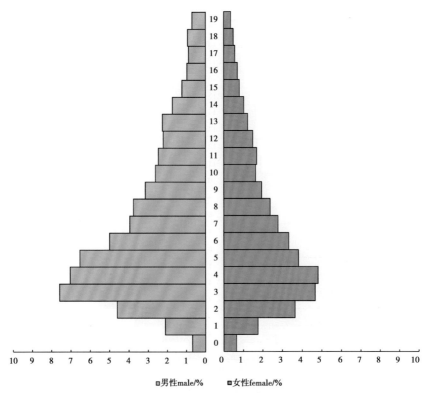

图 8-1-7　2017—2018 年华东地区儿童肿瘤监测机构白血病患儿年龄／性别构成

Figure 8-1-7　Age/gender composition of children with leukemia in pediatric cancer surveillance sites in East China in 2017-2018

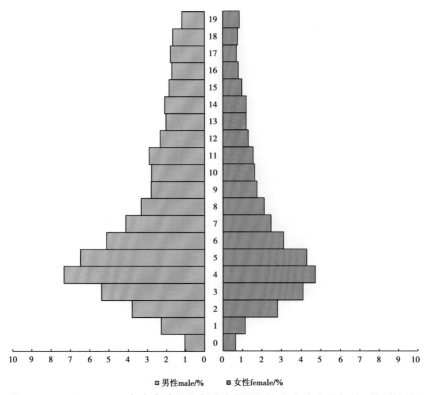

图 8-1-8　2017—2018 年中南地区儿童肿瘤监测机构白血病患儿年龄／性别构成

Figure 8-1-8　Age/gender composition of children with leukemia in pediatric cancer surveillance sites in Central and Southern China in 2017-2018

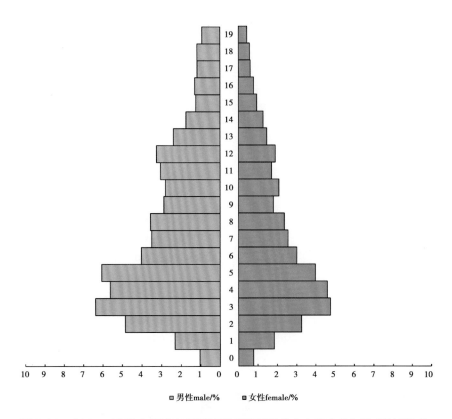

图 8-1-9　2017—2018 年西南地区儿童肿瘤监测机构白血病患儿年龄 / 性别构成

Figure 8-1-9　Age/gender composition of children with leukemia in pediatric cancer surveillance sites in Southwest China in 2017-2018

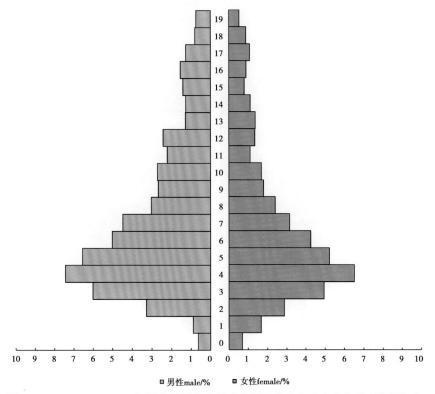

图 8-1-10　2017—2018 年西北地区儿童肿瘤监测机构白血病患儿年龄 / 性别构成

Figure 8-1-10　Age/gender composition of children with leukemia in pediatric cancer surveillance sites in Northwest China in 2017-2018

1.2.3 各省份白血病患儿年龄/性别构成情况

除青海外,其他30个省份出院患儿的性别分布均呈现为男性比例高于女性;除黑龙江、青海和西藏外,其他28个省份出院患儿年龄集中分布在2~7岁年龄组。以河南为例,从性别分布来看,男性患儿占全部出院人次比例为63.08%,女性患儿为36.92%;从年龄分布来看,4岁年龄组所占比例最高(11.14%),其次为5岁(9.86%)和3岁(7.97%)年龄组(图8-1-11~图8-1-40)。

1.2.3 Age/gender composition of children with leukemia in each provincial-level region

Apart from Qinghai, the proportions of discharges among male children with leukemia in other 30 provincial-level regions were higher than those of female. Apart from Heilongjiang, Qinghai and Xizang, the discharges among children with leukemia in other 28 provincial-level regions were concentrated in the 2-7-year age group. Taking Henan as an example, from the perspective of gender distribution, male children accounted for 63.08% of all discharges and female accounted for 36.92%. In terms of age distribution, the 4-year age group accounted for the highest proportion (11.14%), followed by the 5-year age group (9.86%) and the 3-year age group (7.97%) (Figure 8-1-11~Figure 8-1-40).

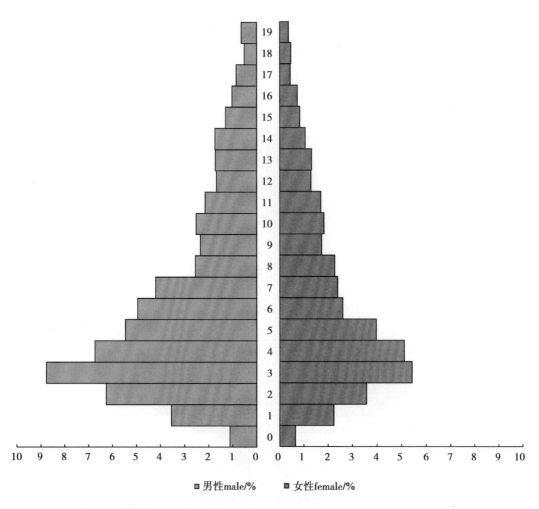

■男性male/%   ■女性female/%

图8-1-11 2017—2018年北京儿童肿瘤监测机构白血病患儿年龄/性别构成

Figure 8-1-11 Age/gender composition of children with leukemia in pediatric cancer surveillance sites in Beijing in 2017-2018

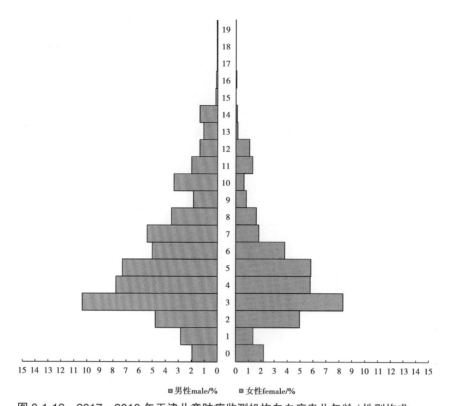

图 8-1-12　2017—2018 年天津儿童肿瘤监测机构白血病患儿年龄 / 性别构成

Figure 8-1-12　Age/gender composition of children with leukemia in pediatric cancer surveillance sites in Tianjin in 2017-2018

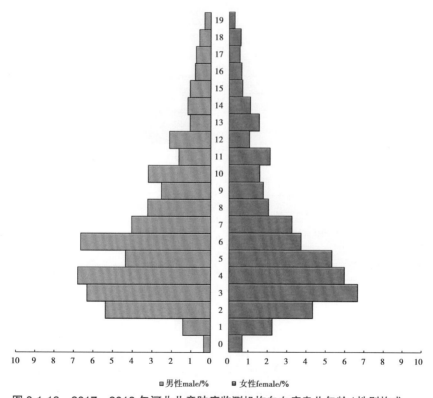

图 8-1-13　2017—2018 年河北儿童肿瘤监测机构白血病患儿年龄 / 性别构成

Figure 8-1-13　Age/gender composition of children with leukemia in pediatric cancer surveillance sites in Hebei in 2017-2018

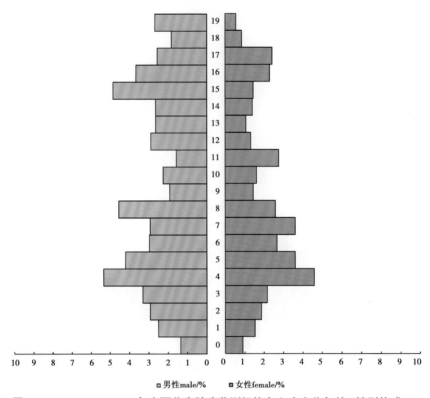

图 8-1-14　2017—2018 年山西儿童肿瘤监测机构白血病患儿年龄／性别构成

Figure 8-1-14　Age/gender composition of children with leukemia in pediatric cancer surveillance sites in Shanxi in 2017-2018

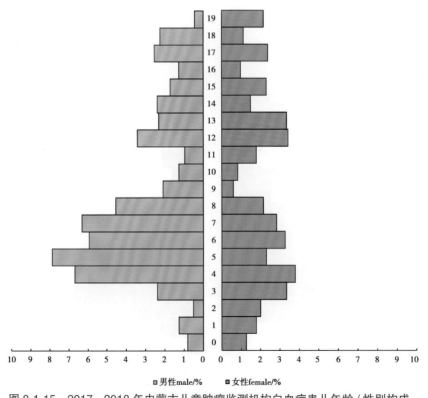

图 8-1-15　2017—2018 年内蒙古儿童肿瘤监测机构白血病患儿年龄／性别构成

Figure 8-1-15　Age/gender composition of children with leukemia in pediatric cancer surveillance sites in Inner Mongolia in 2017-2018

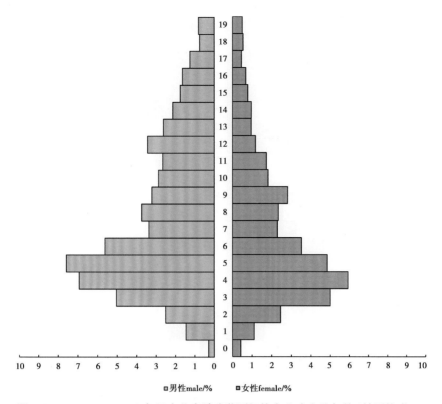

图 8-1-16　2017—2018 年辽宁儿童肿瘤监测机构白血病患儿年龄／性别构成

Figure 8-1-16　Age/gender composition of children with leukemia in pediatric cancer surveillance sites in Liaoning in 2017-2018

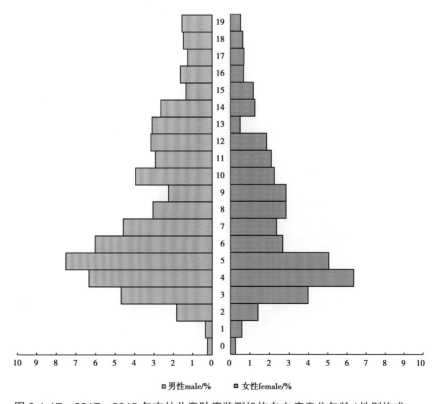

图 8-1-17　2017—2018 年吉林儿童肿瘤监测机构白血病患儿年龄／性别构成

Figure 8-1-17　Age/gender composition of children with leukemia in pediatric cancer surveillance sites in Jilin in 2017-2018

133

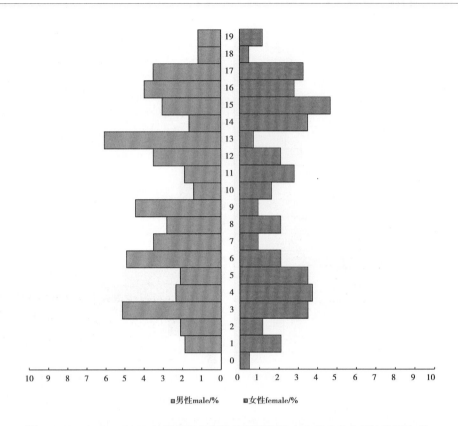

图 8-1-18　2017—2018 年黑龙江儿童肿瘤监测机构白血病患儿年龄／性别构成

Figure 8-1-18　Age/gender composition of children with leukemia in pediatric cancer surveillance sites in Heilongjiang in 2017-2018

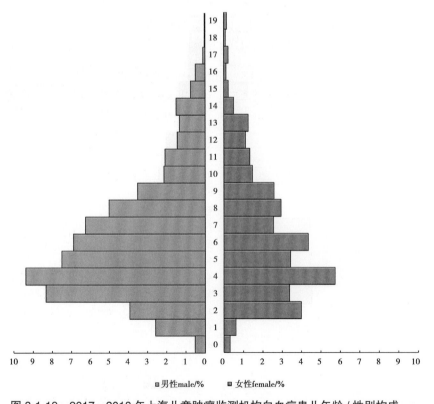

图 8-1-19　2017—2018 年上海儿童肿瘤监测机构白血病患儿年龄／性别构成

Figure 8-1-19　Age/gender composition of children with leukemia in pediatric cancer surveillance sites in Shanghai in 2017-2018

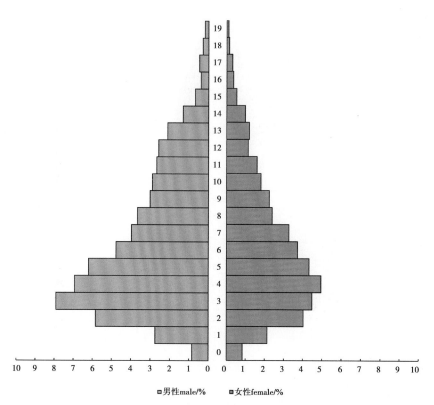

图 8-1-20　2017—2018 年江苏儿童肿瘤监测机构白血病患儿年龄 / 性别构成

Figure 8-1-20　Age/gender composition of children with leukemia in pediatric cancer surveillance sites in Jiangsu in 2017-2018

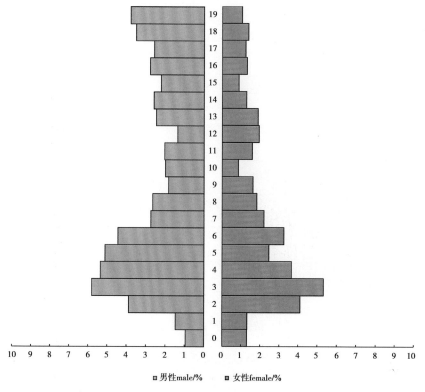

图 8-1-21　2017—2018 年浙江儿童肿瘤监测机构白血病患儿年龄 / 性别构成

Figure 8-1-21　Age/gender composition of children with leukemia in pediatric cancer surveillance sites in Zhejiang in 2017-2018

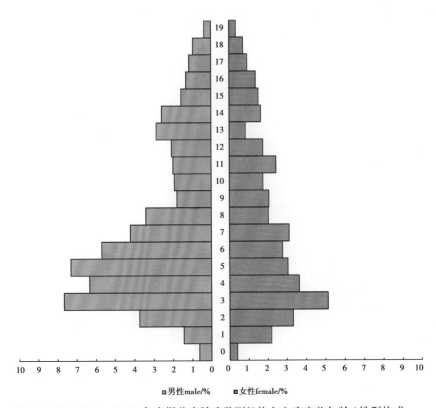

图 8-1-22 2017—2018 年安徽儿童肿瘤监测机构白血病患儿年龄／性别构成

Figure 8-1-22 Age/gender composition of children with leukemia in pediatric cancer surveillance sites in Anhui in 2017-2018

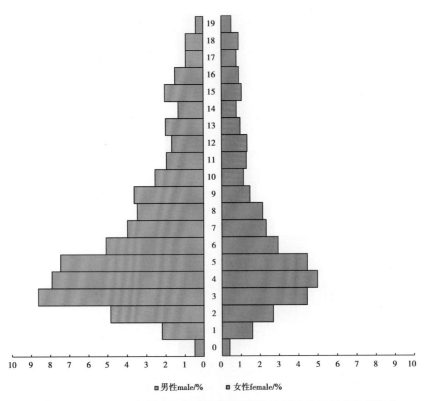

图 8-1-23 2017—2018 年福建儿童肿瘤监测机构白血病患儿年龄／性别构成

Figure 8-1-23 Age/gender composition of children with leukemia in pediatric cancer surveillance sites in Fujian in 2017-2018

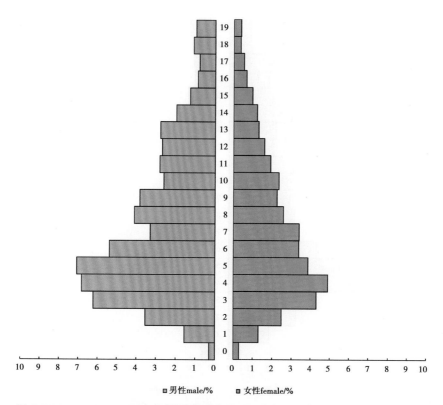

图 8-1-24　2017—2018 年江西儿童肿瘤监测机构白血病患儿年龄 / 性别构成

Figure 8-1-24　Age/gender composition of children with leukemia in pediatric cancer surveillance sites in Jiangxi in 2017-2018

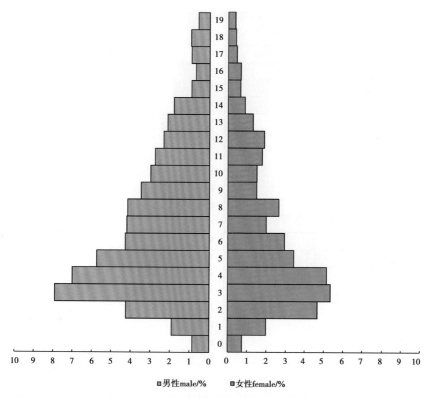

图 8-1-25　2017—2018 年山东儿童肿瘤监测机构白血病患儿年龄 / 性别构成

Figure 8-1-25　Age/gender composition of children with leukemia in pediatric cancer surveillance sites in Shandong in 2017-2018

137

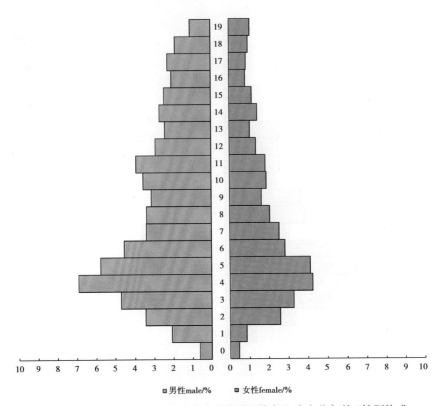

图 8-1-26　2017—2018 年河南儿童肿瘤监测机构白血病患儿年龄／性别构成

Figure 8-1-26　Age/gender composition of children with leukemia in pediatric cancer surveillance sites in Henan in 2017-2018

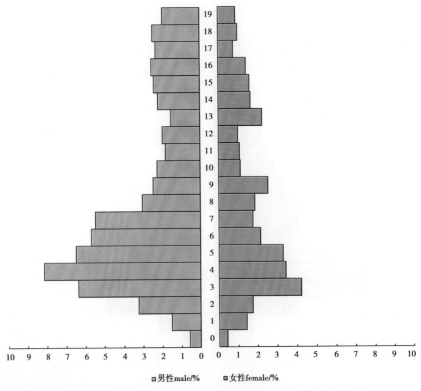

图 8-1-27　2017—2018 年湖北儿童肿瘤监测机构白血病患儿年龄／性别构成

Figure 8-1-27　Age/gender composition of children with leukemia in pediatric cancer surveillance sites in Hubei in 2017-2018

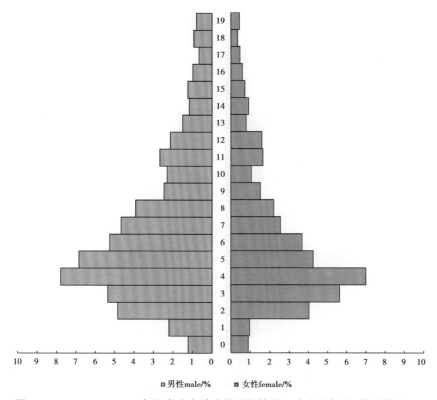

图 8-1-28　2017—2018 年湖南儿童肿瘤监测机构白血病患儿年龄 / 性别构成

Figure 8-1-28　Age/gender composition of children with leukemia in pediatric cancer surveillance sites in Hunan in 2017-2018

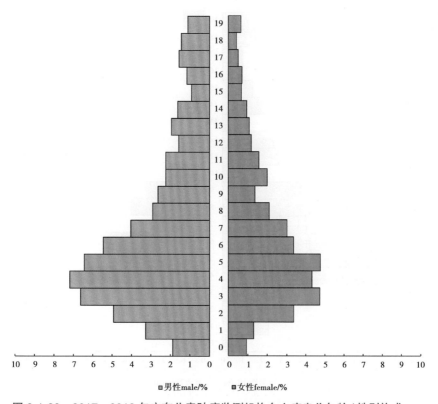

图 8-1-29　2017—2018 年广东儿童肿瘤监测机构白血病患儿年龄 / 性别构成

Figure 8-1-29　Age/gender composition of children with leukemia in pediatric cancer surveillance sites in Guangdong in 2017-2018

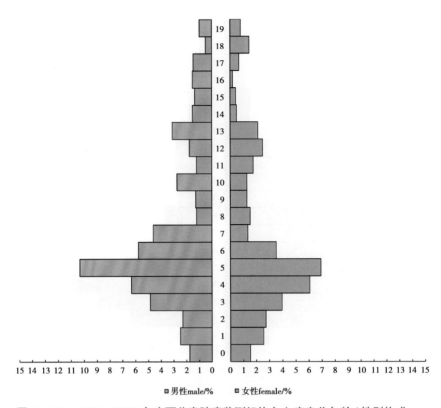

图 8-1-30　2017—2018 年广西儿童肿瘤监测机构白血病患儿年龄／性别构成

Figure 8-1-30　Age/gender composition of children with leukemia in pediatric cancer surveillance sites in Guangxi in 2017-2018

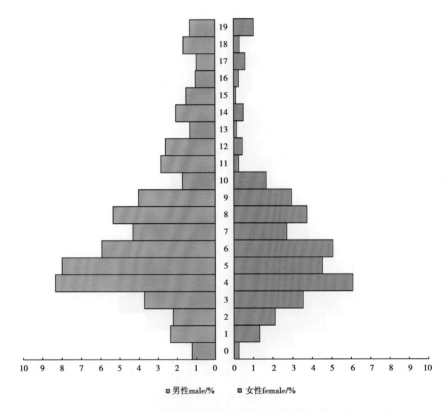

图 8-1-31　2017—2018 年海南儿童肿瘤监测机构白血病患儿年龄／性别构成

Figure 8-1-31　Age/gender composition of children with leukemia in pediatric cancer surveillance sites in Hainan in 2017-2018

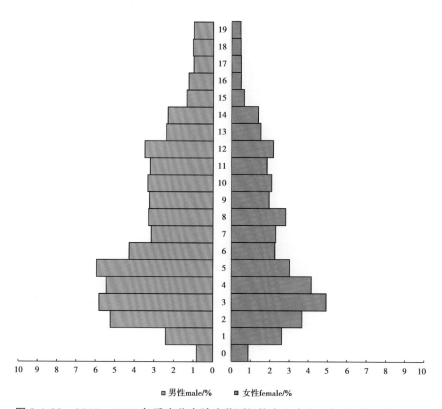

图 8-1-32　2017—2018 年重庆儿童肿瘤监测机构白血病患儿年龄 / 性别构成

Figure 8-1-32　Age/gender composition of children with leukemia in pediatric cancer surveillance sites in Chongqing in 2017-2018

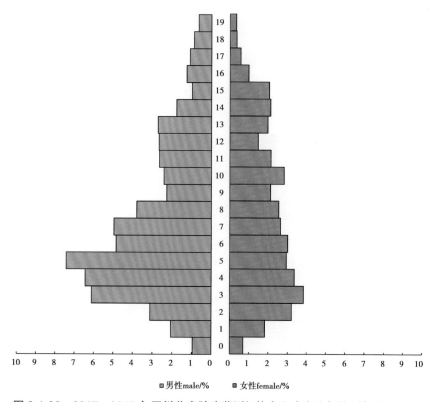

图 8-1-33　2017—2018 年四川儿童肿瘤监测机构白血病患儿年龄 / 性别构成

Figure 8-1-33　Age/gender composition of children with leukemia in pediatric cancer surveillance sites in Sichuan in 2017-2018

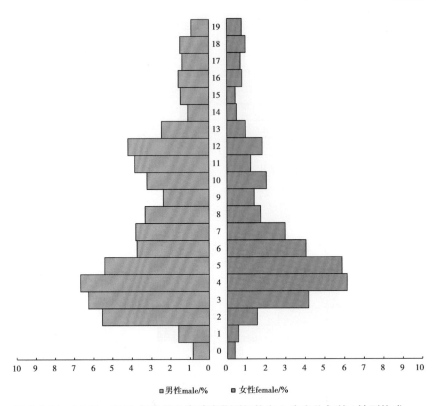

图 8-1-34　2017—2018 年贵州儿童肿瘤监测机构白血病患儿年龄／性别构成

Figure 8-1-34　Age/gender composition of children with leukemia in pediatric cancer surveillance sites in Guizhou in 2017-2018

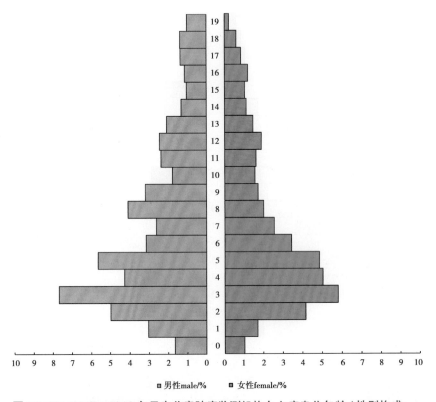

图 8-1-35　2017—2018 年云南儿童肿瘤监测机构白血病患儿年龄／性别构成

Figure 8-1-35　Age/gender composition of children with leukemia in pediatric cancer surveillance sites in Yunnan in 2017-2018

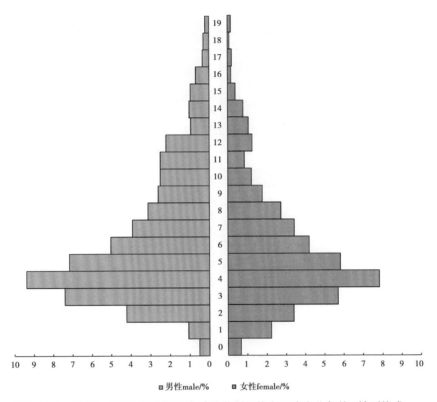

图 8-1-36　2017—2018 年陕西儿童肿瘤监测机构白血病患儿年龄／性别构成

Figure 8-1-36　Age/gender composition of children with leukemia in pediatric cancer surveillance sites in Shaanxi in 2017-2018

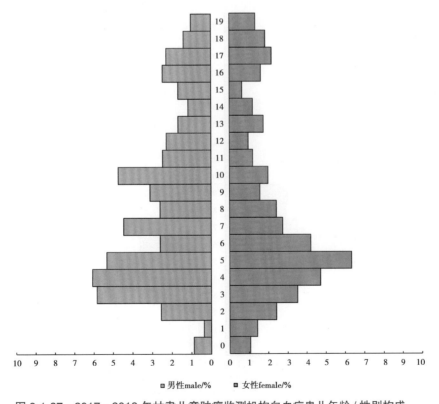

图 8-1-37　2017—2018 年甘肃儿童肿瘤监测机构白血病患儿年龄／性别构成

Figure 8-1-37　Age/gender composition of children with leukemia in pediatric cancer surveillance sites in Gansu in 2017-2018

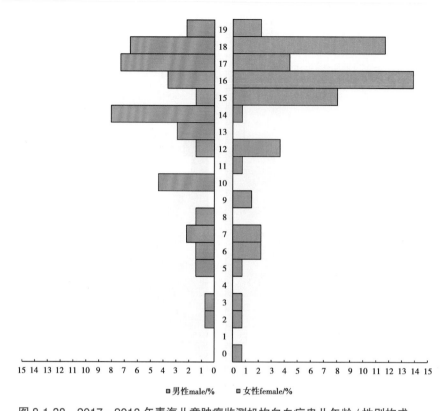

图 8-1-38　2017—2018 年青海儿童肿瘤监测机构白血病患儿年龄／性别构成

Figure 8-1-38　Age/gender composition of children with leukemia in pediatric cancer surveillance sites in Qinghai in 2017-2018

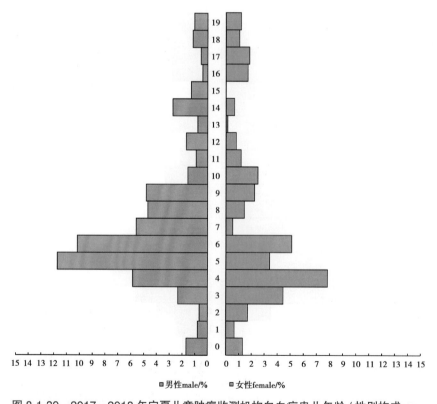

图 8-1-39　2017—2018 年宁夏儿童肿瘤监测机构白血病患儿年龄／性别构成

Figure 8-1-39　Age/gender composition of children with leukemia in pediatric cancer surveillance sites in Ningxia in 2017-2018

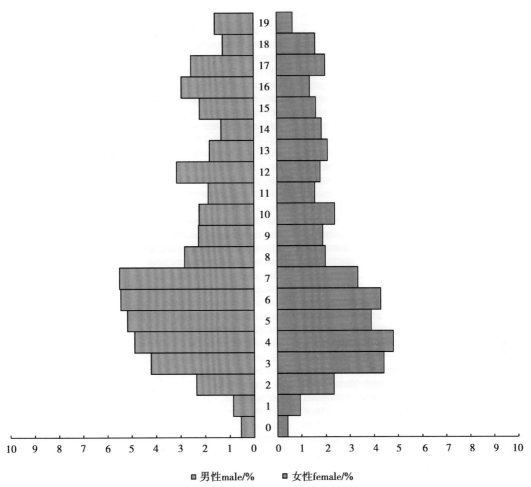

■ 男性male/%   ■ 女性female/%

图 8-1-40   2017—2018 年新疆儿童肿瘤监测机构白血病患儿年龄／性别构成

Figure 8-1-40   Age/gender composition of children with leukemia in pediatric cancer surveillance sites in Xinjiang in 2017-2018

1.3   全国儿童肿瘤监测机构白血病患儿就医省份分布

1.3.1   全国各省份白血病患儿本省就医与省外就医的分布情况

总体而言，白血病患儿本省就医的比例为 73.32%。在所有省份中，本省就医比例前 3 位的省份分别为北京（98.60%）、重庆（94.13%）和江苏（93.41%）。省外就医比例前 3 位分别为西藏（86.60%）、黑龙江（79.62%）和内蒙古（70.25%）（图 8-1-41）。

1.3   Distribution of provincial-level regions visited by children with leukemia in pediatric cancer surveillance sites in China

1.3.1   Distribution of children with leukemia receiving medical treatment in and out of their own provincial-level regions

In general, 73.32% of all children with leukemia sought medical treatment in their own provincial-level regions. Beijing (98.60%), Chongqing (94.13%) and Jiangsu (93.41%) were the top three recipients of patients. Xizang (86.60%), Heilongjiang (79.62%) and Inner Mongolia (70.25%) were the top three provincial-level regions in terms of the proportion of patients going to other provincial-level regions for medical treatment (Figure 8-1-41).

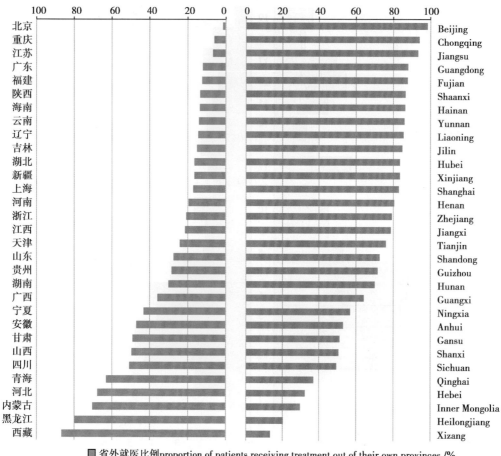

图 8-1-41　2017—2018 年全国各省份白血病患儿本省就医与省外就医比例 /%

Figure 8-1-41　Proportion of children with leukemia receiving medical treatment in and out of their own provincial-level regions in 2017-2018/%

1.3.2　全国各省份白血病患儿省外就医的去向省份分布情况

各省份白血病患儿选择省外就医的去向分布呈现明显的规律,主要的去向省份为北京、江苏、重庆、上海和广东。如户籍地为安徽的白血病患儿,选择省外就医的主要去向为江苏、北京和上海,分别占户籍地为安徽的白血病患儿选择省外就医总数的 65.4%、14.4% 和 11.3%。再如户籍地为四川的白血病患儿,选择省外就医的主要去向为重庆和北京,分别占户籍地为四川的白血病患儿选择省外就医总数的 76.1% 和 8.9%(图 8-1-42,按行方向查看)。

1.3.2　Distribution of provincial-level regions receiving children with leukemia from other provincial-level regions

The distribution of provincial-level regions receiving children with leukemia from outside the provincial-level regions showed obvious regularity. The main destinations were Beijing, Jiangsu, Chongqing, Shanghai and Guangdong. For Anhui children with leukemia, the main destinations were Jiangsu, Beijing, and Shanghai, accounting for 65.4%, 14.4% and 11.3%, respectively, of the total Anhui children with leukemia going outside Anhui. For Sichuan children with leukemia, Chongqing and Beijing were the main destinations, accounting for 76.1% and 8.9%, respectively, of the total Sichuan children with leukemia going outside Sichuan (Figure 8-1-42, view in rows).

収治省外就医肿瘤患儿的医院省份分布 / provincial distribution of hospitals receiving children with cancer from outside the province

外转就医肿瘤患儿的地区分布 / distribution of the provinces of origin of children with cancer receiving treatment out of their own provinces

	北京 Beijing	天津 Tianjin	河北 Hebei	山西 Shanxi	内蒙古 Inner Mongolia	辽宁 Liaoning	吉林 Jilin	黑龙江 Heilongjiang	上海 Shanghai	江苏 Jiangsu	浙江 Zhejiang	安徽 Anhui	福建 Fujian	江西 Jiangxi	山东 Shandong	河南 Henan	湖北 Hubei	湖南 Hunan	广东 Guangdong	广西 Guangxi	海南 Hainan	重庆 Chongqing	四川 Sichuan	贵州 Guizhou	云南 Yunnan	西藏 Xizang	陕西 Shaanxi	甘肃 Gansu	青海 Qinghai	宁夏 Ningxia	新疆 Xinjiang	合计 total
北京 Beijing	97.0	34.5	6.6			1.6	6.6			13.1			1.6					1.6			1.6			6.6			13.1				13.1	100
天津 Tianjin	86.5	11.5	0.4									0.8			0.4	1.4																100
河北 Hebei	81.3	0.8	0.4	0.1	0.1	0.1	0.0	0.0	0.1	0.6	0.1	0.1	0.1		0.1	0.4	0.0		0.0		0.0	0.0	0.4	0.0			7.9	0.0	0.0	0.0		100
山西 Shanxi	82.3	0.3	0.8	0.1	0.9	1.3	0.7	0.3	0.1	0.2	0.1	0.1	0.1		0.0	3.4			0.1		0.3	0.0	0.2		0.0		0.8				0.2	100
内蒙古 Inner Mongolia	80.0	3.1			0.1							0.1			1.3	0.4			0.1		1.4		0.2	1.8	0.0			0.3		1.4		100
辽宁 Liaoning	80.8	1.6			5.8	4.6	5.8	1.5	0.3	3.0	0.3		0.4	0.2	1.3	0.4			1.9		1.4		0.1					0.3			0.7	100
吉林 Jilin	87.4	2.3	0.5			3.1	0.7		0.3	0.9		0.1			4.7				2.3		0.1	0.1	1.1					0.1				100
黑龙江 Heilongjiang	29.4			0.1	0.3	3.1	0.7		0.7	0.5	0.1			0.2	3.2			0.8	2.3		0.1			2.3			0.2					100
上海 Shanghai	35.0		0.2			0.5		0.2		60.9	1.4	0.1	0.1	0.7	3.1	1.1	0.1	0.8		0.1		4.2	0.1	0.4						0.1		100
江苏 Jiangsu	25.1		0.2			0.2		0.1	52.7	10.5		0.6	0.1	0.1	0		0.2		2.3		0.1	0.3	0.8	0.3	0.0		0.2				0.2	100
浙江 Zhejiang	14.3		0.2		0.0	0.5	0.2	0.1	58.7	65.4	1.4		0.2	0.1	3.1	1.1	0.4	0.3	0.9	0.1	0.3	0.4	0.8	0.3	0.1		1.0			0.0	0.0	100
安徽 Anhui	59.3		0.1		0.4	0.9	0.8	0.2	11.3	3.3	2.6		0.2	0	0.8	0.4	0.1	0.3	8.2	0.1	0.0	1.3	0.3	0.0	0.1		0.7			0.1	0.1	100
福建 Fujian	50.1		0.1	0.0					15.8	4.4	9.1	0.1			0.1	0.9	0.9	1.0	10.2	0.2	0.0	0.4	0.0	0.2	0.1		0.1				0.0	100
江西 Jiangxi	88.2		0.2			0.9	0.8	0.1	14.4	2.6	7.5	1.0	7.4		0.0	0.9	0.1	0.0	10.2	0.2	0.0	0.4	0.0	0.0	0.0		0.1			0.1	0.1	100
山东 Shandong	64.8	1.2	0.2	0.0			0.1	0.1	3.2	2.6	7.5	1.6	0.0		1.3		8.8	0.0	0.8	0.0	0.0	0.1	0.5	0.0	0.2		2.7	0.1		0.2	0.7	100
河南 Henan	46.1	1.4	0.1	0.1	0.1	0.5			2.8	5.7	8.9	1.7	6.7		0.1	1.3		2.0	2.5		2.3	3.1	0.3	0.1				0.1				100
湖北 Hubei	50.7				1.6		0.3	0.1	2.5	3.6	2.3	0.8	0.7	0.2	0.1	0.2	2.7	18.5	19.0	0.0	0.1	3.1	0.3	0.1	0.2			0.1			0.4	100
湖南 Hunan	43.3	0.1	0.0			0.8	0.3	0.2	2.5	6.7	1.7	0.8	5.6	2.9	9.5	0.7	3.1	1.0	18.5	0.0	2.5	1.0	0.3	0.9	0.1		0.5	0.5		0.3	0.4	100
广东 Guangdong	45.5	0.3	3.0	0.1		0.8	0.3	0.8	0.3	30.3		0.5	2.3	0.8	0		0.2	2.2	33.2	0.9	1.9	2.6	1.3	0.9	0.1					2.4	0.3	100
广西 Guangxi	53.0								0.3	1.8	0		2.3	0.8	0.3			0.3	46.1	0					0.1							100
海南 Hainan	30.9				1.4	0.7	0.3		5.3	3.8	3.5	0.1	1.7	0.3	8.0	0.3	5.2	0.2	18.7	0.3		13.1	13.1	2.8	0.3		3.1				0.3	100
重庆 Chongqing	8.9		0.1		0.1		0.1		2.7	1.0	0.5	0.1	2.5	0.4	2.7	0.4	0.1	0.2	1.4	0.1	1.2	76.1	1.4	0.1	0.3		0.1	0	0.0		0.8	100
四川 Sichuan	14.5					0.2	0.4		2.4	0.8	3.3	0.5	4.5		0.1	0.4	1.7	0.4	2.1	0.2		52.3	1.1		16.1		0.1					100
贵州 Guizhou	48.0	0.1	1.0			0.4	1.3	0.1	1.4	20.2	5.3	0.5			2.4	1.0	1.6	0.4	1.6			13.4	2.3	1.3						0	0	100
云南 Yunnan	11.8		1.0							14.3	4.8		0.1		1.4			1.2				19.0	22.6	1.2			2.4	17.9				100
西藏 Xizang	82.2	0.4	0.1	0.1	1.6	0.2	0.1		2.9	2.9	0.2	0.1	0.1		1.4	1.3		0.3	0.7		1.1	0.2	2.1	1.5						3.0	0.1	100
陕西 Shaanxi	27.0	1.0				0.2	0.4	0.0	0.2	6.6	0.2		0.0	0.0	0.0	0.8	3.1	0.3	0.5			1.2	2.1	0.4			56.0			0.6	0.7	100
甘肃 Gansu	62.8	1.3				0.2		0.4		3.6	1.9	0.4			0.0	1.8			0.4				1.3		0.2		23.1	7.1			0	100
青海 Qinghai	72.7	0.6								0.2					0.3	0.6							0.2				23.7					100
宁夏 Ningxia	90.8								1.0										0.5			1.2	0.6				3.0	1.3				100
新疆 Xinjiang																																100

图 8-1-42　2017—2018 年全国各省份户籍地肿瘤患儿就诊的省份分布 /%

Figure 8-1-42　Distribution of provincial-level regions receiving children with leukemia from other provincial-level regions in 2017-2018/%

1.3.3　全国各省份收治白血病患儿来源的省份分布情况

各省份儿童肿瘤监测机构收治的省外就医白血病患儿来源分布略有差异,多数省份收治的白血病患儿来源以其相邻省份为主。如天津,其收治的省外就医白血病患儿主要来源于河北,占天津收治的省外就医白血病患儿总数的80.2%。再如重庆,其收治的省外就医白血病患儿主要来源于四川和贵州,分别占重庆收治的省外就医白血病患儿总数的70.7%和21.4%(图8-1-43,按列方向查看)。

1.4　全国儿童肿瘤监测机构白血病患儿住院费用医疗付费方式构成

1.4.1　全国白血病患儿住院费用医疗付费方式构成情况

在全国白血病患儿住院费用的医疗付费方式中,占比最高的前3种类型分别为全自费(33.86%)、新型农村合作医疗(23.07%)和城镇居民基本医疗保险(19.43%)(图8-1-44)。

1.4.2　六大区白血病患儿住院费用医疗付费方式构成情况

六大区的医疗付费方式所占比例各不相同,西南地区、华北地区和华东地区均以全自费占比最高,分别为46.24%、44.50%和35.24%。中南地区、西北地区和东北地区以新型农村合作医疗占比最高,分别为38.34%、35.72%和23.42%(图8-1-45~图8-1-50)。

1.3.3　Distribution of the provincial-level regions of origin of children with leukemia receiving treatment out of their own provincial-level regions

There was a slight difference in the distribution of the provincial-level regions of origin of children with leukemia admitted to surveillance sites in different provincial-level regions, and most of the children were mainly from their neighboring provincial-level regions. For example, in Tianjin, the children hospitalized from other provincial-level regions were mainly from Hebei, accounting for 80.2% of the total children hospitalized from other provincial-level regions in Tianjin. In Chongqing, children hospitalized from other provincial-level regions were mainly from Sichuan and Guizhou, accounting for 70.7% and 21.4%, respectively, of the total children hospitalized from other provincial-level regions in Chongqing (Figure 8-1-43, view in lines).

1.4　Composition of medical payment methods for hospitalization expenses of children with leukemia in pediatric cancer surveillance sites in China

1.4.1　Composition of medical payment methods for hospitalization expenses of children with leukemia nationally

Among the medical payment methods of children with leukemia nationally, the top three methods were 100% self-pay (33.86%), new rural cooperative medical system (23.07%) and basic medical insurance for urban residents (19.43%) (Figure 8-1-44).

1.4.2　Composition of medical payment methods for hospitalization expenses of children with leukemia in the six regions

The proportions of medical payment methods in the six regions were different, and the proportion of 100% self-pay was the highest in Southwest China, North China and East China, which were 46.24%, 44.50% and 35.24%, respectively. In Central and Southern China, Northwest China and Northeast China, the proportion of new rural cooperative medical system was the highest, accounting for 38.34%, 35.72% and 23.42%, respectively (Figure 8-1-45~Figure 8-1-50).

省外就医肿瘤患儿的来源省份分布 distribution of the provinces of origin of children with cancer receiving treatment out of their own provinces	收治省外就医肿瘤患儿的医院省份分布 provincial distribution of hospitals receiving children with cancer from outside the province																													
	北京 Beijing	天津 Tianjin	河北 Hebei	山西 Shanxi	内蒙古 Inner Mongolia	辽宁 Liaoning	吉林 Jilin	黑龙江 Heilongjiang	上海 Shanghai	江苏 Jiangsu	浙江 Zhejiang	安徽 Anhui	福建 Fujian	江西 Jiangxi	山东 Shandong	河南 Henan	湖北 Hubei	湖南 Hunan	广东 Guangdong	广西 Guangxi	海南 Hainan	重庆 Chongqing	四川 Sichuan	贵州 Guizhou	云南 Yunnan	西藏 Xizang	陕西 Shaanxi	甘肃 Gansu	青海 Qinghai	宁夏 Ningxia	新疆 Xinjiang
北京Beijing		1.7	4.5	0	0	0.3	1.1	0	0	0.2	0	0	0.2	0	0	0	0	0.8	0	0	0.7	0	0	3.6	0	0	0.4	0	0	0	7.8
天津Tianjin	0.9		1.2	0	0	0	0	0	0	0	0	1.2	0	0	0.2	1.3	0	0	0	0	0	0	0	0	0	0	0	0	0	0	0
河北Hebei	24.0	80.2		28.6	10.8	1.4	1.1	6.4	0.1	1.1	0	0.5	0.8	0	1.4	11.4	0.2	0	0.2	0	1.3	0	0.6	0.9	0	0	1.7	0	0	2.8	0
山西Shanxi	6.0	1.6	20.0		32.8	4.9	5.0	0	0.0	0.4	0.1	1.1	0.2	0	0.3	28.0	0	0	0.2	0	4.7	0.0	2.7	11.0	0	0	10.3	2.1	0	0	4.9
内蒙古Inner Mongolia	8.1	0.8	4.4	14.3		56.9	27.4	21.3	0	0.1	0.2	1.6	0	0	0.2	0	0	0	0.1	0	0	0	0	0	0.3	0	1.3	0	0	39.8	0
辽宁Liaoning	2.8	2.9	1.1	0	1.6		18.6	0	0	0.7	0.3	0	0.6	1.7	2.3	1.3	0	0	1.1	0	10.0	0	0.6	17.4	0	0	0	0	0	0	0
吉林Jilin	2.0	1.0	4.4	0	0	5.8		23.4	0.1	0.1	0	0.5	2.7	0	5.7	0	0	0	0.9	0	0	0	0.3	0	0	0	0	4.3	0	0	0
黑龙江Heilongjiang	4.3	2.9	0	7.1	6.3	7.8	3.3		0.4	0.2	0.1	0	0	0	7.7	0	0	0	0.1	0	0.7	0.1	5.7	0	0	0	0.2	0	0	0	0
上海Shanghai	0.1	0	0	0	0	0	0	0		1.7	0	0	0	0	0	0	0	0.8	0.5	0	0	0	0	2.8	0	0	0	0	0	0	0
江苏Jiangsu	1.2	0.1	2.2	0	0	0.8	0	4.3	18.5		1.5	0.5	0.2	5.8	5.3	0	0.2	0	0.5	4.1	0	1.0	0.4	3.7	0	0	0	0	0	0	1.0
浙江Zhejiang	0.9	0	2.2	0	0	0.3	0	2.1	22.7	2.5		3.7	0.2	0.8	0	4.7	0.4	1.6	0.7	0	0	0.1	3.2	2.8	0	0	0.1	0	0	0	2.0
安徽Anhui	2.2	0.4	10.0	0	1.6	3.7	2.7	0	18.1	64.9	13.1		1.4	3.3	6.3	6.1	4.0	10.5	2.3	0	0	0.5	13.1	0.9	0.9	0	2.6	0	50.0	0	1.0
福建Fujian	2.6	0.1	1.1	0	9.4	0	3.3	0	7.1	0.9	12.8	0.5		0	0.3	0	0.2	0	5.9	8.2	0	0.4	1.4	0	0.6	0	0.6	0	0	1.0	0
江西Jiangxi	4.6	0.1	0	0	0	4.4	0	0	13.7	2.6	21.8	14.9	32.6		0.2	9.0	4.8	23.4	15.1	25.0	0.7	0.3	0.4	4.6	0.6	0	0.1	0	0	0	0
山东Shandong	12.1	4.2	7.8	7.1	0	7.6	1.8	10.6	4.5	2.3	1.5	18.1	0.2	0.8		2.9	0	0	1.7	0	0	0.2	7.4	0	0.3	0	0.3	0	25.0	7.8	2.9
河南Henan	7.8	0.3	2.2	10.7	3.1	3.4	24.9	4.3	4.1	4.4	13.4	31.4	7.3	0.8	7.7		61.7	0.8	4.8	4.2	0.7	0.1	1.8	0	2.8	0	5.6	4.3	0	0	23.5
湖北Hubei	1.5	1.2	0	0	0	0	1.5	0	1.0	0.8	9.5	9.0	10.7	0	0.2	4.7		16.1	10.3	0	15.3	0.7	1.1	0.9	0	0	0	2.1	0	0	0
湖南Hunan	3.8	0.1	1.1	3.6	0	0	2.4	8.5	1.9	3.2	5.6	9.6	2.5	55.7	36.6	1.8	11.8		22.8	4.2	1.3	0.5	2.5	2.8	0	0	0	0	0	0	8.8
广东Guangdong	1.1	0.2	25.6	0	0	1.0	0	12.8	0.2	4.8	1.4	2.1	6.8	10.7	0	1.8	4.6	6.5		29.2	12.7	0.0	2.5	6.4	0	0	0.2	0	0	1.9	0
广西Guangxi	1.6	0	0	3.6	0	0	0	0	0.1	0.3	0.2	0	3.3	5.7	0	0	0.4	16.1	15.8		11.3	0.5	4.2	0	0.3	0	0	0	0	0	0
海南Hainan	0.4	0	0	0	0	0	0	0	0.0	0.3	0	0	0	0	0.2	0	0	0.8	7.2	0		0	0	0	0	0	0	0	0	6.8	0
重庆Chongqing	0.3	0	0	0	6.3	0.3	0.3	0	0.5	0.2	1.0	0	0.8	0.8	3.8	0.4	2.9	0	2.9	4.2	0		13.4	7.3	0.3	0	0.5	0	0	0	1.0
四川Sichuan	1.2	0	2.2	21.4	3.1	0	0.9	0	3.7	0.8	2.3	0.5	16.1	12.3	18.3	5.4	0.6	8.1	3.1	4.2	33.3	70.7		3.7	4.3	0	0.3	0	25.0	0	31.4
贵州Guizhou	0.8	0	0	0	0	0	0	0	1.5	0.3	6.3	0	12.8	0	0.2	2.5	5.9	6.5	2.0	16.7	0	21.4	7.1		89.2	0	0.1	0	0	0	0
云南Yunnan	1.2	0.1	8.9	0	0	0.5	3.0	2.1	0.4	3.2	4.3	2.1	0.2	0	0	2.9	2.3	2.4	0.6	0	0	2.3	6.4	9.2		0	0	0	0	0	0
西藏Xizang	0.1	0	0	0	0	0	0	0	0	0.3	0.4	0	0	1.6	0.3	0	0	0.8	0	0	0	0.4	6.7	0.9	0		0.1	31.9	0	0	0
陕西Shaanxi	2.6	0.2	1.1	3.6	25.0	0	0.3	0	0.9	0.6	0.2	0.5	0.2	0	2.3	4.7	0	0	0.4	0	7.3	0.1	0	13.8	0	0		0	0	28.2	1.0
甘肃Gansu	1.8	1.5	0	0	0	0.7	2.4	2.1	0.2	2.8	4.0	1.1	0.2	0	0.2	6.1	0	4.8	0.5	0	0	0.5	15.2	7.3	0	0	64.5		0	11.7	14.7
青海Qinghai	0.5	0.2	0	0	0	0	0	2.1	0	0.2	0	0	0	0	0	0	0	0	0.1	0	0	0	1.1	0	0	0	3.0	34.0		0	0
宁夏Ningxia	1.2	0.2	0	0	0	0.2	0	0	0	0.0	0	1.1	0	0	0	3.2	0	0	0	0	0	0	0.4	0	0.3	0	6.8	0	0		0
新疆Xinjiang	2.3	0	0	0	0	0	0	0	0.3	0.1	0	0	0	0	0.3	1.8	0	0	0.2	0	0	0.2	1.8	0	0	0	1.3	21.3	0	0	
合计total	100	100	100	100	100	100	100	100	100	100	100	100	100	100	100	100	100	100	100	100	100	100	100	100	100	0	100	100	100	100	100

图 8-1-43 2017—2018 年全国各省份儿童肿瘤监测机构省外就医白血病患儿来源分布 /%

Figure 8-1-43 Distribution of provincial-level regions of origin of children with leukemia receiving treatment out of their own provincial-level regions in 2017-2018/%

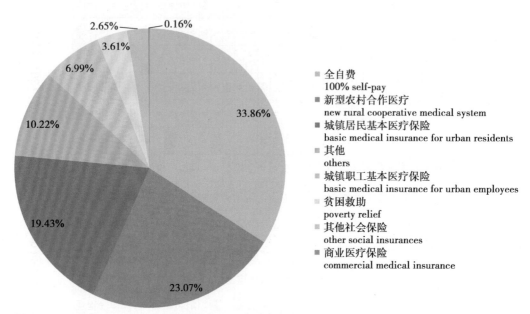

图 8-1-44　2017—2018 年全国白血病患儿住院费用医疗付费方式构成

Figure 8-1-44　Composition of medical payment methods for hospitalization expenses of children with leukemia nationally in 2017-2018

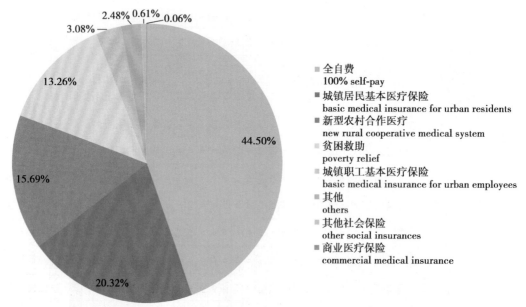

图 8-1-45　2017—2018 年华北地区白血病患儿住院费用医疗付费方式构成

Figure 8-1-45　Composition of medical payment methods for hospitalization expenses of children with leukemia in North China in 2017-2018

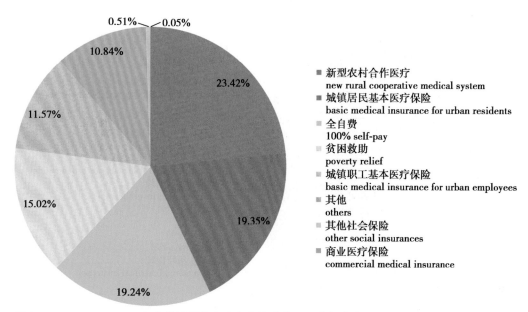

图 8-1-46　2017—2018 年东北地区白血病患儿住院费用医疗付费方式构成

Figure 8-1-46　Composition of medical payment methods for hospitalization expenses of children with leukemia in Northeast China in 2017-2018

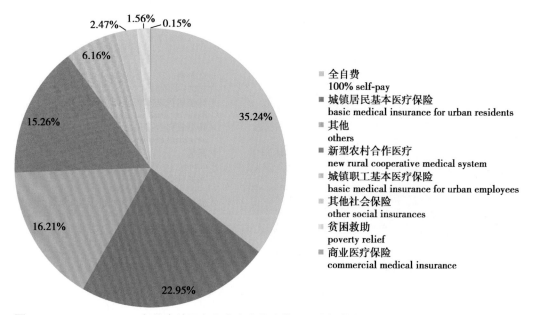

图 8-1-47　2017—2018 年华东地区白血病患儿住院费用医疗付费方式构成

Figure 8-1-47　Composition of medical payment methods for hospitalization expenses of children with leukemia in East China in 2017-2018

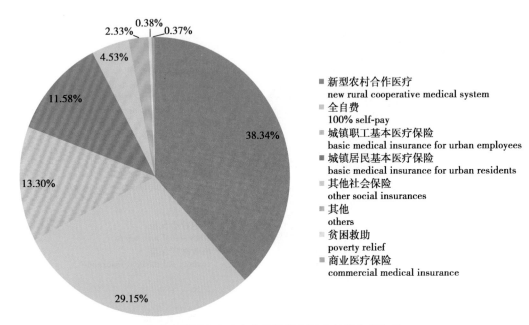

新型农村合作医疗
new rural cooperative medical system
全自费
100% self-pay
城镇职工基本医疗保险
basic medical insurance for urban employees
城镇居民基本医疗保险
basic medical insurance for urban residents
其他社会保险
other social insurances
其他
others
贫困救助
poverty relief
商业医疗保险
commercial medical insurance

图 8-1-48　2017—2018 年中南地区白血病患儿住院费用医疗付费方式构成

Figure 8-1-48　Composition of medical payment methods for hospitalization expenses of children with leukemia in Central and Southern China in 2017-2018

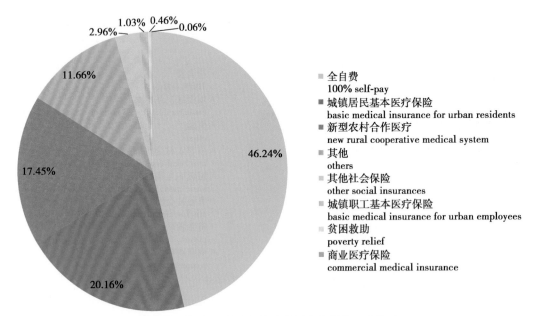

全自费
100% self-pay
城镇居民基本医疗保险
basic medical insurance for urban residents
新型农村合作医疗
new rural cooperative medical system
其他
others
其他社会保险
other social insurances
城镇职工基本医疗保险
basic medical insurance for urban employees
贫困救助
poverty relief
商业医疗保险
commercial medical insurance

图 8-1-49　2017—2018 年西南地区白血病患儿住院费用医疗付费方式构成

Figure 8-1-49　Composition of medical payment methods for hospitalization expenses of children with leukemia in Southwest China in 2017-2018

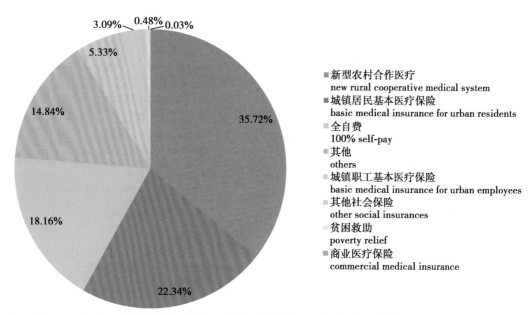

图 8-1-50   2017—2018 年西北地区白血病患儿住院费用医疗付费方式构成

Figure 8-1-50   Composition of medical payment methods for hospitalization expenses of children with leukemia in Northwest China in 2017-2018

图例：
- 新型农村合作医疗 new rural cooperative medical system
- 城镇居民基本医疗保险 basic medical insurance for urban residents
- 全自费 100% self-pay
- 其他 others
- 城镇职工基本医疗保险 basic medical insurance for urban employees
- 其他社会保险 other social insurances
- 贫困救助 poverty relief
- 商业医疗保险 commercial medical insurance

1.4.3   各省份白血病患儿住院费用医疗付费方式构成情况

河北、内蒙古、黑龙江、江苏、福建、湖南、广东、广西、四川、云南、西藏和青海 12 个省份均以全自费所占比例最高。山西、吉林、安徽、河南、海南、贵州、陕西和甘肃 8 个省份的新型农村合作医疗占比最高。天津、上海、山东、重庆、宁夏和新疆 6 个省份的城镇居民基本医疗保险占比最高（图 8-1-51~图 8-1-81）。

1.4.3   Composition of medical payment methods for hospitalization expenses of children with leukemia in each provincial-level region

The proportion of 100% self-pay was the highest in the following 12 provincial-level regions: Hebei, Inner Mongolia, Heilongjiang, Jiangsu, Fujian, Hunan, Guangdong, Guangxi, Sichuan, Yunnan, Xizang and Qinghai. Shanxi, Jilin, Anhui, Henan, Hainan, Guizhou, Shaanxi and Gansu had the highest proportion of new rural cooperative medical system payment method. The following 6 provincial-level regions—Tianjin, Shanghai, Shandong, Chongqing, Ningxia and Xinjiang—had the highest proportion of payment by basic medical insurance for urban residents (Figure 8-1-51~Figure 8-1-81).

153

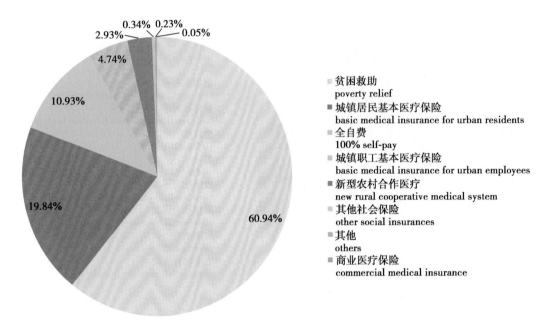

图 8-1-51　2017—2018 年北京白血病患儿住院费用医疗付费方式构成

Figure 8-1-51　Composition of medical payment methods for hospitalization expenses of children with leukemia in Beijing in 2017-2018

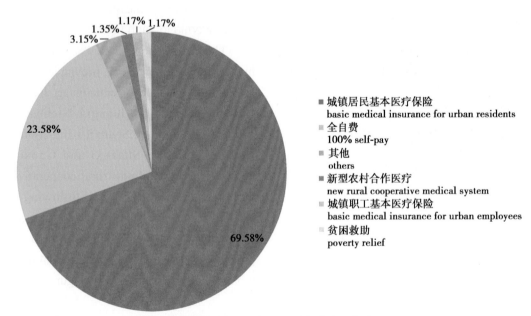

图 8-1-52　2017—2018 年天津白血病患儿住院费用医疗付费方式构成

Figure 8-1-52　Composition of medical payment methods for hospitalization expenses of children with leukemia in Tianjin in 2017-2018

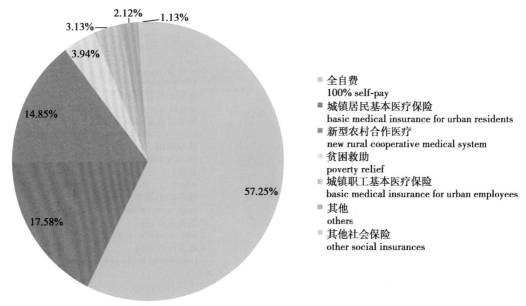

图 8-1-53　2017—2018 年河北白血病患儿住院费用医疗付费方式构成

Figure 8-1-53　Composition of medical payment methods for hospitalization expenses of children with leukemia in Hebei in 2017-2018

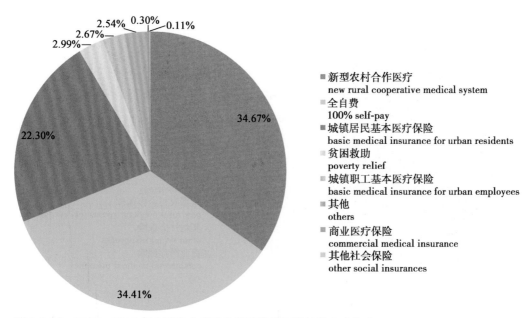

图 8-1-54　2017—2018 年山西白血病患儿住院费用医疗付费方式构成

Figure 8-1-54　Composition of medical payment methods for hospitalization expenses of children with leukemia in Shanxi in 2017-2018

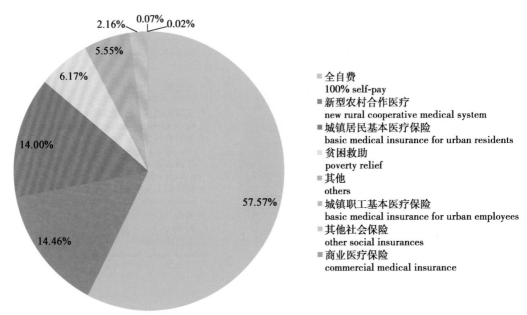

图 8-1-55　2017—2018 年内蒙古白血病患儿住院费用医疗付费方式构成

Figure 8-1-55　Composition of medical payment methods for hospitalization expenses of children with leukemia in Inner Mongolia in 2017-2018

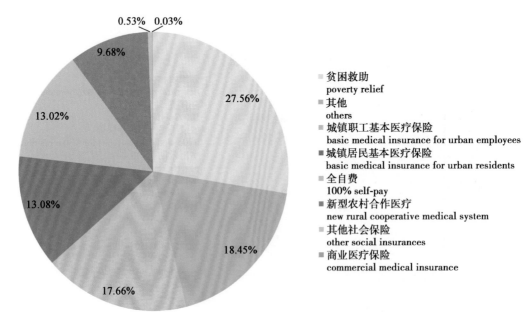

图 8-1-56　2017—2018 年辽宁白血病患儿住院费用医疗付费方式构成

Figure 8-1-56　Composition of medical payment methods for hospitalization expenses of children with leukemia in Liaoning in 2017-2018

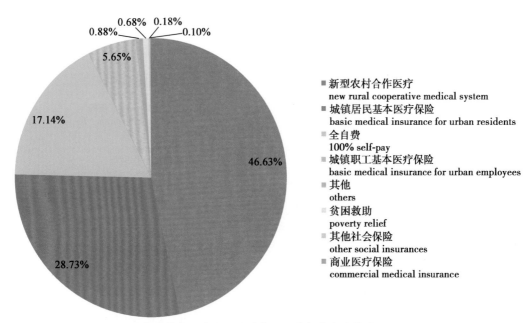

图 8-1-57　2017—2018 年吉林白血病患儿住院费用医疗付费方式构成

Figure 8-1-57　Composition of medical payment methods for hospitalization expenses of children with leukemia in Jilin in 2017-2018

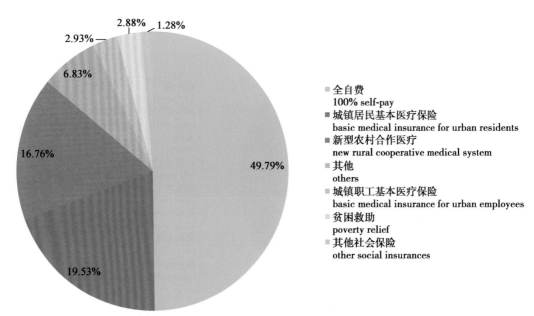

图 8-1-58　2017—2018 年黑龙江白血病患儿住院费用医疗付费方式构成

Figure 8-1-58　Composition of medical payment methods for hospitalization expenses of children with leukemia in Heilongjiang in 2017-2018

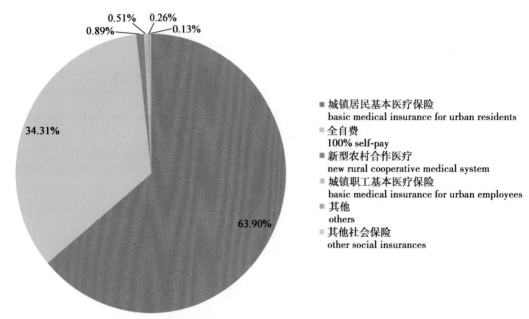

图 8-1-59　2017—2018 年上海白血病患儿住院费用医疗付费方式构成

Figure 8-1-59　Composition of medical payment methods for hospitalization expenses of children with leukemia in Shanghai in 2017-2018

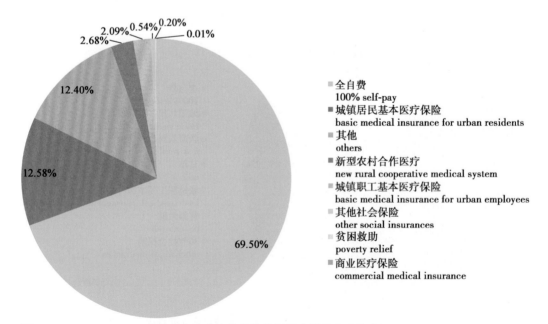

图 8-1-60　2017—2018 年江苏白血病患儿住院费用医疗付费方式构成

Figure 8-1-60　Composition of medical payment methods for hospitalization expenses of children with leukemia in Jiangsu in 2017-2018

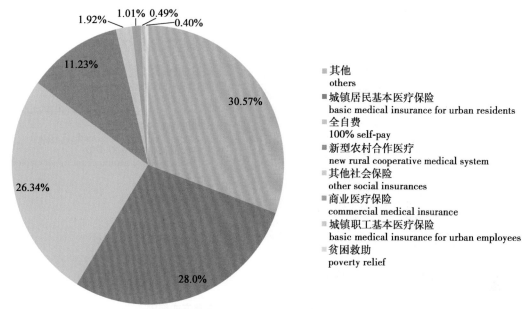

图 8-1-61　2017—2018 年浙江白血病患儿住院费用医疗付费方式构成

Figure 8-1-61　Composition of medical payment methods for hospitalization expenses of children with leukemia in Zhejiang in 2017-2018

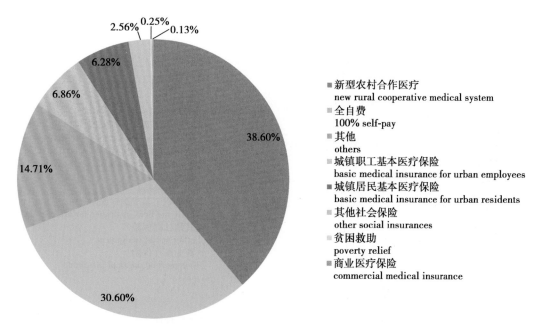

图 8-1-62　2017—2018 年安徽白血病患儿住院费用医疗付费方式构成

Figure 8-1-62　Composition of medical payment methods for hospitalization expenses of children with leukemia in Anhui in 2017-2018

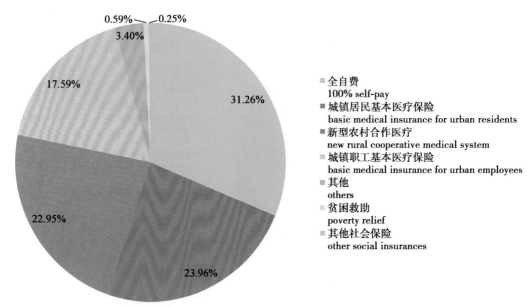

图 8-1-63 2017—2018 年福建白血病患儿住院费用医疗付费方式构成

Figure 8-1-63 Composition of medical payment methods for hospitalization expenses of children with leukemia in Fujian in 2017-2018

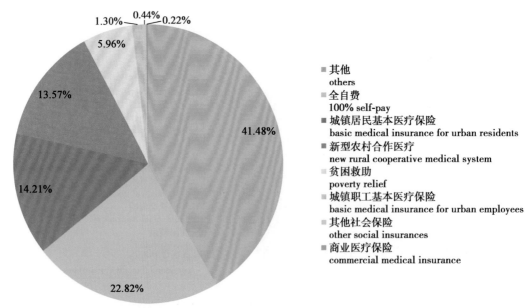

图 8-1-64 2017—2018 年江西白血病患儿住院费用医疗付费方式构成

Figure 8-1-64 Composition of medical payment methods for hospitalization expenses of children with leukemia in Jiangxi in 2017-2018

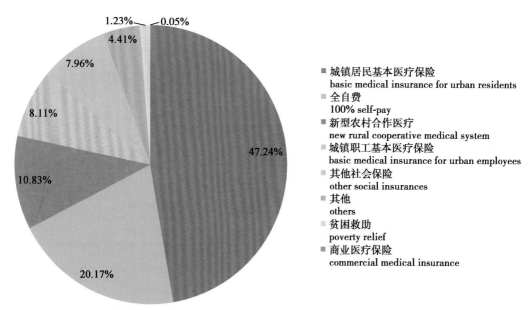

图 8-1-65　2017—2018 年山东白血病患儿住院费用医疗付费方式构成

Figure 8-1-65　Composition of medical payment methods for hospitalization expenses of children with leukemia in Shandong in 2017-2018

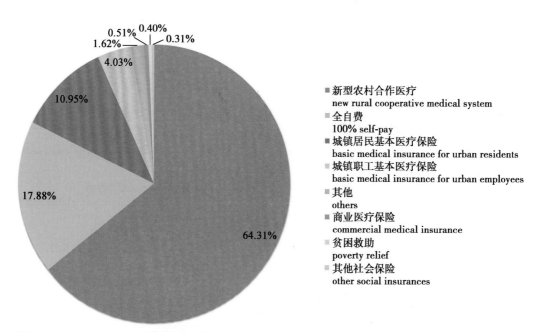

图 8-1-66　2017—2018 年河南白血病患儿住院费用医疗付费方式构成

Figure 8-1-66　Composition of medical payment methods for hospitalization expenses of children with leukemia in Henan in 2017-2018

161

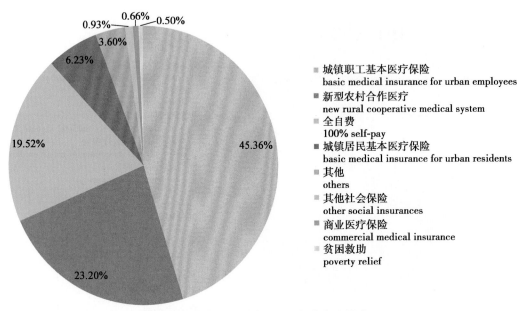

图 8-1-67 2017—2018 年湖北白血病患儿住院费用医疗付费方式构成

Figure 8-1-67 Composition of medical payment methods for hospitalization expenses of children with leukemia in Hubei in 2017-2018

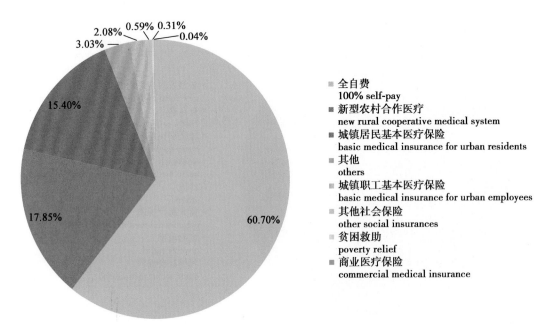

图 8-1-68 2017—2018 年湖南白血病患儿住院费用医疗付费方式构成

Figure 8-1-68 Composition of medical payment methods for hospitalization expenses of children with leukemia in Hunan in 2017-2018

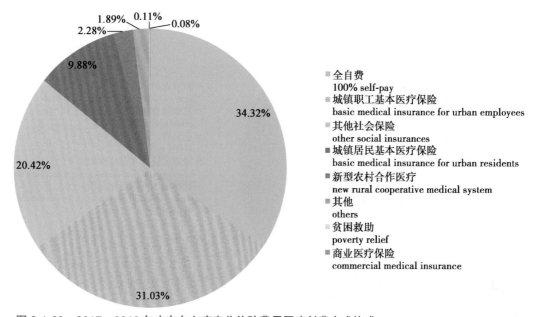

图 8-1-69　2017—2018 年广东白血病患儿住院费用医疗付费方式构成

Figure 8-1-69　Composition of medical payment methods for hospitalization expenses of children with leukemia in Guangdong in 2017-2018

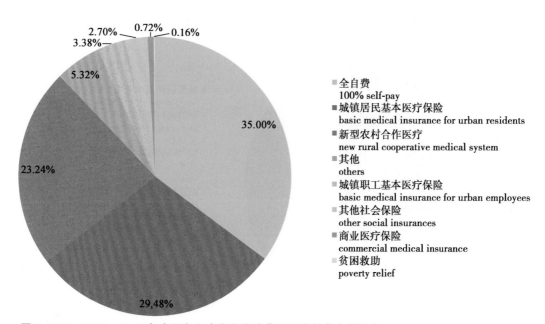

图 8-1-70　2017—2018 年广西白血病患儿住院费用医疗付费方式构成

Figure 8-1-70　Composition of medical payment methods for hospitalization expenses of children with leukemia in Guangxi in 2017-2018

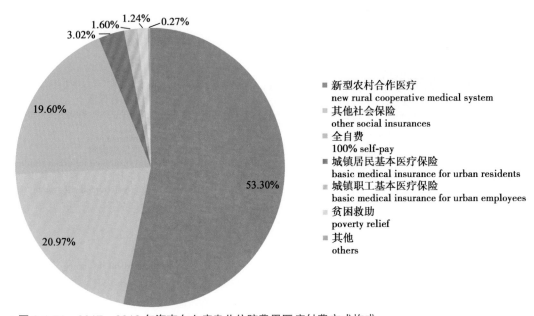

图 8-1-71　2017—2018 年海南白血病患儿住院费用医疗付费方式构成

Figure 8-1-71　Composition of medical payment methods for hospitalization expenses of children with leukemia in Hainan in 2017-2018

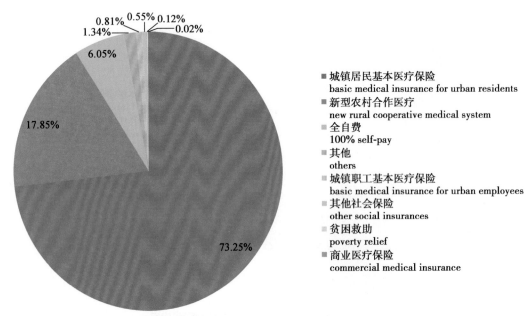

图 8-1-72　2017—2018 年重庆白血病患儿住院费用医疗付费方式构成

Figure 8-1-72　Composition of medical payment methods for hospitalization expenses of children with leukemia in Chongqing in 2017-2018

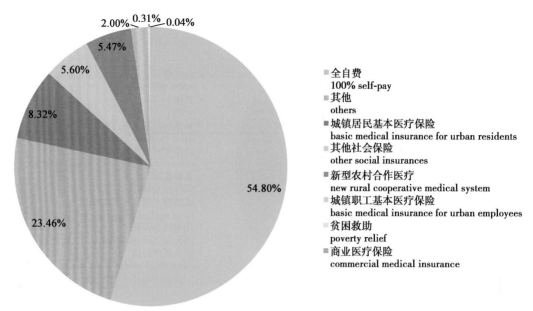

图 8-1-73   2017—2018 年四川白血病患儿住院费用医疗付费方式构成

Figure 8-1-73   Composition of medical payment methods for hospitalization expenses of children with leukemia in Sichuan in 2017-2018

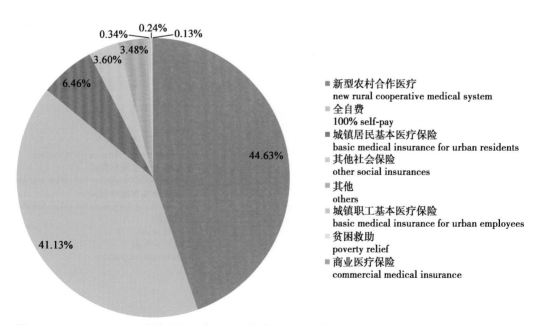

图 8-1-74   2017—2018 年贵州白血病患儿住院费用医疗付费方式构成

Figure 8-1-74   Composition of medical payment methods for hospitalization expenses of children with leukemia in Guizhou in 2017-2018

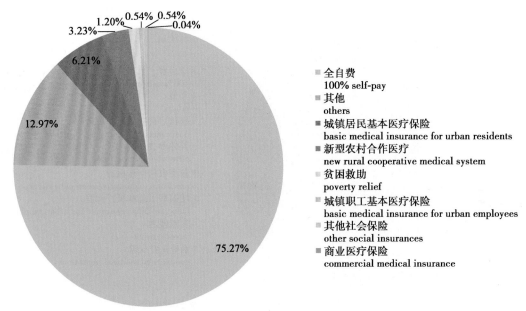

图 8-1-75　2017—2018 年云南白血病患儿住院费用医疗付费方式构成

Figure 8-1-75　Composition of medical payment methods for hospitalization expenses of children with leukemia in Yunnan in 2017-2018

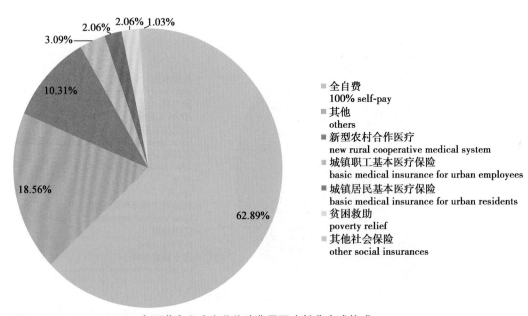

图 8-1-76　2017—2018 年西藏白血病患儿住院费用医疗付费方式构成

Figure 8-1-76　Composition of medical payment methods for hospitalization expenses of children with leukemia in Xizang in 2017-2018

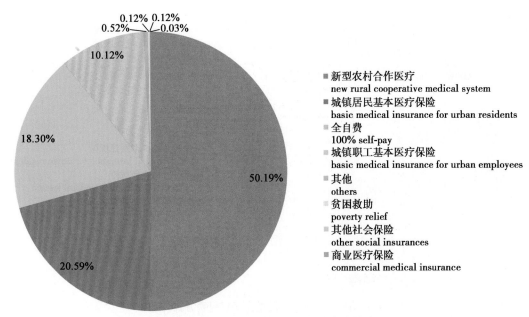

图 8-1-77   2017—2018 年陕西白血病患儿住院费用医疗付费方式构成

Figure 8-1-77   Composition of medical payment methods for hospitalization expenses of children with leukemia in Shaanxi in 2017-2018

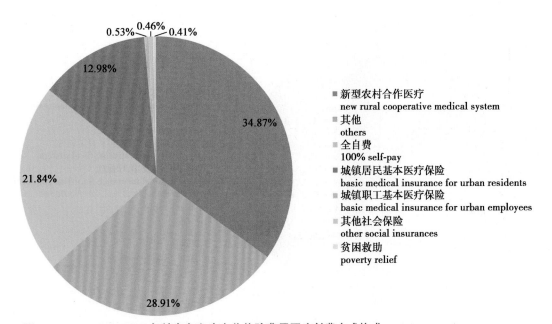

图 8-1-78   2017—2018 年甘肃白血病患儿住院费用医疗付费方式构成

Figure 8-1-78   Composition of medical payment methods for hospitalization expenses of children with leukemia in Gansu in 2017-2018

167

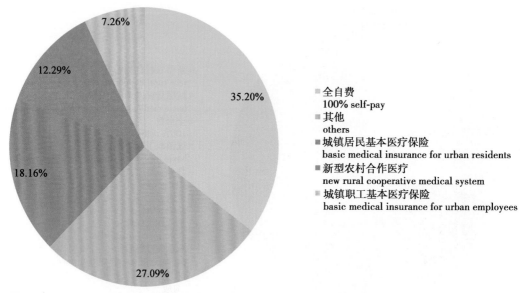

图 8-1-79　2017—2018 年青海白血病患儿住院费用医疗付费方式构成

Figure 8-1-79　Composition of medical payment methods for hospitalization expenses of children with leukemia in Qinghai in 2017-2018

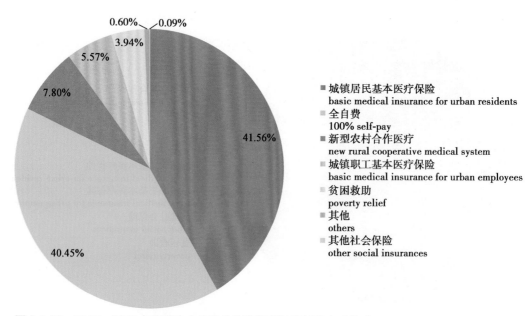

图 8-1-80　2017—2018 年宁夏白血病患儿住院费用医疗付费方式构成

Figure 8-1-80　Composition of medical payment methods for hospitalization expenses of children with leukemia in Ningxia in 2017-2018

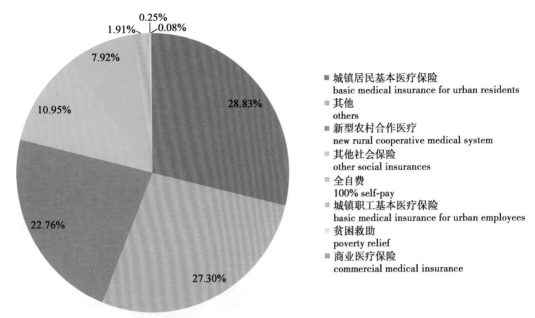

图 8-1-81　2017—2018 年新疆白血病患儿住院费用医疗付费方式构成

Figure 8-1-81　Composition of medical payment methods for hospitalization expenses of children with leukemia in Xinjiang in 2017-2018

1.5　全国儿童肿瘤监测机构白血病患儿住院费用分析

1.5.1　全国儿童肿瘤监测机构白血病患儿次均住院费用情况

1.5.1.1　全国及六大区白血病患儿次均住院费用情况　全国白血病患儿次均住院费用（中位数）为 5 332.30 元。高于全国中位数水平的地区分别为中南地区（8 133.77 元）和西南地区（6 133.23 元），低于全国中位数水平的地区分别为西北地区（3 844.19 元）、华北地区（4 716.28 元）、华东地区（4 754.43 元）和东北地区（5 119.80 元）（图 8-1-82）。

1.5　Analysis of hospitalization expenses of children with leukemia in pediatric cancer surveillance sites in China

1.5.1　Expenses per hospitalization of children with leukemia in pediatric cancer surveillance sites in China

1.5.1.1　Expenses per hospitalization of children with leukemia in the six regions and the whole country　Nationally, the median expense per hospitalization was 5, 332.30 CNY. The regions above the national median were Central and Southern China (8, 133.77 CNY), and Southwest China (6, 133.23 CNY), while those below the national median were Northeast China (5, 119.80 CNY), East China (4, 754.43 CNY), North China (4, 716.28 CNY) and Northwest China (3, 844.19 CNY) (Figure 8-1-82).

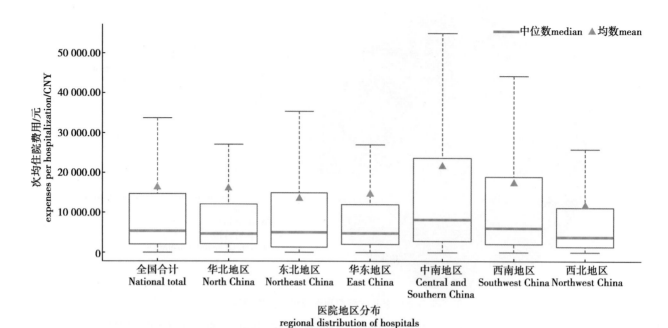

图 8-1-82　2017—2018 年全国及六大区白血病患儿次均住院费用

Figure 8-1-82　Expenses per hospitalization of children with leukemia in the six regions and the whole country in 2017-2018

1.5.1.2　各省份白血病患儿次均住院费用情况　根据白血病患儿次均住院费用（中位数），前 3 位的省份分别为青海（12 025.19 元）、西藏（11 068.28 元）和河南（10 687.66 元），后 3 位分别为上海（2 078.21 元）、陕西（2 185.41 元）和福建（3 042.94 元）（图 8-1-83）。

1.5.1.2　Expenses per hospitalization of children with leukemia in each provincial-level region　In terms of the median expenses per hospitalization of children with leukemia, the top three provincial-level regions were Qinghai (12, 025.19 CNY), Xizang (11, 068.28 CNY) and Henan (10, 687.66 CNY), while the last three were Shanghai (2, 078.21 CNY), Shaanxi (2, 185.41 CNY) and Fujian (3, 042.94 CNY) (Figure 8-1-83).

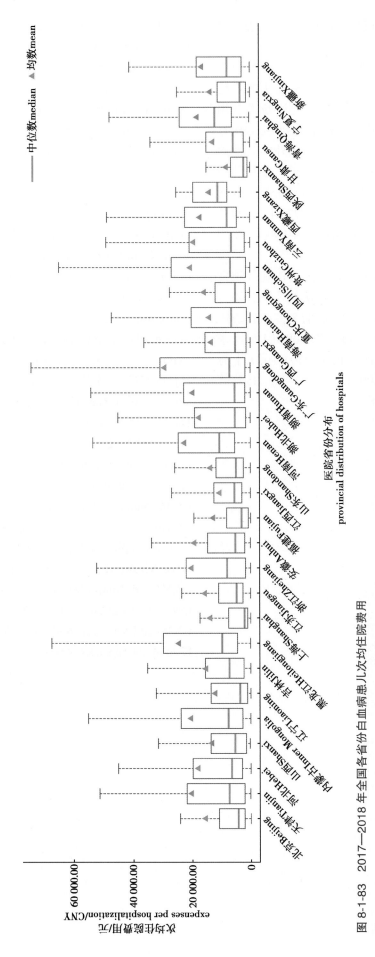

图 8-1-83　2017—2018 年全国各省份白血病患儿次均住院费用

Figure 8-1-83　Expenses per hospitalization of children with leukemia in each provincial-level region in 2017-2018

1.5.2 全国儿童肿瘤监测机构白血病患儿次均住院分项费用情况

1.5.2.1 全国及六大区白血病患儿次均住院分项费用情况 根据全国白血病患儿次均住院分项费用（中位数），前 3 位分别为诊断类费用（1 356.50 元）、西药类费用（1 116.50 元）和综合医疗服务类费用（726.30 元）。除华北地区外的其他地区分项费用中位数的顺位与全国相同。如东北地区，次均住院分项费用（中位数）前 3 位分别为诊断类费用（1 282.00 元）、西药类费用（777.64 元）和综合医疗服务类费用（776.36 元）（图 8-1-84）。按均数统计的结果详见图 8-1-85。

1.5.2.2 各省份白血病患儿次均住院分项费用情况 根据各省份白血病患儿次均住院分项费用（中位数），以诊断类费用为例，前 3 位的省份依次为西藏（5 477.00 元）、青海（2 795.00 元）和广东（2 385.57 元），后 3 位依次为福建（230.00 元）、上海（295.00 元）和陕西（600.00 元）（图 8-1-86）。按均数统计的结果详见图 8-1-87。

1.5.2 Expenses of each item per hospitalization of children with leukemia in pediatric cancer surveillance sites in China

1.5.2.1 Expenses of each item per hospitalization of children with leukemia in the six regions and the whole country In terms of the median expenses of each item per hospitalization of children with leukemia, the top three items were diagnostic expenses (1, 356.50 CNY), western medication expenses (1, 116.50 CNY) and comprehensive medical services expenses (726.30 CNY). Apart from North China, the rank of the median expenses of each item in other five regions were the same with that of the national median. For example, in Northeast China, the top three median expenses of each item per hospitalization were the cost of diagnostic expenses (1, 282.00 CNY), western medication expenses (777.64 CNY), and comprehensive medical services expenses (777.36 CNY) (Figure 8-1-84). Data by the mean expenses in Figure 8-1-85.

1.5.2.2 Expenses of each item per hospitalization of children with leukemia in each provincial-level region In terms of the median expenses of each item per hospitalization of children with leukemia in each provincial-level region, taking diagnoses expenses as an example, the top three provincial-level regions were Xizang (5, 477.00 CNY), Qinghai (2, 795.00 CNY) and Guangdong (2, 385.57 CNY). The last three were Fujian (230.00 CNY), Shanghai (295.00 CNY) and Shaanxi (600.00 CNY) (Figure 8-1-86). Data by the mean expenses in Figure 8-1-87.

分项费用/元 expenses of each item/CNY

regional distribution of hospitals	综合医疗服务类费用 comprehensive medical service expenses	诊断类费用 diagnostic expenses	治疗类费用 treatment expenses	康复类费用 rehabilitation expenses	中医类费用 traditional chinese medicine service expenses	西药类费用 western medication expenses	中药类费用 traditional chinese medication expenses	血液和血液制品类费用 blood and blood product expenses	耗材类费用 medical consumable expenses	其他类费用 others
全国合计 National total	726.30	1 356.50	37.00	0	0	1 116.50	0	0	217.55	5.58
华北地区 North China	373.50	1 386.00	0	0	0	1 018.57	0	0	395.41	0
东北地区 Northeast China	776.36	1 282.00	83.49	0	0	777.64	0	0	329.90	27.39
华东地区 East China	704.00	1 268.50	60.00	0	0	1 122.89	0	0	216.24	30.00
中南地区 Central and Southern China	880.40	1 726.00	105.10	0	0	1 405.44	0	0	216.93	8.00
西南地区 Southwest China	1 229.65	1 686.00	55.00	0	0	1 669.12	0	0	121.76	1.00
西北地区 Northwest China	671.00	1 025.80	120.00	0	0	812.34	0	0	67.82	0

图 8-1-84　2017—2018 年全国及六大区白血病患儿次均住院分项费用（按中位数计）

Figure 8-1-84　Expenses of each item per hospitalization of children with leukemia in the six regions and the whole country in 2017-2018 (by the median)

分项费用/元 expenses of each item/CNY

regional distribution of hospitals	综合医疗服务类费用 comprehensive medical service expenses	诊断类费用 diagnostic expenses	治疗类费用 treatment expenses	康复类费用 rehabilitation expenses	中医类费用 traditional chinese medicine service expenses	西药类费用 western medication expenses	中药类费用 traditional chinese medication expenses	血液和血液制品类费用 blood and blood product expenses	耗材类费用 medical consumable expenses	其他类费用 others
全国合计 National total	2 231.07	3 409.17	372.38	11.80	20.24	5 421.99	105.37	1 700.11	958.06	759.02
华北地区 North China	1 974.25	3 702.81	148.73	0.32	1.97	5 090.75	45.75	2 152.38	1 182.02	663.64
东北地区 Northeast China	2 093.59	2 855.23	302.69	9.50	12.93	4 227.09	73.98	1 876.61	1 020.31	1 453.59
华东地区 East China	2 099.44	2 938.44	367.92	26.48	0.58	5 425.20	107.96	1 406.15	860.69	577.64
中南地区 Central and Southern China	2 659.89	4 405.08	743.96	3.45	80.62	6 566.65	204.30	1 529.40	1 266.01	1 614.47
西南地区 Southwest China	2 986.71	3 804.70	421.72	16.60	26.97	6 084.80	145.41	2 052.96	759.67	183.35
西北地区 Northwest China	1 723.27	2 360.25	352.59	1.76	18.33	4 237.24	52.65	1 111.74	362.65	355.82

图 8-1-85　2017—2018 年全国及六大区白血病患儿次均住院分项费用（按均数计）

Figure 8-1-85　Expenses of each item per hospitalization of children with leukemia in the six regions and the whole country in 2017-2018 (by the mean)

省份分布 provincial distribution of hospitals	综合医疗服务类费用 comprehensive medical service expenses	诊断类费用 diagnostic expenses	治疗类费用 treatment expenses	康复类费用 rehabilitation expenses	中医类费用 traditional chinese medicine service expenses	西药类费用 western medication expenses	中药类费用 traditional chinese medication expenses	血液和血液制品类费用 blood and blood product expenses	耗材类费用 medical consumable expenses	其他类费用 others
北京Beijing	321.50	1 320.00	0	0	0	891.54	0	0	433.48	0
天津Tianjin	1 351.65	1 700.30	15.00	0	0	1 470.81	0	0	347.78	20.00
河北Hebei	843.00	1 474.50	120.00	0	0	1 727.68	0	186.30	347.48	0
山西Shanxi	842.00	1 537.00	40.00	0	0	779.51	0	0	223.15	6.60
内蒙古Inner Mongolia	682.34	1 397.00	415.10	0	0	2 443.84	0	0	146.28	36.00
辽宁Liaoning	506.05	1 045.00	79.70	0	0	634.85	44.40	714.00	243.60	548.55
吉林Jilin	1 441.50	2 217.00	129.00	0	0	1 550.69	0	0	764.00	0
黑龙江Heilongjiang	1 069.00	1 862.00	100.00	0	0	2 409.89	0	308.75	752.50	449.00
上海Shanghai	277.00	295.00	140.00	0	0	724.14	0	0	221.64	0
江苏Jiangsu	568.70	1 364.85	22.00	9.00	0	1 197.45	46.84	0	298.31	383.10
浙江Zhejiang	773.25	1 762.00	169.00	0	0	1 966.14	0	0	305.35	7.00
安徽Anhui	1 155.40	1 208.50	90.00	88.00	0	906.01	40.23	1 438.00	151.36	48.82
福建Fujian	537.67	230.00	0	0	0	505.46	0	0	0	9.00
江西Jiangxi	749.00	1 753.00	72.00	30.00	0	1 628.42	126.45	240.00	212.01	30.00
山东Shandong	946.00	1 255.00	130.00	0	0	970.20	0	0	365.60	0
河南Henan	1 239.75	1 447.55	291.00	0	0	4 107.93	0	0	59.33	21.70
湖北Hubei	459.00	1 837.00	0	0	0	1 133.12	0	0	269.14	6.00
湖南Hunan	818.50	1 615.75	92.00	0	0	1 020.34	0	0	400.77	48.00
广东Guangdong	868.00	2 385.57	171.34	0	0	598.79	0	0	199.00	0
广西Guangxi	776.95	1 494.70	203.00	0	0	892.08	0	0	125.23	0
海南Hainan	839.00	1 228.71	195.00	0	0	921.29	123.74	0	264.52	0
重庆Chongqing	1 001.31	2 352.90	0	0	9	893.10	0	0	130.67	5.00
四川Sichuan	1 293.90	1 112.00	140.00	0	0	1 472.78	15.00	0	421.47	0
贵州Guizhou	1 055.43	1 751.48	118.30	0	0	1 313.77	0	0	0	49.00
云南Yunnan	1 900.00	1 581.00	180.00	0	0	4 193.84	76.50	1 860.00	93.38	0.04
西藏Xizang	1 706.00	5 477.00	0	0	0	693.80	0	100.00	0	0
陕西Shaanxi	385.00	600.00	100.00	0	0	485.94	0	0	466.58	0
甘肃Gansu	1 255.00	1 382.50	60.00	6.00	0	1 292.53	0	0	72.12	0
青海Qinghai	1 141.00	2 795.00	162.00	0	0	2 569.80	0	674.50	379.63	0
宁夏Ningxia	618.55	739.50	190.10	0	0	740.66	161.97	1 195.25	224.13	1.95
新疆Xinjiang	999.00	2 250.00	250.50	0	0	2 306.32	0	0	6.36	38.00

分项费用/元　expenses of each item/CNY

图 8-1-86　2017—2018 年全国各省份白血病患儿次均住院分项费用（按中位数计）

Figure 8-1-86　Expenses of each item per hospitalization of children with leukemia in each provincial-level region in 2017-2018 (by the median)

医院省份分布 provincial distribution of hospitals	分项费用/元 expenses of each item/CNY									
	综合医疗服务类费用 comprehensive medical service expenses	诊断类费用 diagnostic expenses	治疗类费用 treatment expenses	康复类费用 rehabilitation expenses	中医类费用 traditional chinese medicine service expenses	西药类费用 western medication expenses	中药类费用 traditional chinese medication expenses	血液和血液制品类费用 blood and blood product expenses	耗材类费用 medical consumable expenses	其他类费用 others
北京Beijing	1 780.86	3 778.43	42.18	0.19	0.97	4 780.03	38.82	2 281.14	1 255.95	727.15
天津Tianjin	4 336.91	4 063.26	401.23	0.27	0.76	6 412.60	58.38	1 075.64	1 122.93	191.61
河北Hebei	2 103.59	3 432.05	315.74	1.10	13.69	6 578.32	97.97	2 255.67	1 040.44	723.45
山西Shanxi	2 419.35	3 116.78	336.19	1.54	0.49	4 183.83	52.59	1 122.27	678.17	140.31
内蒙古Inner Mongolia	2 201.58	3 031.16	1 698.97	0.08	7.46	8 167.97	65.04	1 854.78	668.80	429.86
辽宁Liaoning	1 642.39	2 062.22	311.36	34.05	0	3 648.01	99.65	2 997.63	639.83	2 287.60
吉林Jilin	2 741.08	3 819.29	288.54	0.40	18.69	4 664.30	40.35	1 135.30	1 565.68	14.59
黑龙江Heilongjiang	2 560.60	3 862.72	347.00	0	0	8 647.67	328.89	2 670.01	1 404.13	5 109.82
上海Shanghai	1 970.75	3 576.87	250.86	2.27	0.36	5 314.30	38.81	552.10	1 079.54	18.70
江苏Jiangsu	1 814.20	3 560.52	337.06	26.11	0.05	5 734.06	122.98	1 624.99	1 290.02	1 134.02
浙江Zhejiang	2 441.96	3 383.81	834.03	19.88	0.51	8 747.83	56.06	1 689.92	1 039.63	413.76
安徽Anhui	3 458.59	3 267.18	268.36	168.62	8.96	6 669.30	155.93	3 366.63	722.21	301.41
福建Fujian	2 106.64	1 488.85	210.94	0.03	0.03	5 482.59	6.50	563.14	74.60	322.57
江西Jiangxi	1 557.46	2 592.46	261.93	18.60	1.25	3 655.36	288.38	1 713.51	543.49	132.15
山东Shandong	2 293.05	2 751.44	504.14	0.63	1.34	4 427.22	69.29	1 374.30	911.57	663.11
河南Henan	2 633.32	2 796.40	1 263.21	2.73	36.51	8 737.10	98.78	1 403.27	435.74	751.07
湖北Hubei	2 160.08	4 587.67	462.30	1.74	0.46	5 867.01	64.76	1 047.88	974.72	116.79
湖南Hunan	2 662.71	4 100.47	438.65	6.89	343.63	5 861.83	717.89	1 811.81	1 454.80	842.71
广东Guangdong	3 439.72	7 157.90	914.88	4.25	3.10	7 249.35	14.82	1 898.01	2 143.45	4 633.19
广西Guangxi	1 981.14	3 265.11	600.19	0.09	1.14	4 032.59	26.79	1 670.88	770.78	99.88
海南Hainan	1 825.58	1 696.60	551.24	0.01	15.74	4 433.09	251.42	889.11	822.60	52.38
重庆Chongqing	2 661.21	4 170.80	117.81	16.87	48.90	3 641.20	25.66	1 564.11	724.91	22.75
四川Sichuan	4 031.69	3 405.03	902.96	29.91	16.00	6 049.39	88.42	2 216.20	1 328.55	246.68
贵州Guizhou	2 723.20	4 380.33	521.54	1.34	1.85	7 202.43	304.93	2 022.39	697.00	461.86
云南Yunnan	2 844.97	3 042.19	390.23	47.24	3.25	8 779.49	276.02	3 564.26	386.45	81.60
西藏Xizang	1 812.00	5 360.69	7.50	0	0	4 053.99	3.04	316.92	873.11	5.28
陕西Shaanxi	1 382.20	1 503.10	219.05	0.04	17.09	2 980.17	14.86	694.91	290.69	328.68
甘肃Gansu	2 184.21	2 344.47	306.02	12.76	42.41	4 540.37	96.70	1 625.04	370.36	309.20
青海Qinghai	1 855.57	3 884.59	324.78	4.09	0	5 992.99	24.67	2 831.64	649.59	873.84
宁夏Ningxia	1 994.61	2 508.44	531.51	11.73	12.29	3 315.07	453.48	4 827.01	955.97	29.61
新疆Xinjiang	2 107.10	3 932.61	619.84	0.04	11.73	6 574.85	68.03	1 240.64	379.99	418.21

图 8-1-87　2017—2018 年全国各省份白血病患儿次均住院分项费用（按均数计）

Figure 8-1-87　Expenses of each item per hospitalization of children with leukemia in each provincial-level region in 2017-2018（by the mean）

175

1.6 全国儿童肿瘤监测机构白血病患儿平均住院日分析

1.6.1 全国及六大区白血病患儿平均住院日情况

全国白血病患儿平均住院日的中位数为 4 天。高于全国中位数水平的地区为中南地区(7 天),西南地区(6 天)、东北地区(5 天)和西北地区(5 天),与全国中位数水平相同的地区为华东地区(4 天),低于全国中位数水平的地区为华北地区(2 天)(图 8-1-88)。

1.6.2 各省份白血病患儿平均住院日情况

根据各省份白血病患儿平均住院日的中位数,白血病患儿平均住院日最长的省份是青海(11 天),其次是内蒙古(9 天)、黑龙江(9 天)和河南(9 天),最短的是北京和上海(1 天)(图 8-1-89)。

1.6 Analysis of the average length of hospitalization of children with leukemia in pediatric cancer surveillance sites in China

1.6.1 Average length of hospitalization of children with leukemia in the six regions and the whole country

Nationally, the median of average length of hospitalization was 4 days. Central and Southern China (7 days), Southwest China (6 days), Northeast China (5 days) and Northwest China (5 days) were higher than the national median, East China (4 days) was the same with the national median, and North China (2 days) was lower than the national median (Figure 8-1-88).

1.6.2 Average length of hospitalization of children with leukemia in each provincial-level region

In terms of the median of average length of hospitalization of children with leukemia in each provincial-level region, the provincial-level region with the longest average hospital stay was Qinghai (11 days), followed by Inner Mongolia (9 days), Heilongjiang (9 days) and Henan (9 days), and the shortest were Beijing and Shanghai (1 day) (Figure 8-1-89).

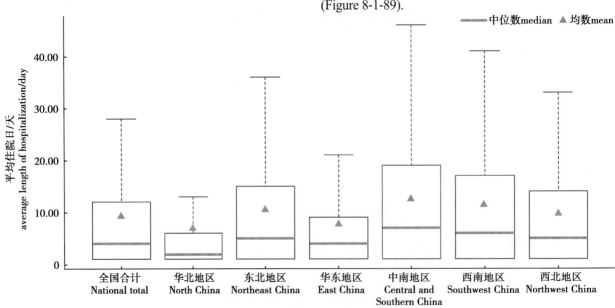

图 8-1-88 2017—2018 年全国及六大区白血病患儿平均住院日

Figure 8-1-88 Average length of hospitalization of children with leukemia in the six regions and the whole country in 2017-2018

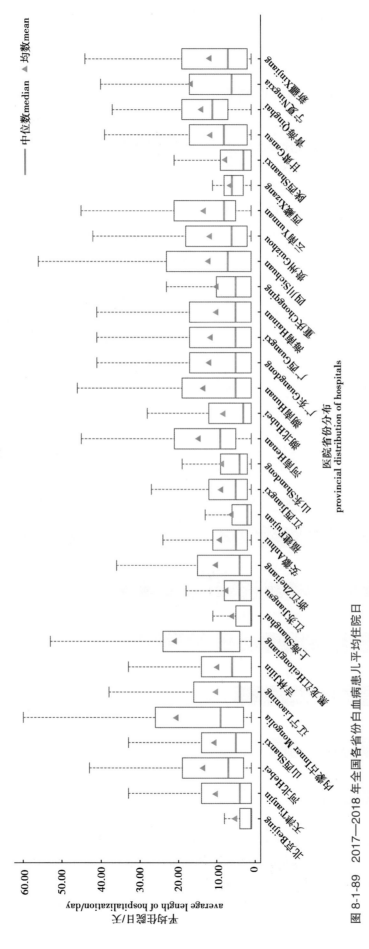

图 8-1-89　2017—2018 年全国各省份白血病患儿平均住院日

Figure 8-1-89　Average length of hospitalization of children with leukemia in each provincial-level region in 2017-2018

2 淋巴瘤

2.1 全国儿童肿瘤监测机构淋巴瘤患儿出院人次分析

2.1.1 六大区淋巴瘤患儿出院人次构成情况

在淋巴瘤患儿出院人次中,各大区出院人次占全部出院人次的比例由高到低依次为华北地区(32.97%)、华东地区(21.64%)、中南地区(20.40%)、西南地区(11.40%)、西北地区(8.44%)和东北地区(5.15%)(图 8-2-1)。

2 Lymphoma

2.1 Analysis of discharges among children with lymphoma in pediatric cancer surveillance sites in China

2.1.1 Composition of discharges among children with lymphoma in the six regions

In terms of the discharges among children with lymphoma, the regions with the highest to the lowest proportions of discharges among children with lymphoma in all discharges were North China (32.97%), East China (21.64%), Central and Southern China (20.40%), Southwest China (11.40%), Northwest China (8.44%) and Northeast China (5.15%) (Figure 8-2-1).

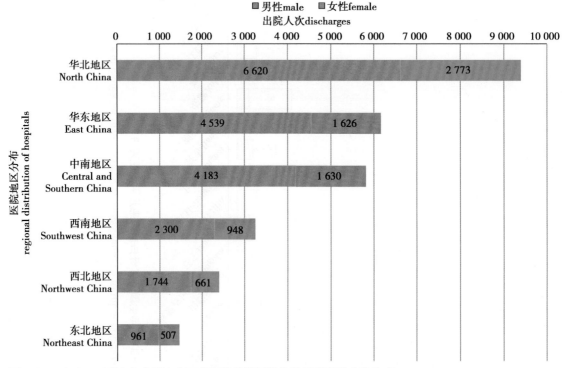

图 8-2-1 2017—2018 年全国六大区儿童肿瘤监测机构淋巴瘤出院人次构成

Figure 8-2-1 Composition of discharges among children with lymphoma in pediatric cancer surveillance sites in the six regions in 2017-2018

2.1.2 各省份淋巴瘤患儿出院人次构成情况

在所有省份中,淋巴瘤患儿出院人次占全部出院人次比例前 3 位的省份分别为北京(29.17%)、河南(9.96%)和山东(5.25%),后 3 位分别为西藏(0.00%)、青海(0.24%)和内蒙古(0.32%)(图 8-2-2,图 8-2-3)。

2.1.2 Composition of discharges among children with lymphoma in each provincial-level region

Among all provincial-level regions, Beijing (29.17%), Henan (9.96%) and Shandong (5.25%) were the three provincial-level regions with the highest proportions of discharges among children with lymphoma in all discharges, and Xizang (0.00%), Qinghai (0.24%) and Inner Mongolia (0.32%) had the lowest proportions of discharges among children with lymphoma (Figure 8-2-2~Figure 8-2-3).

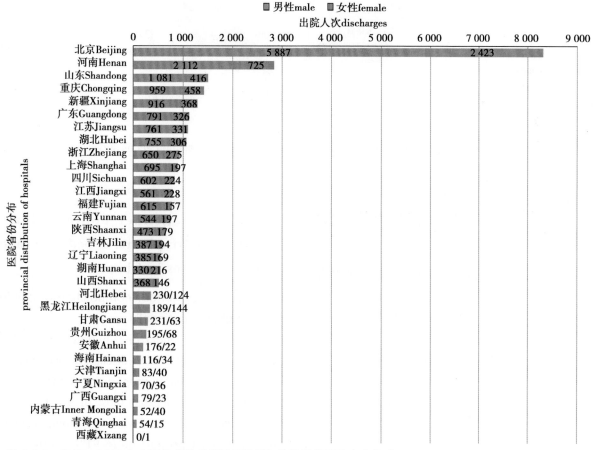

图 8-2-2   2017—2018 年全国各省份儿童肿瘤监测机构淋巴瘤出院人次构成

Figure8-2-2   Composition of discharges among children with lymphoma in pediatric cancer surveillance sites in each provincial-level region in 2017-2018

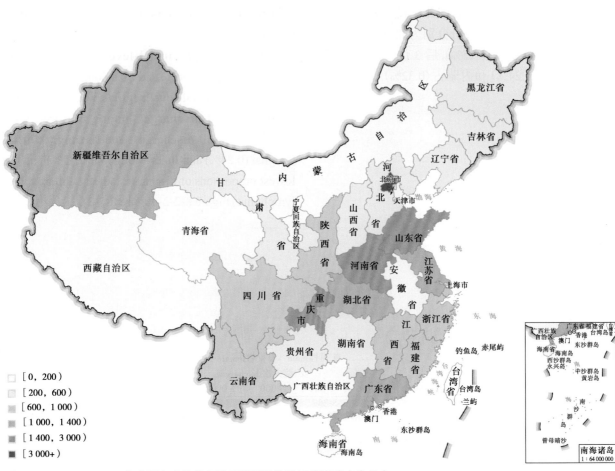

图 8-2-3　2017—2018 年全国各省份儿童肿瘤监测机构淋巴瘤出院人次分布

Figure 8-2-3　Distribution of discharges among children with lymphoma in pediatric cancer surveillance sites in each provincial-level region in 2017-2018

2.2　全国儿童肿瘤监测机构淋巴瘤患儿年龄／性别构成

2.2.1　全国淋巴瘤患儿年龄／性别构成情况

从性别分布来看,男性患儿占全部出院人次比例为 71.41%,女性患儿为 28.59%;男性患儿各年龄段的出院人次比例均高于女性患儿。从年龄分布来看,5 岁年龄组所占比例最高(6.91%),其次为 10 岁(6.86%)和 9 岁(6.83%)年龄组(图 8-2-4)。

2.2　Age/gender composition of children with lymphoma in pediatric cancer surveillance sites in China

2.2.1　Age/gender composition of children with lymphoma nationally

In terms of gender distribution, male children accounted for 71.41% of all discharges, and female for 28.59%. The discharge proportions of male children at all ages were higher than those of female. In terms of age distribution, the 5-year age group accounted for the highest proportion (6.91%), followed by the 10-year age group (6.86%) and the 9-year age group (6.83%)(Figure 8-2-4).

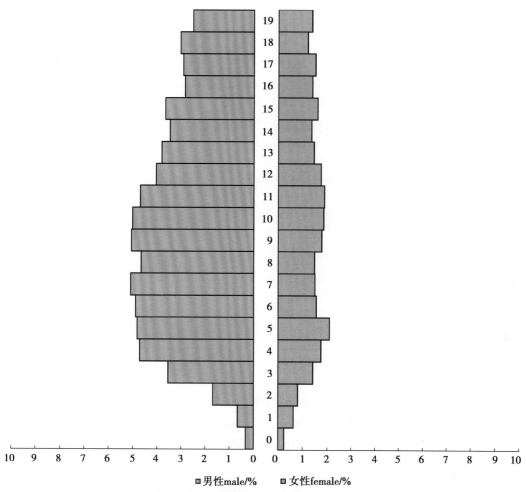

□男性male/%　　□女性female/%

图 8-2-4　2017—2018 年全国儿童肿瘤监测机构淋巴瘤患儿年龄 / 性别构成

Figure 8-2-4　Age/gender composition of children with lymphoma in pediatric cancer surveillance sites in China in 2017-2018

2.2.2　六大区淋巴瘤患儿年龄 / 性别构成情况

从性别分布来看,六大区均显示男性患儿占全部出院人次比例高于女性。从年龄分布来看,六大区的比例各有不同,其中华北地区和华东地区的 10 岁年龄组所占比例最高;东北地区的 11 岁年龄组所占比例最高;中南地区的 17 岁年龄组所占比例最高;西南地区的 7 岁年龄组所占比例最高;西北地区的 4 岁年龄组所占比例最高(图 8-2-5~图 8-2-10)。

2.2.2　Age/gender composition of children with lymphoma in the six regions

In terms of gender distribution, male children accounted for a higher proportion of all discharges than female in all the six regions. In terms of age distribution, the proportions of the six regions were different, among which the proportions of the 10-year age group in North China and East China were the highest. The proportions of the 11-year age group in Northeast China, the 17-year age group in Central and Southern China, the 7-year age group in Southwest China, and the 4-year age group in Northwest China were the highest in their respective regions (Figure 8-2-5~Figure 8-2-10).

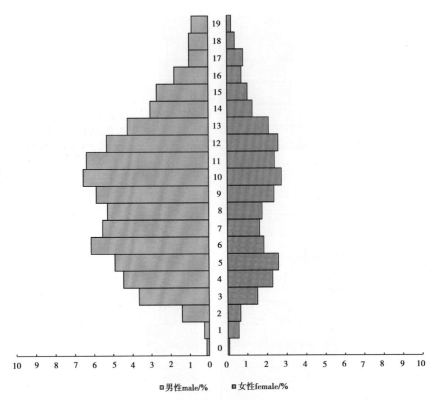

图 8-2-5 2017—2018 年华北地区儿童肿瘤监测机构淋巴瘤患儿年龄／性别构成

Figure 8-2-5 Age/gender composition of children with lymphoma in pediatric cancer surveillance sites in North China in 2017-2018

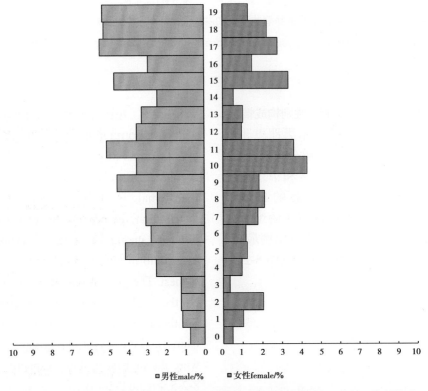

图 8-2-6 2017—2018 年东北地区儿童肿瘤监测机构淋巴瘤患儿年龄／性别构成

Figure 8-2-6 Age/gender composition of children with lymphoma in pediatric cancer surveillance sites in Northeast China in 2017-2018

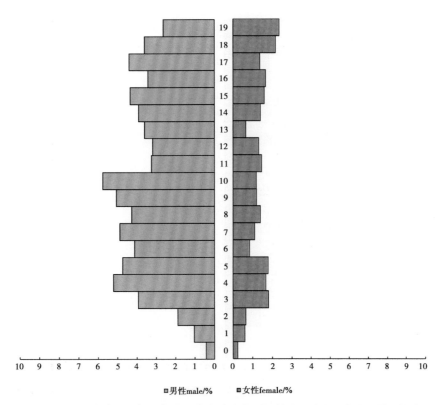

图 8-2-7　2017—2018 年华东地区儿童肿瘤监测机构淋巴瘤患儿年龄／性别构成

Figure 8-2-7　Age/gender composition of children with lymphoma in pediatric cancer surveillance sites in East China in 2017-2018

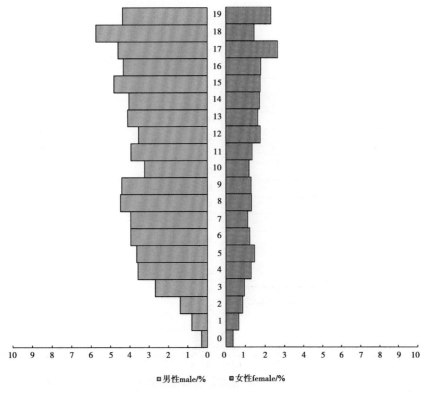

图 8-2-8　2017—2018 年中南地区儿童肿瘤监测机构淋巴瘤患儿年龄／性别构成

Figure 8-2-8　Age/gender composition of children with lymphoma in pediatric cancer surveillance sites in Central and Southern China in 2017-2018

183

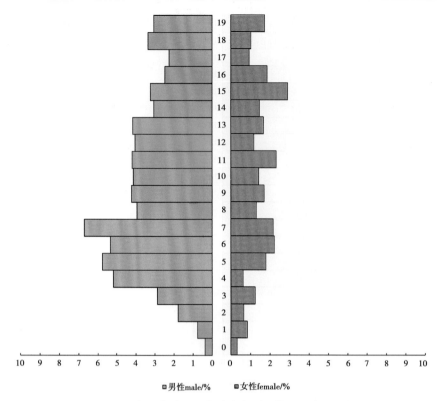

图 8-2-9　2017—2018 年西南地区儿童肿瘤监测机构淋巴瘤患儿年龄 / 性别构成

Figure 8-2-9　Age/gender composition of children with lymphoma in pediatric cancer surveillance sites in Southwest China in 2017-2018

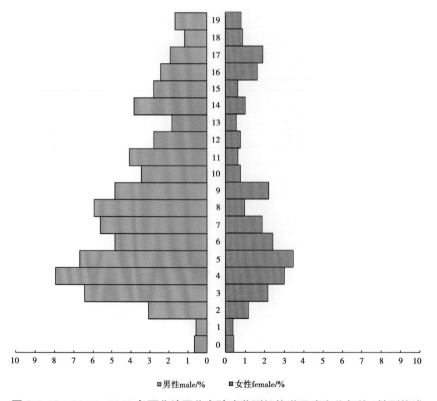

图 8-2-10　2017—2018 年西北地区儿童肿瘤监测机构淋巴瘤患儿年龄 / 性别构成

Figure 8-2-10　Age/gender composition of children with lymphoma in pediatric cancer surveillance sites in Northwest China in 2017-2018

2.2.3 各省份淋巴瘤患儿年龄/性别构成情况

从性别分布来看,除西藏外的其他30个省份出院患儿的性别分布均呈现男性比例高于女性;从年龄分布来看,各省份出院患儿的年龄分布各有不同。以北京为例,从性别分布来看,男性患儿占全部出院人次比例为70.84%,女性患儿为29.16%;从年龄分布来看,10岁年龄组所占比例最高(9.59%),其次为11岁(9.06%)和9岁(8.54%)年龄组(图8-2-11~图8-2-38)。

2.2.3 Age/gender composition of children with lymphoma in each provincial-level region

In terms of gender distribution, male children accounted for a higher proportion of all discharges than female in all 30 provincial-level regions except for Xizang. In terms of age distribution, it varies a lot among all provincial-level regions. Taking Beijing as an example, in terms of gender distribution, male children accounted for 70.84%, and female 29.16% of the total discharges. In terms of age distribution, the 10-year age group accounted for the highest proportion (9.59%), followed by the 11-year age group (9.06%) and the 9-year age group (8.54%) (Figure 8-2-11~Figure 8-2-38).

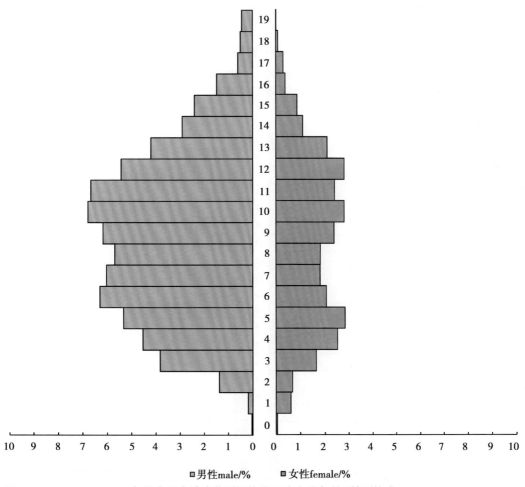

□男性male/%　　□女性female/%

图 8-2-11　2017—2018 年北京儿童肿瘤监测机构淋巴瘤患儿年龄/性别构成

Figure 8-2-11　Age/gender composition of children with lymphoma in pediatric cancer surveillance sites in Beijing in 2017-2018

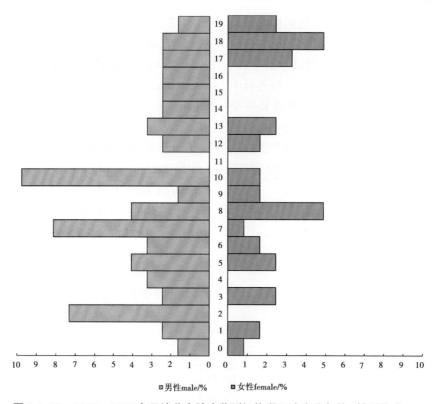

图 8-2-12　2017—2018 年天津儿童肿瘤监测机构淋巴瘤患儿年龄／性别构成

Figure 8-2-12　Age/gender composition of children with lymphoma in pediatric cancer surveillance sites in Tianjin in 2017-2018

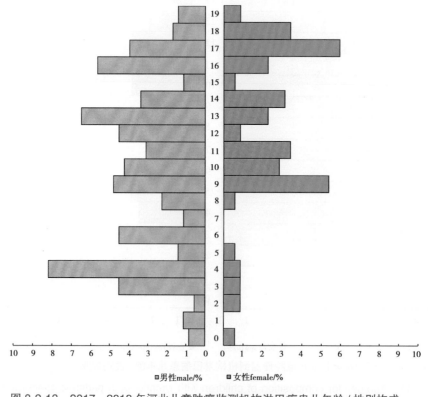

图 8-2-13　2017—2018 年河北儿童肿瘤监测机构淋巴瘤患儿年龄／性别构成

Figure 8-2-13　Age/gender composition of children with lymphoma in pediatric cancer surveillance sites in Hebei in 2017-2018

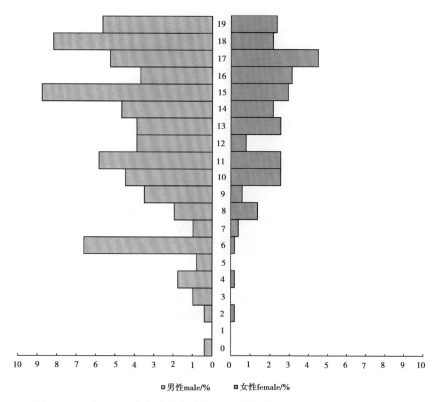

图 8-2-14　2017—2018 年山西儿童肿瘤监测机构淋巴瘤患儿年龄 / 性别构成

Figure 8-2-14　Age/gender composition of children with lymphoma in pediatric cancer surveillance sites in Shanxi in 2017-2018

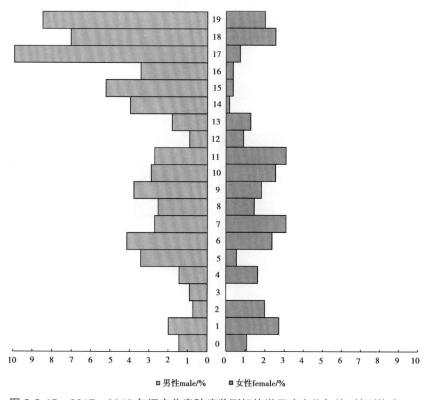

图 8-2-15　2017—2018 年辽宁儿童肿瘤监测机构淋巴瘤患儿年龄 / 性别构成

Figure 8-2-15　Age/gender composition of children with lymphoma in pediatric cancer surveillance sites in Liaoning in 2017-2018

187

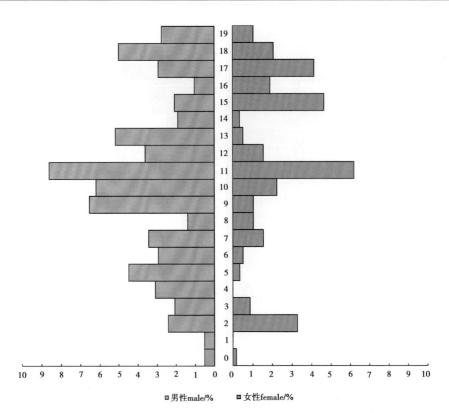

图 8-2-16　2017—2018 年吉林儿童肿瘤监测机构淋巴瘤患儿年龄／性别构成

Figure 8-2-16　Age/gender composition of children with lymphoma in pediatric cancer surveillance sites in Jilin in 2017-2018

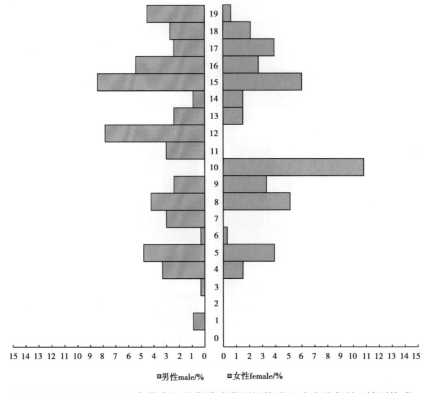

图 8-2-17　2017—2018 年黑龙江儿童肿瘤监测机构淋巴瘤患儿年龄／性别构成

Figure 8-2-17　Age/gender composition of children with lymphoma in pediatric cancer surveillance sites in Heilongjiang in 2017-2018

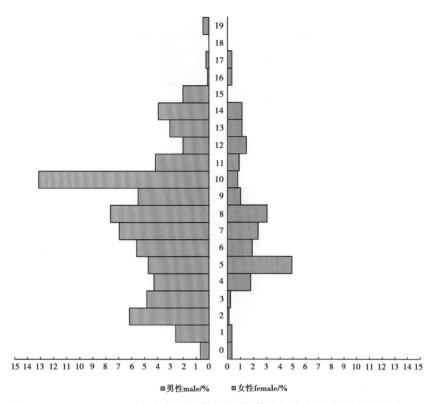

图 8-2-18　2017—2018 年上海儿童肿瘤监测机构淋巴瘤患儿年龄 / 性别构成

Figure 8-2-18　Age/gender composition of children with lymphoma in pediatric cancer surveillance sites in Shanghai in 2017-2018

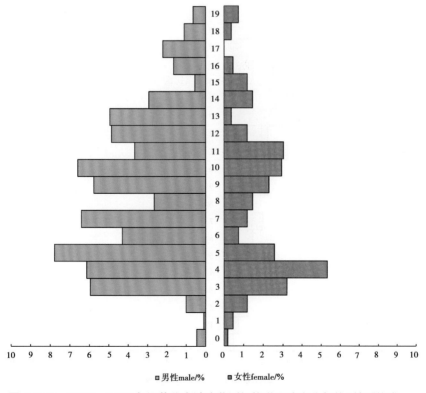

图 8-2-19　2017—2018 年江苏儿童肿瘤监测机构淋巴瘤患儿年龄 / 性别构成

Figure 8-2-19　Age/gender composition of children with lymphoma in pediatric cancer surveillance sites in Jiangsu in 2017-2018

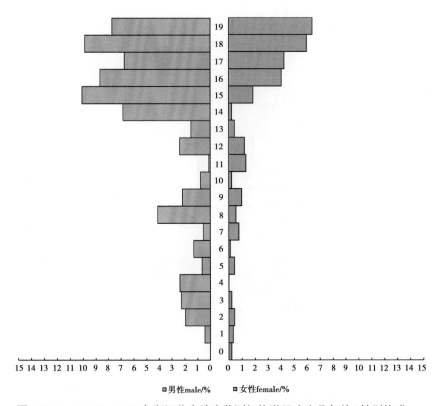

图 8-2-20　2017—2018 年浙江儿童肿瘤监测机构淋巴瘤患儿年龄／性别构成

Figure 8-2-20　Age/gender composition of children with lymphoma in pediatric cancer surveillance sites in Zhejiang in 2017-2018

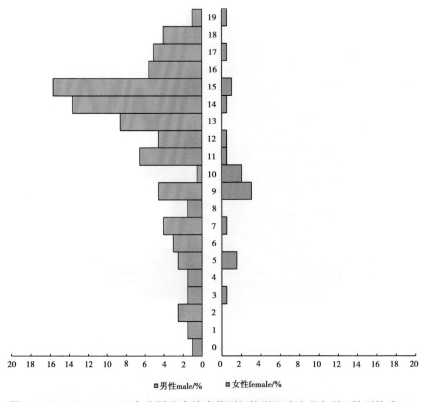

图 8-2-21　2017—2018 年安徽儿童肿瘤监测机构淋巴瘤患儿年龄／性别构成

Figure 8-2-21　Age/gender composition of children with lymphoma in pediatric cancer surveillance sites in Anhui in 2017-2018

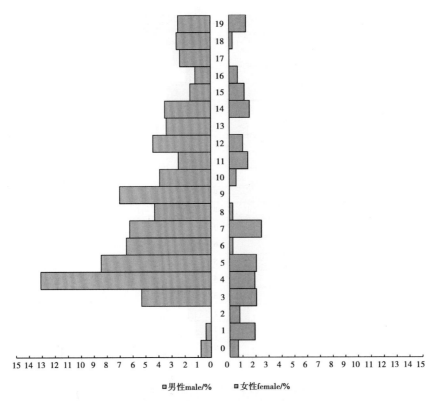

图 8-2-22　2017—2018 年福建儿童肿瘤监测机构淋巴瘤患儿年龄 / 性别构成

Figure 8-2-22　Age/gender composition of children with lymphoma in pediatric cancer surveillance sites in Fujian in 2017-2018

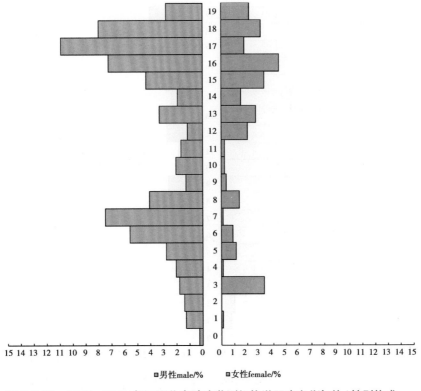

图 8-2-23　2017—2018 年江西儿童肿瘤监测机构淋巴瘤患儿年龄 / 性别构成

Figure 8-2-23　Age/gender composition of children with lymphoma in pediatric cancer surveillance sites in Jiangxi in 2017-2018

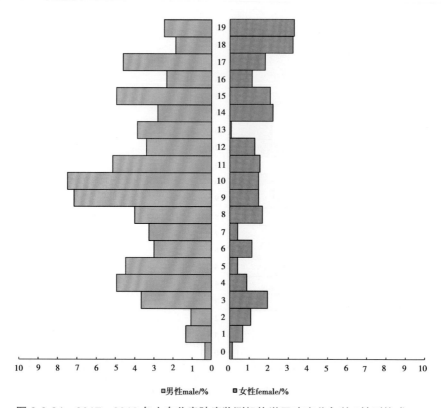

图 8-2-24　2017—2018 年山东儿童肿瘤监测机构淋巴瘤患儿年龄 / 性别构成

Figure 8-2-24　Age/gender composition of children with lymphoma in pediatric cancer surveillance sites in Shandong in 2017-2018

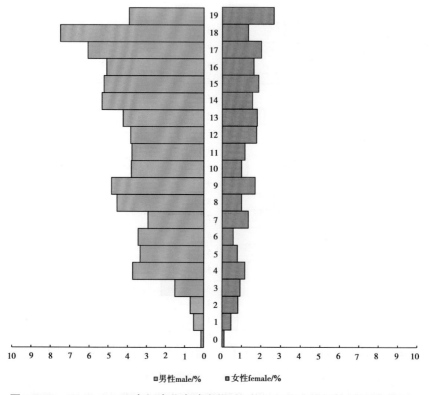

图 8-2-25　2017—2018 年河南儿童肿瘤监测机构淋巴瘤患儿年龄 / 性别构成

Figure 8-2-25　Age/gender composition of children with lymphoma in pediatric cancer surveillance sites in Henan in 2017-2018

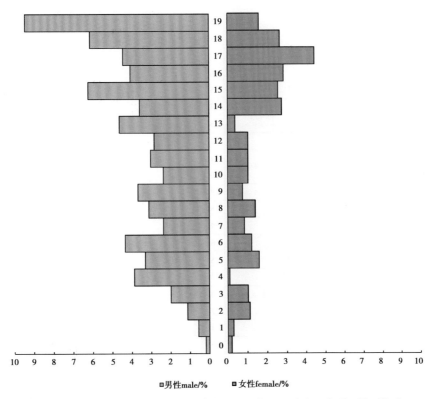

图 8-2-26　2017—2018 年湖北儿童肿瘤监测机构淋巴瘤患儿年龄／性别构成

Figure 8-2-26　Age/gender composition of children with lymphoma in pediatric cancer surveillance sites in Hubei in 2017-2018

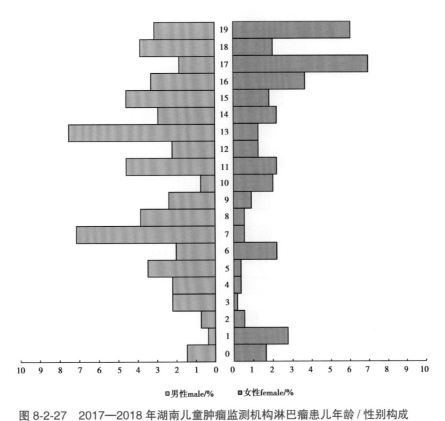

图 8-2-27　2017—2018 年湖南儿童肿瘤监测机构淋巴瘤患儿年龄／性别构成

Figure 8-2-27　Age/gender composition of children with lymphoma in pediatric cancer surveillance sites in Hunan in 2017-2018

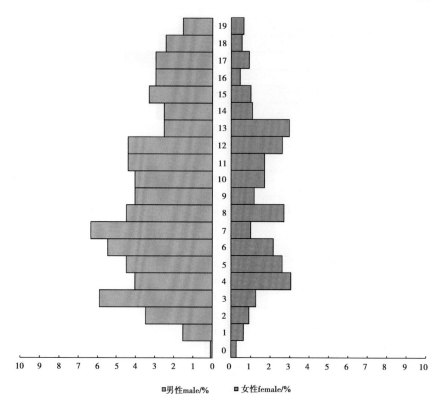

图 8-2-28　2017—2018 年广东儿童肿瘤监测机构淋巴瘤患儿年龄／性别构成

Figure 8-2-28　Age/gender composition of children with lymphoma in pediatric cancer surveillance sites in Guangdong in 2017-2018

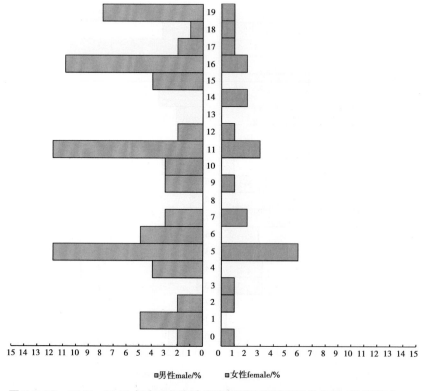

图 8-2-29　2017—2018 年广西儿童肿瘤监测机构淋巴瘤患儿年龄／性别构成

Figure 8-2-29　Age/gender composition of children with lymphoma in pediatric cancer surveillance sites in Guangxi in 2017-2018

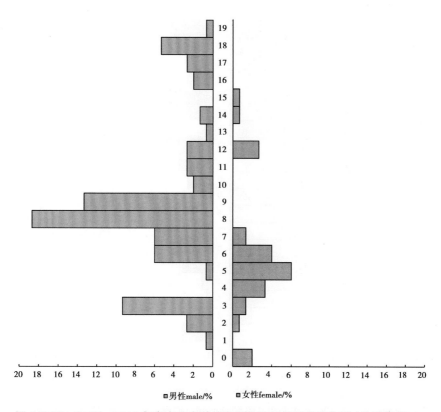

图 8-2-30　2017—2018 年海南儿童肿瘤监测机构淋巴瘤患儿年龄／性别构成

Figure 8-2-30　Age/gender composition of children with lymphoma in pediatric cancer surveillance sites in Hainan in 2017-2018

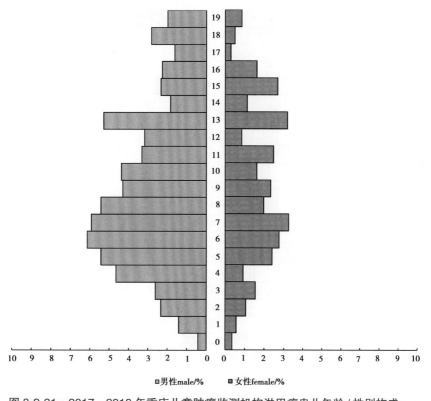

图 8-2-31　2017—2018 年重庆儿童肿瘤监测机构淋巴瘤患儿年龄／性别构成

Figure 8-2-31　Age/gender composition of children with lymphoma in pediatric cancer surveillance sites in Chongqing in 2017-2018

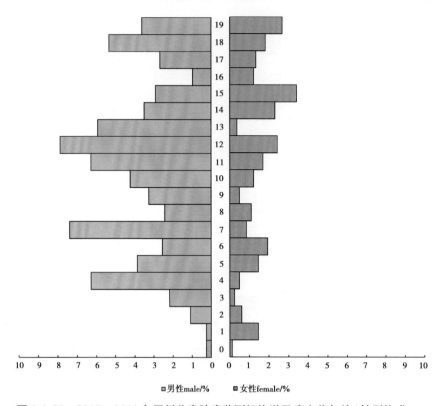

图 8-2-32　2017—2018 年四川儿童肿瘤监测机构淋巴瘤患儿年龄／性别构成

Figure 8-2-32　Age/gender composition of children with lymphoma in pediatric cancer surveillance sites in Sichuan in 2017-2018

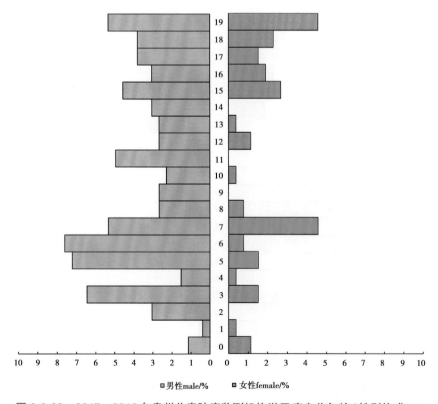

图 8-2-33　2017—2018 年贵州儿童肿瘤监测机构淋巴瘤患儿年龄／性别构成

Figure 8-2-33　Age/gender composition of children with lymphoma in pediatric cancer surveillance sites in Guizhou in 2017-2018

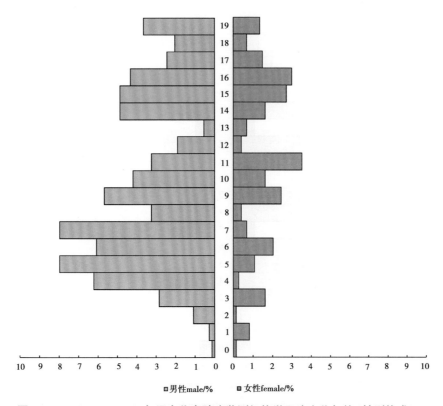

图 8-2-34   2017—2018 年云南儿童肿瘤监测机构淋巴瘤患儿年龄 / 性别构成

Figure 8-2-34   Age/gender composition of children with lymphoma in pediatric cancer surveillance sites in Yunnan in 2017-2018

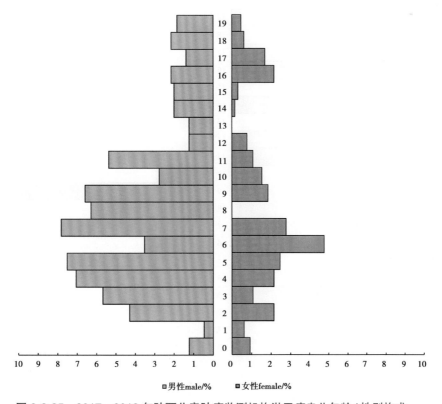

图 8-2-35   2017—2018 年陕西儿童肿瘤监测机构淋巴瘤患儿年龄 / 性别构成

Figure 8-2-35   Age/gender composition of children with lymphoma in pediatric cancer surveillance sites in Shaanxi in 2017-2018

197

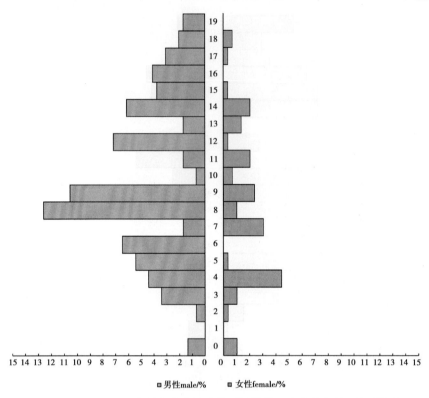

图 8-2-36　2017—2018 年甘肃儿童肿瘤监测机构淋巴瘤患儿年龄 / 性别构成

Figure 8-2-36　Age/gender composition of children with lymphoma in pediatric cancer surveillance sites in Gansu in 2017-2018

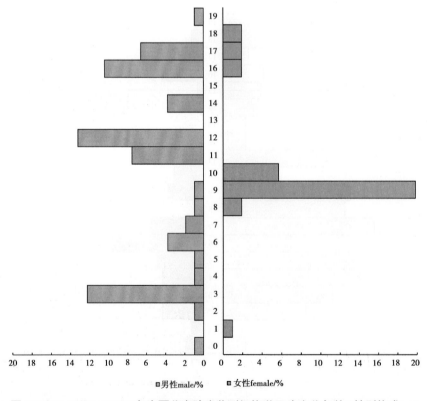

图 8-2-37　2017—2018 年宁夏儿童肿瘤监测机构淋巴瘤患儿年龄 / 性别构成

Figure 8-2-37　Age/gender composition of children with lymphoma in pediatric cancer surveillance sites in Ningxia in 2017-2018

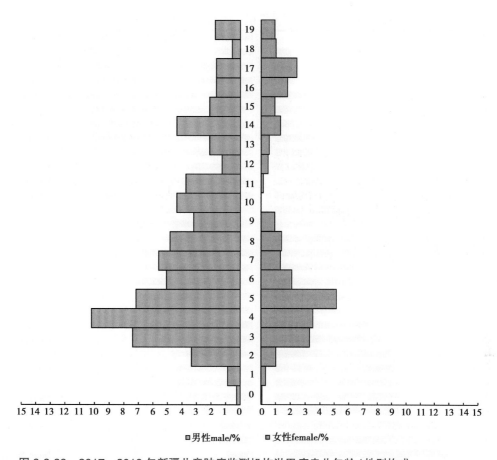

图 8-2-38　2017—2018 年新疆儿童肿瘤监测机构淋巴瘤患儿年龄 / 性别构成

Figure 8-2-38　Age/gender composition of children with lymphoma in pediatric cancer surveillance sites in Xinjiang in 2017-2018

2.3　全国儿童肿瘤监测机构淋巴瘤患儿就医省份分布

2.3.1　全国各省份淋巴瘤患儿本省就医与省外就医的分布情况

总体而言,淋巴瘤患儿本省就医的比例为61.34%。在所有省份中,本省就医比例前 3 位的省份分别为北京(99.82%)、新疆(92.07%)和上海(91.43%)。省外就医比例前 3 位分别为西藏(94.44%)、内蒙古(87.02%)和安徽(82.92%)(图8-2-39)。

2.3　Distribution of provincial-level regions visited by children with lymphoma in pediatric cancer surveillance sites in China

2.3.1　Distribution of children with lymphoma receiving medical treatment in and out of their own provincial-level regions

In general, 61.34% of all children with lymphoma sought medical treatment in their own provincial-level regions. Beijing (99.82%), Xinjiang (92.07%) and Shanghai (91.43%) were the top three recipients of patients from other provincial-level regions. Xizang (94.44%), Inner Mongolia (87.02%) and Anhui (82.92%) were the top three provincial-level regions in terms of the proportion of patients going to other provincial-level regions for medical treatment (Figure 8-2-39).

199

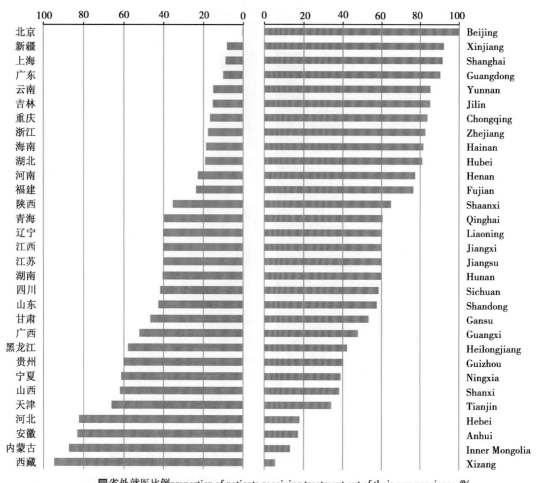

省外就医比例 proportion of patients receiving treatment out of their own provinces /%

本省就医比例 proportion of patients receiving treatment in their own provinces/%

图 8-2-39　2017—2018 年全国各省份淋巴瘤患儿本省就医与省外就医比例 /%

Figure 8-2-39　Proportion of children with lymphoma receiving medical treatment in and out of their own provincial-level regions in 2017-2018/%

2.3.2 全国各省份淋巴瘤患儿省外就医的去向省份分布情况

各省份淋巴瘤患儿选择省外就医的去向分布呈现明显的规律,主要的去向省份为北京、上海、重庆、江苏和广东。如户籍地为江西的淋巴瘤患儿,选择省外就医的主要去向为上海、北京和广东,分别占户籍地为江西的淋巴瘤患儿选择省外就医总数的 39.5%、30.3% 和 14.4%。再如户籍地为云南的肿瘤患儿,选择省外就医的主要去向为重庆、北京和上海,分别占户籍地为云南的淋巴瘤患儿选择省外就医总数的 41.7%、36.7% 和 12.5%(图 8-2-40,按行方向查看)。

2.3.2 Distribution of provincial-level regions receiving children with lymphoma from outside the provincial-level regions

The distribution of provincial-level regions receiving children with lymphoma from outside their provincial-level regions showed obvious regularity, and the main destinations were Beijing, Shanghai, Chongqing, Jiangsu and Guangdong. For Jiangxi children with lymphoma, the main destinations were Shanghai, Beijing and Guangdong, accounting for 39.5%, 30.3% and 14.4%, respectively, of the total number of Jiangxi children with lymphoma going outside Jiangxi. For Yunnan children with lymphoma, Chongqing, Beijing and Shanghai were the main destinations, accounting for 41.7%, 36.7% and 12.5%, respectively, of the total number of Yunnan children with lymphoma going outside Yunnan (Figure 8-2-40, view in linesview in rows).

收治外省肿瘤患儿的医院省份分布
provincial distribution of hospitals receiving children with cancer from outside the province

	北京 Beijing	天津 Tianjin	河北 Hebei	山西 Shanxi	内蒙古 Inner Mongolia	辽宁 Liaoning	吉林 Jilin	黑龙江 Heilongjiang	上海 Shanghai	江苏 Jiangsu	浙江 Zhejiang	安徽 Anhui	福建 Fujian	江西 Jiangxi	山东 Shandong	河南 Henan	湖北 Hubei	湖南 Hunan	广东 Guangdong	广西 Guangxi	海南 Hainan	重庆 Chongqing	四川 Sichuan	贵州 Guizhou	云南 Yunnan	西藏 Xizang	陕西 Shaanxi	甘肃 Gansu	青海 Qinghai	宁夏 Ningxia	新疆 Xinjiang	合计 total
北京 Beijing	100.00	0	0	0	0	0	0	0	0	0	0	0	0	0	0	0	0	0	100.0	0	0	0	0	0	0	0	0	0	0	0	0	100
天津 Tianjin	97.1	2.5	0	0	0	0	0	0	0	0	0	0	0	0	0	0	0	0	0	0	0	0	0	0	0	0	0	0	0	0	0	100
河北 Hebei	96.1	0		0	0	0	0	0	0	0.1	0	0	0	0	0	0.1	0.2	0	0	0	0	0	0	0	0	0	0	0	0	0	0	100
山西 Shanxi	89.2	0.8	0.1	0.2	0	1.2	0.1	0	0.6	0.4	0	0	0	0	0.5	0	0	0	0.2	0	0	0.5	0	0	0	0	1.0	0	0	0	0	100
内蒙古 Inner Mongolia	97.3	0.3	0	0		2.1	0	0	0	0	0.3	0	0	0	1.5	0.6	0	0	0.2	0	0	0	0	0	0	0	0	0	0	0.3	0	100
辽宁 Liaoning	85.8	0.3	0	0	0		6.7	0	0	0	0.3	0	0	0	2.4	0.6	0	1.2	0	0	0	0.5	0	0	0	0	0	0	0	0	0	100
吉林 Jilin	88.6	0	0	0	0	10.6		0	0	0	0	0	0	0	0	0	0	0	0	0	0	0	0	0	0	0	0	0	0	0	0	100
黑龙江 Heilongjiang	100.00	2.2	0	0	0	1.6	6.7		0	0.7	0	0.2	0	0	0	0	0	0	0	0	0	0	0	0	0	0	0	0	0	0	0.2	100
上海 Shanghai	48.3	0	0	0	0	0	0	0	44.0	0	0	0	0.5	0	0	0	7.2	0	11.5	0	0	2.4	0	0	0	0	0.5	0	0	0	0.5	100
江苏 Jiangsu	35.7	1.2	0	1.3	0.1	1.1	0.2	0.6	60.7	1.2	0.2	0	0	1.9	2.0	6.5	8.1	0	24.2	0.3	8.2	3.1	7.1	0.3	0.3	0	0.3	0	0	0	0	100
浙江 Zhejiang	47.5	0.1	0	0.3	0.1	0.5	0	0	13.2	34.6	4.2	0	0	0	0.1	0.3	1.6	0	1.2	1.2	0	1.2	1.0	0	0	0	0.1	0	0.1	0.6	0	100
安徽 Anhui	30.4	0	2.3	0	0	0	5.0	0	29.4	3.2	0.9		0.4	0	0	0.6	7.2	0.9	4.5	0	0	1.2	0	0	0	0	1.7	0.6	0	0	0	100
福建 Fujian	96.1	1.2	0.1	0	0	0	0	0	39.5	0.8	9.0	0.2	0.2	0	0	0	1.3	1.7	14.4	0	0	3.1	0	0	0	0	0	0	0	0	0	100
江西 Jiangxi	82.8	1.2	0	0.4	0	0.1	0.1	0	1.1	0.2	0.5	0.2	0	0	0	0.4	0	0	0.2	0	0	0	0	0	0	0	0	0	0	0	0	100
山东 Shandong	82.7	0.2	0	0	0	0	0	0	3.0	2.5	0.2	0	0.5	0	0	0	7.2	0	0.2	0	0.1	2.4	0	0	0	0	1.1	0	0	0	0.2	100
河南 Henan	52.4	0	0	0	0	0	0	0	0	0	2.5	0	0	0	2.0		8.1	0	0	0.3	0	3.1	0	0.3	0.3	0	0.5	0	0	0	0	100
湖北 Hubei	48.1	0	0	0	0	1.2	1.2	1.2	1.2	11.7	0	0	1.2	0	0	9.4	7.1	0	24.2	1.2	0	1.2	7.1	0	0	0	0.3	0	0	0	0	100
湖南 Hunan	41.2	0	0	0	0	0	0	0	1.2	0	0	0	0	0	0	0	3.7	0.9	54.2	1.2	0	1.2	0	1.3	0	0	0.6	0	0	0	0	100
广东 Guangdong	65.7	0	0	0	0	0	0	0	0	0	3.1	0	9.0	0	0	0	3.7	0	28.1	0	0	3.1	0	0	0	0	0	0	0	0	0	100
广西 Guangxi	47.9	0	0	0	0	0	0	0	1.4	0.7	0	0	9.0	0	8.3	0	17.4	0	11.8	0	0	0	2.1	0	0	0	0.7	0	0	0	0	100
海南 Hainan	10.6	0	0	0	0	0	0	0	1.8	1.6	1.6	0	0.2	0	2.0	0	0	0	2.7	0.3	0	73.4	0	1.3	0	0	0.5	0.4	0	0	2.2	100
重庆 Chongqing	17.6	0	0.4	0	0	0	0	0	10.0	0	0.5	0	7.9	0	0	0.3	0	0.3	0.8	0	0	48.3	3.7	0	1.1	0	0	0	0	0	0	100
四川 Sichuan	36.6	0	0	0	0	0	0	0	12.5	1.7	2.5	0	0.8	0	0	2.3	0	0	2.5	0	0	41.7	1.7	0	10.6	0	0	0	0	0	0	100
贵州 Guizhou	29.4	0	0	0	0	0	0	0	3.4	0	0	0	0	0	0	0	0.3	0	11.8	0	0	0	58.8	0	0	0	0	0	0	0	0	100
云南 Yunnan	86.6	0.4	0	0	0.3	0	4.1	0	0	0	1.6	0	0	0	0	2.4	0.4	0	1.0	0	0	0.4	3.6	0	0	0	0	0	0	0.3	0	100
西藏 Xizang	59.7	0	0.3	0	0	0	0	0	0	0	0	0	0	0	0	2.4	0	0	0	0	0	0	3.7	0	0	0	23.4	0	0.8	0.8	3.7	100
陕西 Shaanxi	93.0	0	0	0	0	0	0	0	0	0	0	0	0	0	0	2.3	0	0	0	0	0	0	1.7	0	0	0	4.7	0	0	0	6.5	100
甘肃 Gansu	84.5	0	0	0	0	0	0	0	0	0	0	0	0	0	0	5.4	0.3	0	0	0	0	0	0	0	0	0	4.7		0	0	0	100
青海 Qinghai	77.6	0	0	0	0	0	0	0	7.5	0.9	0	0	2.8	0	0	5.6	0.9	4.7	0	0	0	0.4	0	0	0	0	0	5.4	0	0	0	100

distribution of the provinces of origin of children with cancer receiving treatment out of their own provinces

图 8-2-40　2017—2018 年全国各省省份户籍地淋巴瘤患儿选择省外就医的省份分布 /%

Figure 8-2-40　Distribution of provincial-level regions receiving children with lymphoma from other provincial-level regions in 2017-2018/%

2.3.3 全国各省份收治淋巴瘤患儿来源的省份分布情况

各省份儿童肿瘤监测机构收治的省外就医淋巴瘤患儿来源分布略有差异,多数省份收治的淋巴瘤患儿来源以其相邻省份为主。如浙江,其收治的省外就医淋巴瘤患儿主要来源于江西和安徽,分别占浙江收治的省外就医淋巴瘤患儿总数的 37.3%和 31.7%。再如安徽,其收治的省外就医淋巴瘤患儿来源于河南和江西,分别占安徽收治的省外就医淋巴瘤患儿总数的 66.7% 和 33.3%(图 8-2-41,按列方向查看)。

2.4 全国儿童肿瘤监测机构淋巴瘤患儿住院费用医疗付费方式构成

2.4.1 全国淋巴瘤患儿住院费用医疗付费方式构成情况

全国淋巴瘤患儿住院费用的医疗付费方式中,占比最高的前 3 种类型分别为全自费(39.88%)、新型农村合作医疗(20.05%)和城镇居民基本医疗保险(15.53%)(图 8-2-42)。

2.3.3 Distribution of the provincial-level regions of origin of children with lymphoma receiving treatment out of their own provincial-level regions

There was a slight difference in the distribution of the provincial-level regions of origin of children with lymphoma admitted to surveillance sites in different provincial-level regions, and most of the children were mainly from their neighboring provincial-level regions. For example, in Zhejiang, the children hospitalized from other provincial-level regions were mainly from Jiangxi and Anhui, accounting for 37.3% and 31.7%, respectively, of the total number of children hospitalized from other provincial-level regions in Zhejiang. In Anhui, children hospitalized from other provincial-level regions were mainly from Henan and Jiangxi, accounting for 66.7% and 33.3% of the total number of children hospitalized from other provincial-level regions in Anhui, respectively (Figure 8-2-41, view in lines).

2.4 Composition of medical payment methods for hospitalization expenses of children with lymphoma in pediatric cancer surveillance sites in China

2.4.1 Composition of medical payment methods for hospitalization expenses of children with lymphoma nationally

Among the medical payment methods of children with lymphoma nationally, the top three methods were 100% self-pay (39.88%), new rural cooperative medical system (20.05%) and basic medical insurance for urban residents (15.53%)(Figure 8-2-42).

收治省外就医肿瘤患儿的医院省份分布 / provincial distribution of hospitals receiving children with cancer from outside the province

患儿就医省份来源分布 / distribution of the provinces of origin of children with cancer receiving treatment out of their own provinces

来源\就医 Origin\Treatment	北京Beijing	天津Tianjin	河北Hebei	山西Shanxi	内蒙古Inner Mongolia	辽宁Liaoning	吉林Jilin	黑龙江Heilongjiang	上海Shanghai	江苏Jiangsu	浙江Zhejiang	安徽Anhui	福建Fujian	江西Jiangxi	山东Shandong	河南Henan	湖北Hubei	湖南Hunan	广东Guangdong	广西Guangxi	海南Hainan	重庆Chongqing	四川Sichuan	贵州Guizhou	云南Yunnan	西藏Xizang	陕西Shaanxi	甘肃Gansu	青海Qinghai	宁夏Ningxia	新疆Xinjiang
北京Beijing	1.2	0	0	0	0	0	0	0	0	0	0	0	0	0	0	0	0	0	0.4	0	0	0.5	0	0	0	0	0	0	0	0	0
天津Tianjin	19.7	52.1	0	0	0	0	0	0	0	0	0	0	0	0	0	0	0	0	0	0	0	0	0	0	0	0	0	0	0	0	0
河北Hebei	10.0	0	0	0	0	0	0	0	0.6	0.2	0	0	0	0	0	1.6	1.9	0	0	0	0	0	0	0	0	0	0	0	0	0	0
山西Shanxi	7.0	0	10.0	0	0	19.6	1.1	0	0	0.7	0	0	0	0	9.4	0	0	0	0	0	0	0	0	0	0	0	7.5	0	0	18.2	0
内蒙古Inner Mongolia	4.2	6.7	0	7.6	0	25.5	41.9	0	0	0	0	0	0	0	0	3.1	0	0	0.3	0	0	0	0	0	0	0	0	0	0	0	0
辽宁Liaoning	0.9	1.3	0	0	0	0	0	0	0	0	0	0	0	0	11.9	0	0	0	0	0	0	0	0	0	0	0	0	0	0	0	0
吉林Jilin	5.2	0	0	0	0	17.6	0	0	0	0	0	0	0	0	0	0	0	0	0	0	0	0	0	0	0	0	0	0	0	0	0
黑龙江Heilongjiang	0.1	13.3	0	0	0	13.7	30.6	0	0.8	0.8	0	0	0	0	4.8	0	0	5.9	0	0	0	0	0	0	0	0	0	0	0	0	0
上海Shanghai	2.9	0	0	46.2	0	9.8	0	75.0	24.8	0	0.8	0	0	0	0	0	9.0	0	0	0	0	1.9	0	0	0	0	6.5	0	0	0	0
江苏Jiangsu	0.8	0	0	0	0	0	0	0	12.3	83.5	0.6	0	0	0	0	0	0	0	0	0	0	0	0	0	0	0	0.9	0	0	0	0
浙江Zhejiang	5.1	1.3	0	0	0	0	0	0	15.1	1.8	31.7	0	3.7	0	0	0	9.6	0	3.4	0	0	0	17.0	0	0	0	0.9	0	33.3	54.5	0
安徽Anhui	1.4	0	50.0	23.1	100.0	9.8	11.2	0	7.9	0	0	33.3	1.8	0	2.4	4.5	0	0	0	0	0	0	0	0	0	0	0	0	0	0	0
福建Fujian	2.0	0	0	0	0	0	0	0	24.9	0.5	37.3	0	0	0	0	4.5	4.2	0	3.0	0	0	0	0	0	0	0	0	0	0	0	0
江西Jiangxi	13.3	0	0	0	0	0	0	0	0	0	4.0	0	3.6	100.0	0	0	0	52.9	22.9	0	0	0.2	0	0	0	0	0	0	0	0	0
山东Shandong	8.6	17.3	10.0	0	0	0	1.0	0	1.4	5.1	1.6	0	0	0	0	6.1	0	0	0.6	0	0	0	0	0	0	0	0	0	0	0	0
河南Henan	2.2	2.7	0	23.1	0	2.0	0	0	2.9	0	0	66.7	0	0	0	0	34.9	0	2.4	0	12.5	1.0	0	0	0	0	8.3	9.1	0	0	4.7
湖北Hubei	2.4	0	0	0	0	0	1.0	0	0	2.5	7.1	0	0	0	16.7	34.8	0	5.9	7.3	25.0	0	0.7	11.2	0	2.1	0	8.3	0	0	0	2.4
湖南Hunan	0.5	0	0	0	0	0	0	0	0.1	0	0	0	0	0	0	12.1	17.5	0	26.2	0	0	1.6	0	0	2.1	0	0	0	0	0	0
广东Guangdong	0.6	0	0	0	0	0	1.0	0	0.2	0.3	0	0	23.6	0	28.6	0	3.6	5.9	0	25.0	0	0.1	0	0	0	0	0.9	0	0	0	0
广西Guangxi	0.3	0	0	0	0	2.0	0	25.0	0	0	0.8	0	1.8	0	26.2	0	2.4	0	17.7	0	87.5	0.1	0	0	0	0	0.9	0	0	0	0
海南Hainan	0.9	0	0	0	0	0	0	0	0	0	0	0	0	0	0	0	0	0	2.7	0	0	0	0	0	0	0	0	0	0	0	0
重庆Chongqing	0.7	0	20.0	0	0	0	0	0	1.2	2.3	0	0	0	0	0	0	15.1	0	5.2	25.0	0	59.4	5.7	87.5	0	0	2.8	0	0	0	28.6
四川Sichuan	0.9	1.3	0	0	0	0	0	0	0	0	7.1	0	0	0	0	0	0	0	4.6	25.0	0	27.0	26.4	0	0	0	0.9	18.2	0	0	0
贵州Guizhou	0.6	0	0	0	0	0	0	0	4.6	1.6	1.6	0	54.5	0	0	0	0	0	0.9	0	0	7.4	3.8	0	12.5	0	0	0	0	0	0
云南Yunnan	0.1	0	0	0	0	0	0	0	1.8	0.5	2.4	0	1.8	0	0	0	0	0	0.9	0	0	0.1	18.9	12.5	83.3	0	0	0	0	0	0
西藏Xizang	3.3	0	0	0	0	0	12.2	0	0	0	0	0	0	0	0	0	0	0	0	0	0	0	0	0	0	0	0	0	0	0	0
陕西Shaanxi	1.9	0	10.0	0	0	0	0	0	1.2	0	0	0	0	0	0	1.5	0.6	0	0.9	0	0	0	17.0	0	0	0	53.7	0	0	9.1	26.2
甘肃Gansu	0.5	1.3	0	0	0	0	0	0	0	0	0	0	0	0	0	9.1	0.6	0	0.9	0	0	0	0	0	0	0	1.9	72.7	0	18.2	0
青海Qinghai	1.6	0	0	0	0	0	0	0	0	0	0	0	0	0	0	1.5	0	0	0	0	0	0	0	0	0	0	0	0	66.7	0	0
宁夏Ningxia	0	0	0	0	0	0	0	0	0	0	3.2	0	0	0	0	12.1	0	0	0	0	0	0	0	0	0	0	0	0	0	0	0
新疆Xinjiang	1.1	0	0	0	0	0	0	0	1.0	0.3	0	0	0	0	0	9.1	0.6	29.4	0	0	0	0.1	0	0	0	0	6.5	0	0	0	38.1
合计Total	100	100	100	100	100	100	100	100	100	100	100	100	100	100	100	100	100	100	100	100	100	100	100	100	100	0	100	100	100	100	100

图 8-2-41　2017—2018 年全国各省省份儿童肿瘤监测机构省外就医淋巴瘤患儿来源分布 /%

Figure 8-2-41　Distribution of provincial-level regions of origin of children with lymphoma going outside their provincial-level regions for medical treatment in 2017-2018/%

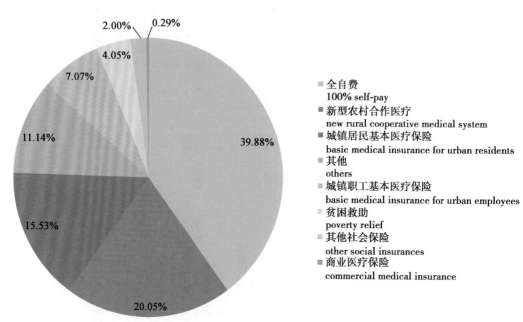

图 8-2-42　2017—2018 年全国淋巴瘤患儿住院费用医疗付费方式构成

Figure 8-2-42　Composition of medical payment methods for hospitalization expenses of children with lymphoma in China in 2017-2018

2.4.2　六大区淋巴瘤患儿住院费用医疗付费方式构成情况

六大区的医疗付费方式所占比例各不相同，华北地区、东北地区、华东地区和西南地区均以全自费占比最高，分别为 59.11%、42.83%、42.04% 和 40.01%。中南地区则以新型农村合作医疗占比最高，为 35.67%，西北地区以其他占比最高，为 25.50%（图 8-2-43~ 图 8-2-48）。

2.4.2　Composition of medical payment methods for hospitalization expenses of children with lymphoma in the six regions

The proportions of medical payment methods in the six regions were different, and the proportion of 100% self-pay was the highest in North China, Northeast China, East China and Southwest China, which were 59.11%, 42.83%, 42.04% and 40.01%, respectively. In Central and Southern China, the proportion of new rural cooperative medical system was the highest, accounting for 35.67%, while in Northwest China, that of other payment methods was the highest, which was 25.50% (Figure 8-2-43~Figure 8-2-48).

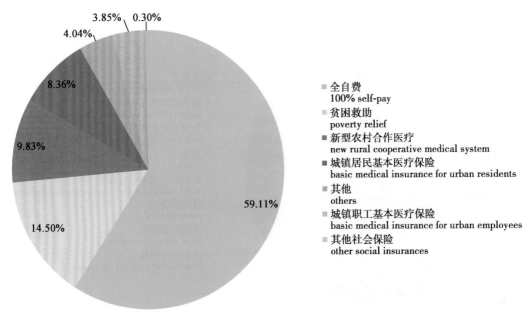

图 8-2-43　2017—2018 年华北地区淋巴瘤患儿住院费用医疗付费方式构成

Figure 8-2-43　Composition of medical payment methods for hospitalization expenses of children with lymphoma in North China in 2017-2018

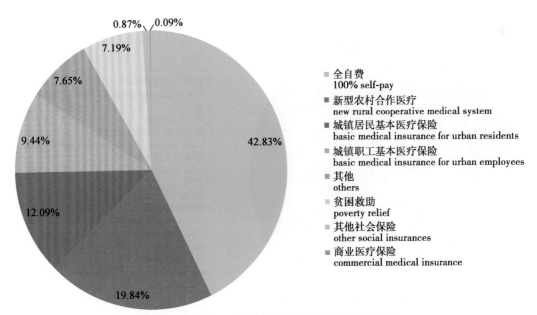

图 8-2-44　2017—2018 年东北地区淋巴瘤患儿住院费用医疗付费方式构成

Figure 8-2-44　Composition of medical payment methods for hospitalization expenses of children with lymphoma in Northeast China in 2017-2018

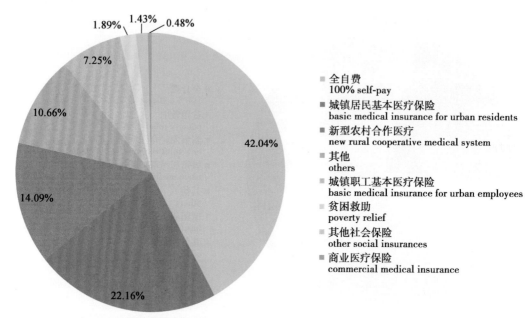

图 8-2-45　2017—2018 年华东地区淋巴瘤患儿住院费用医疗付费方式构成

Figure 8-2-45　Composition of medical payment methods for hospitalization expenses of children with lymphoma in East China in 2017-2018

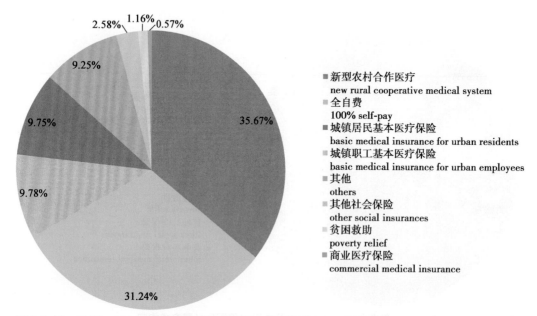

图 8-2-46　2017—2018 年中南地区淋巴瘤患儿住院费用医疗付费方式构成

Figure 8-2-46　Composition of medical payment methods for hospitalization expenses of children with lymphoma in Central and Southern China in 2017-2018

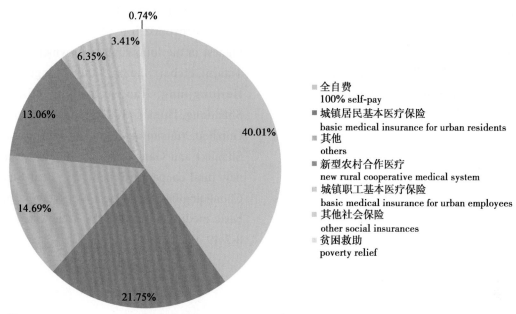

图 8-2-47　2017—2018 年西南地区淋巴瘤患儿住院费用医疗付费方式构成

Figure 8-2-47　Composition of medical payment methods for hospitalization expenses of children with lymphoma in Southwest China in 2017-2018

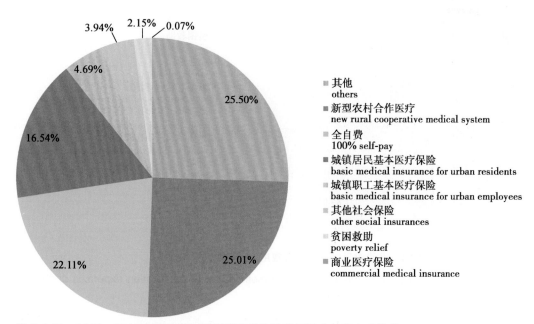

图 8-2-48　2017—2018 年西北地区淋巴瘤患儿住院费用医疗付费方式构成

Figure 8-2-48　Composition of medical payment methods for hospitalization expenses of children with lymphoma in Northwest China in 2017-2018

2.4.3 各省份淋巴瘤患儿住院费用医疗付费方式构成情况

天津、河北、山西、内蒙古、辽宁、黑龙江、江苏、安徽、福建、江西、山东、湖南、广东、广西、四川、贵州、云南和宁夏18个省份均以全自费所占比例最高。吉林、河南、海南、陕西和甘肃5个省份的新型农村合作医疗占比最高。上海和重庆2个省份的城镇居民基本医疗保险占比最高（图8-2-49~图8-2-79）。

2.4.3 Composition of medical payment methods for hospitalization expenses of children with lymphoma in each provincial-level region

The proportion of 100% self-pay was the highest in the following 18 provincial-level regions: Tianjin, Hebei, Shanxi, Inner Mongolia, Liaoning, Heilongjiang, Jiangsu, Anhui, Fujian, Jiangxi, Shandong, Hunan, Guangdong, Guangxi, Sichuan, Guizhou, Yunnan and Ningxia. Jilin, Henan, Hainan, Shaanxi and Gansu had the highest proportion of new rural cooperative medical system. Shanghai and Chongqing had the highest proportion of payment by basic medical insurance for urban residents.(Figure 8-2-49~Figure 8-2-79).

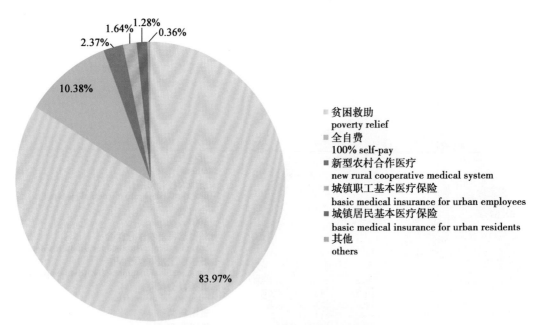

图 8-2-49　2017—2018 年北京淋巴瘤患儿住院费用医疗付费方式构成

Figure 8-2-49　Composition of medical payment methods for hospitalization expenses of children with lymphoma in Beijing in 2017-2018

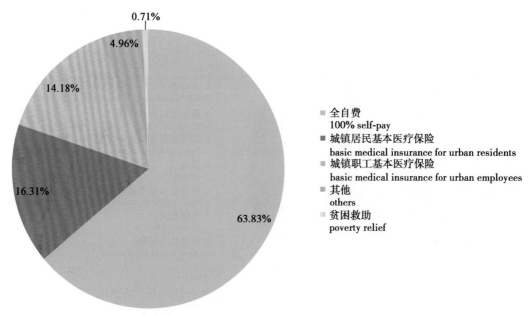

图 8-2-50　2017—2018 年天津淋巴瘤患儿住院费用医疗付费方式构成

Figure 8-2-50　Composition of medical payment methods for hospitalization expenses of children with lymphoma in Tianjin in 2017-2018

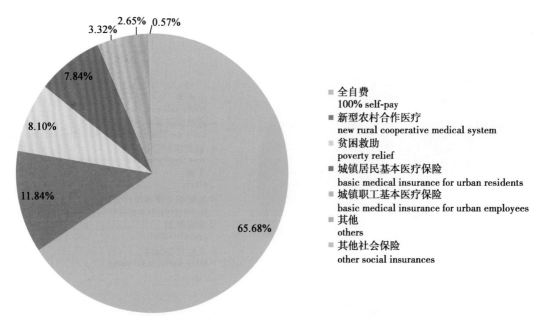

图 8-2-51　2017—2018 年河北淋巴瘤患儿住院费用医疗付费方式构成

Figure 8-2-51　Composition of medical payment methods for hospitalization expenses of children with lymphoma in Hebei in 2017-2018

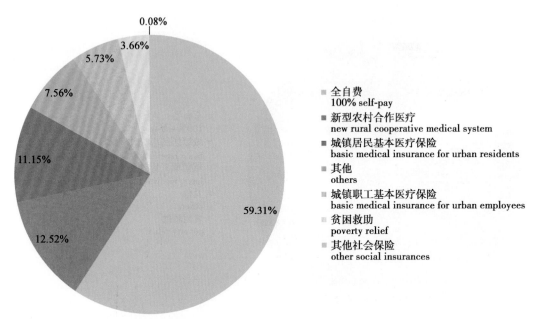

图 8-2-52　2017—2018 年山西淋巴瘤患儿住院费用医疗付费方式构成

Figure 8-2-52　Composition of medical payment methods for hospitalization expenses of children with lymphoma in Shanxi in 2017-2018

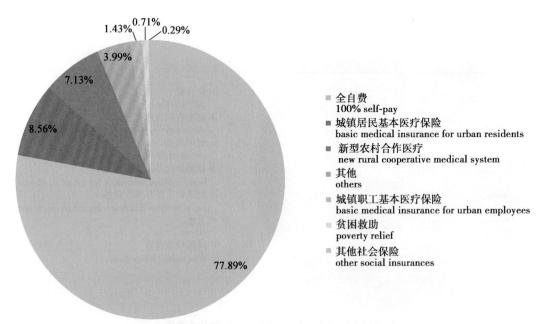

图 8-2-53　2017—2018 年内蒙古淋巴瘤患儿住院费用医疗付费方式构成

Figure 8-2-53　Composition of medical payment methods for hospitalization expenses of children with lymphoma in Inner Mongolia in 2017-2018

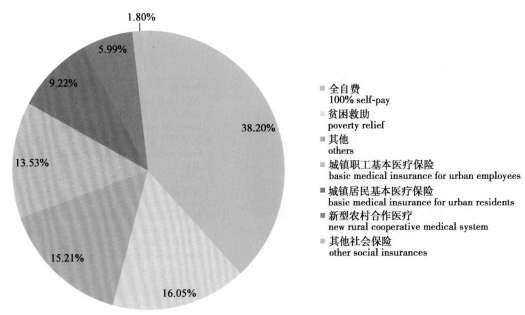

全自费
100% self-pay

贫困救助
poverty relief

其他
others

城镇职工基本医疗保险
basic medical insurance for urban employees

城镇居民基本医疗保险
basic medical insurance for urban residents

新型农村合作医疗
new rural cooperative medical system

其他社会保险
other social insurances

图 8-2-54　2017—2018 年辽宁淋巴瘤患儿住院费用医疗付费方式构成

Figure 8-2-54　Composition of medical payment methods for hospitalization expenses of children with lymphoma in Liaoning in 2017-2018

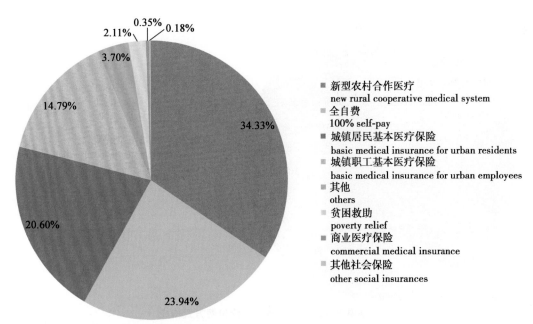

新型农村合作医疗
new rural cooperative medical system

全自费
100% self-pay

城镇居民基本医疗保险
basic medical insurance for urban residents

城镇职工基本医疗保险
basic medical insurance for urban employees

其他
others

贫困救助
poverty relief

商业医疗保险
commercial medical insurance

其他社会保险
other social insurances

图 8-2-55　2017—2018 年吉林淋巴瘤患儿住院费用医疗付费方式构成

Figure 8-2-55　Composition of medical payment methods for hospitalization expenses of children with lymphoma in Jilin in 2017-2018

211

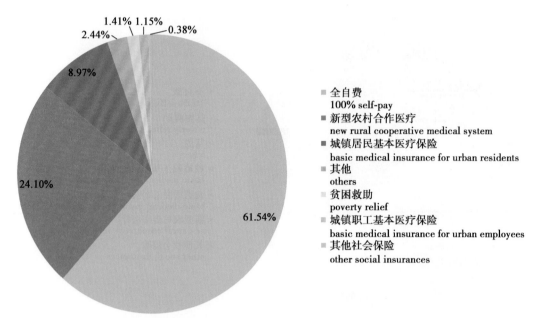

图 8-2-56 2017—2018 年黑龙江淋巴瘤患儿住院费用医疗付费方式构成

Figure 8-2-56 Composition of medical payment methods for hospitalization expenses of children with lymphoma in Heilongjiang in 2017-2018

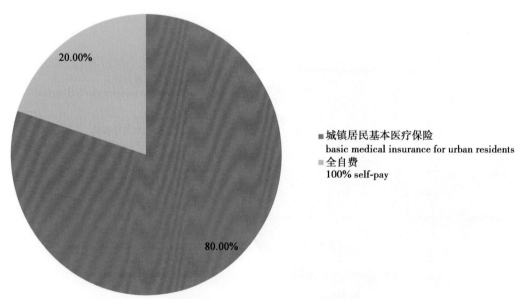

图 8-2-57 2017—2018 年上海淋巴瘤患儿住院费用医疗付费方式构成

Figure 8-2-57 Composition of medical payment methods for hospitalization expenses of children with lymphoma in Shanghai in 2017-2018

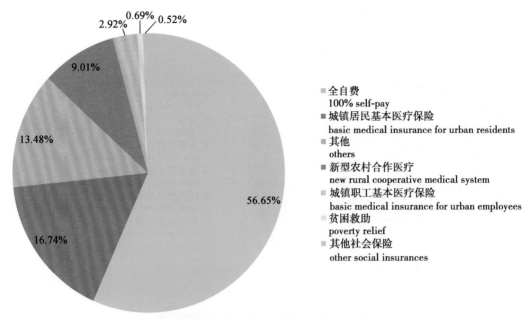

图 8-2-58　2017—2018 年江苏淋巴瘤患儿住院费用医疗付费方式构成

Figure 8-2-58　Composition of medical payment methods for hospitalization expenses of children with lymphoma in Jiangsu in 2017-2018

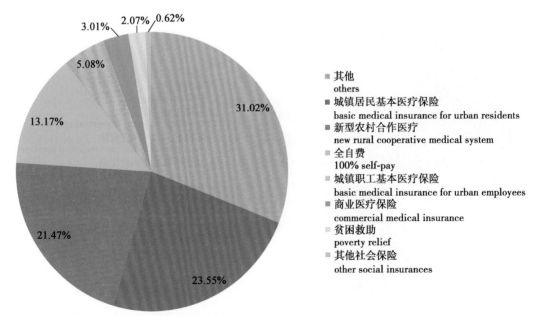

图 8-2-59　2017—2018 年浙江淋巴瘤患儿住院费用医疗付费方式构成

Figure 8-2-59　Composition of medical payment methods for hospitalization expenses of children with lymphoma in Zhejiang in 2017-2018

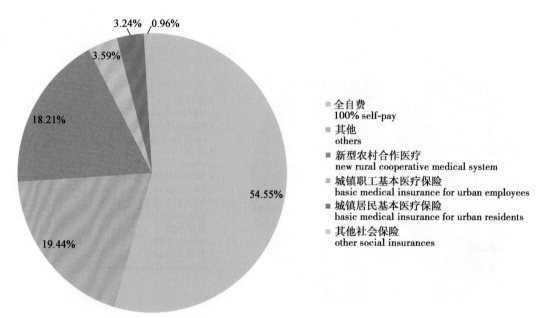

图 8-2-60 2017—2018 年安徽淋巴瘤患儿住院费用医疗付费方式构成

Figure 8-2-60 Composition of medical payment methods for hospitalization expenses of children with lymphoma in Anhui in 2017-2018

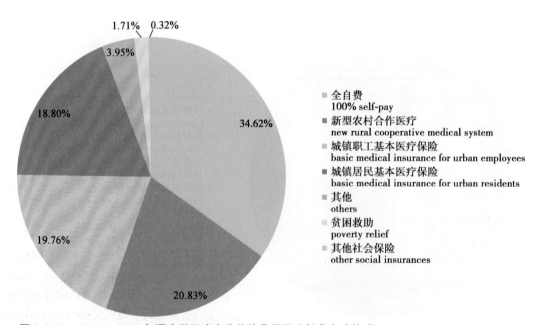

图 8-2-61 2017—2018 年福建淋巴瘤患儿住院费用医疗付费方式构成

Figure 8-2-61 Composition of medical payment methods for hospitalization expenses of children with lymphoma in Fujian in 2017-2018

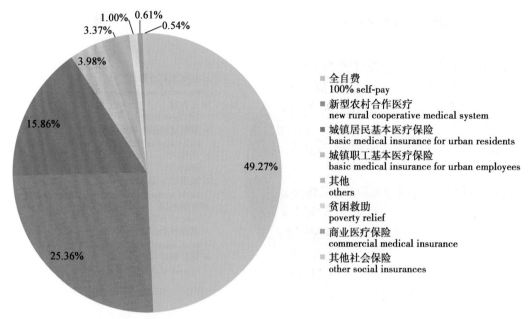

图 8-2-62　2017—2018 年江西淋巴瘤患儿住院费用医疗付费方式构成

Figure 8-2-62　Composition of medical payment methods for hospitalization expenses of children with lymphoma in Jiangxi in 2017-2018

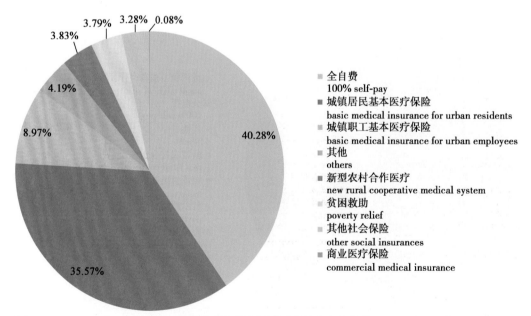

图 8-2-63　2017—2018 年山东淋巴瘤患儿住院费用医疗付费方式构成

Figure 8-2-63　Composition of medical payment methods for hospitalization expenses of children with lymphoma in Shandong in 2017-2018

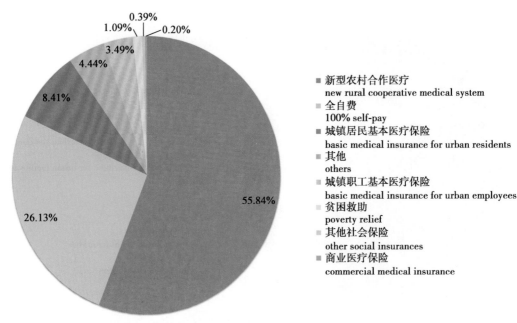

图 8-2-64　2017—2018 年河南淋巴瘤患儿住院费用医疗付费方式构成

Figure 8-2-64　Composition of medical payment methods for hospitalization expenses of children with lymphoma in Henan in 2017-2018

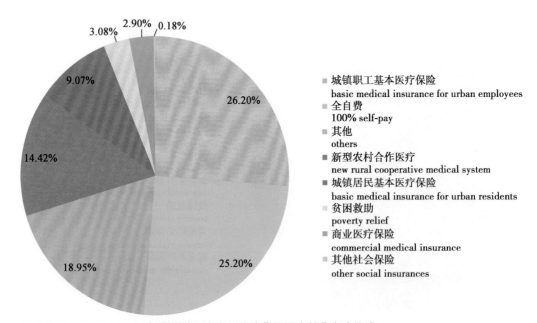

图 8-2-65　2017—2018 年湖北淋巴瘤患儿住院费用医疗付费方式构成

Figure 8-2-65　Composition of medical payment methods for hospitalization expenses of children with lymphoma in Hubei in 2017-2018

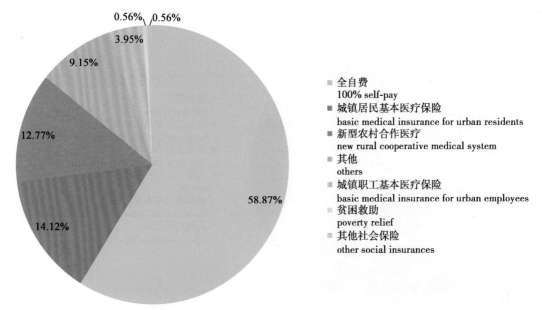

图 8-2-66　2017—2018 年湖南淋巴瘤患儿住院费用医疗付费方式构成

Figure 8-2-66　Composition of medical payment methods for hospitalization expenses of children with lymphoma in Hunan in 2017-2018

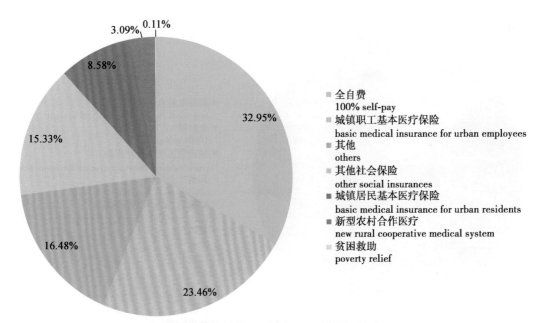

图 8-2-67　2017—2018 年广东淋巴瘤患儿住院费用医疗付费方式构成

Figure 8-2-67　Composition of medical payment methods for hospitalization expenses of children with lymphoma in Guangdong in 2017-2018

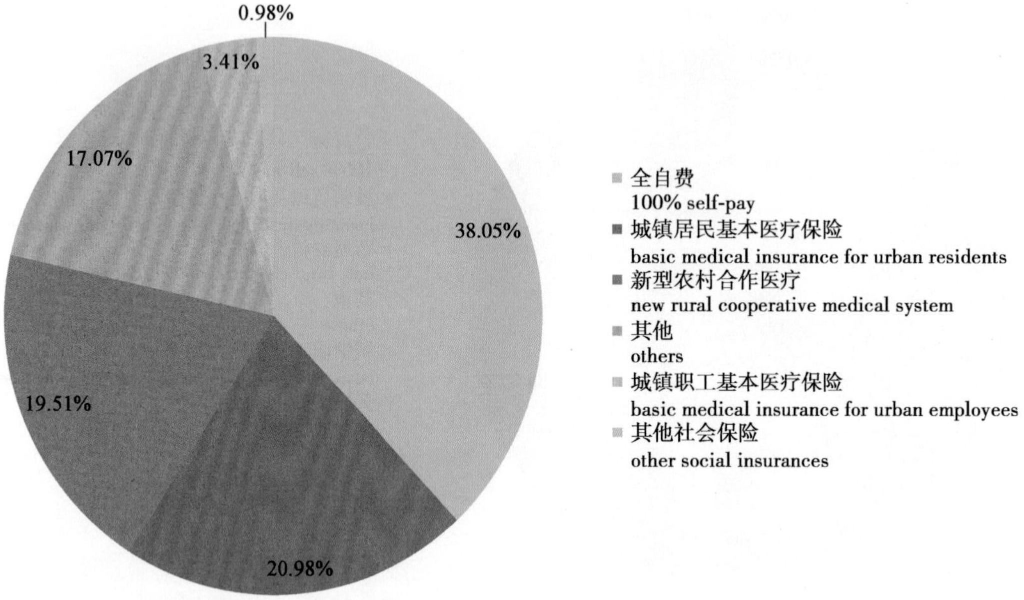

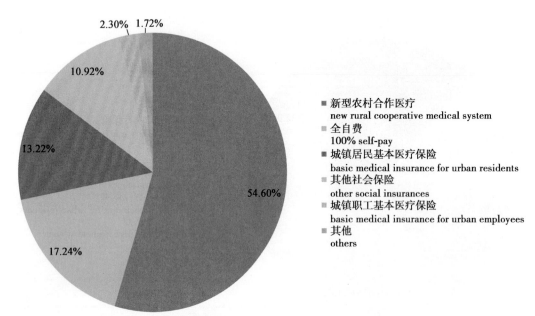

图 8-2-68　2017—2018 年广西淋巴瘤患儿住院费用医疗付费方式构成

Figure 8-2-68　Composition of medical payment methods for hospitalization expenses of children with lymphoma in Guangxi in 2017-2018

图 8-2-69　2017—2018 年海南淋巴瘤患儿住院费用医疗付费方式构成

Figure 8-2-69　Composition of medical payment methods for hospitalization expenses of children with lymphoma in Hainan in 2017-2018

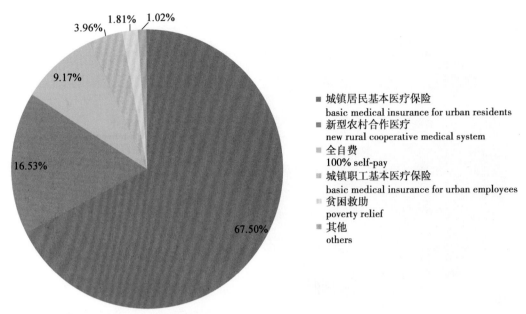

图 8-2-70　2017—2018 年重庆淋巴瘤患儿住院费用医疗付费方式构成

Figure 8-2-70　Composition of medical payment methods for hospitalization expenses of children with lymphoma in Chongqing in 2017-2018

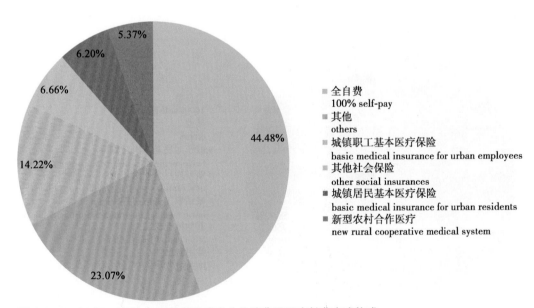

图 8-2-71　2017—2018 年四川淋巴瘤患儿住院费用医疗付费方式构成

Figure 8-2-71　Composition of medical payment methods for hospitalization expenses of children with lymphoma in Sichuan in 2017-2018

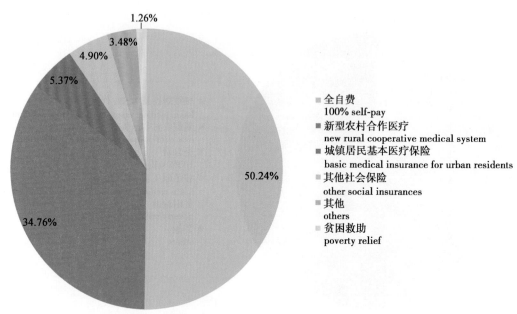

图 8-2-72　2017—2018 年贵州淋巴瘤患儿住院费用医疗付费方式构成

Figure 8-2-72　Composition of medical payment methods for hospitalization expenses of children with lymphoma in Guizhou in 2017-2018

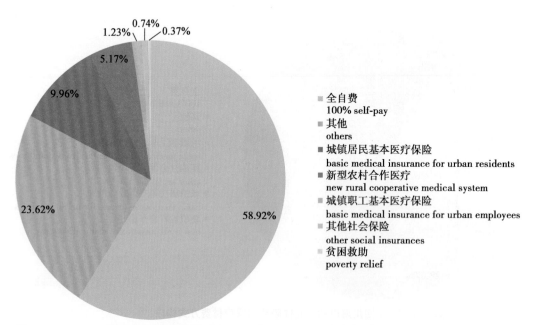

图 8-2-73　2017—2018 年云南淋巴瘤患儿住院费用医疗付费方式构成

Figure 8-2-73　Composition of medical payment methods for hospitalization expenses of children with lymphoma in Yunnan in 2017-2018

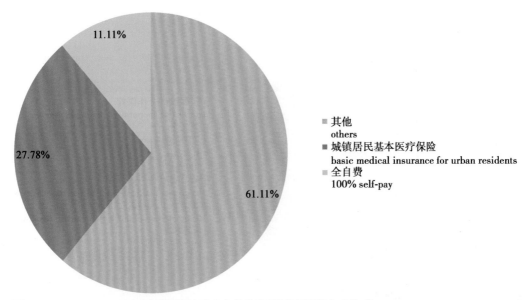

图 8-2-74　2017—2018 年西藏淋巴瘤患儿住院费用医疗付费方式构成

Figure 8-2-74　Composition of medical payment methods for hospitalization expenses of children with lymphoma in Xizang in 2017-2018

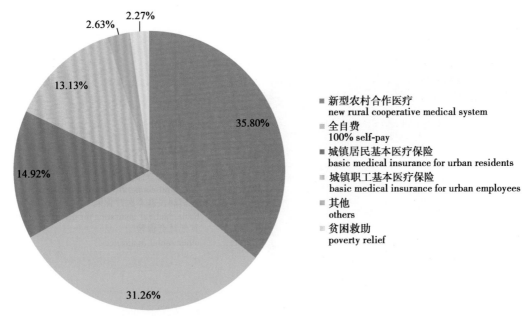

图 8-2-75　2017—2018 年陕西淋巴瘤患儿住院费用医疗付费方式构成

Figure 8-2-75　Composition of medical payment methods for hospitalization expenses of children with lymphoma in Shaanxi in 2017-2018

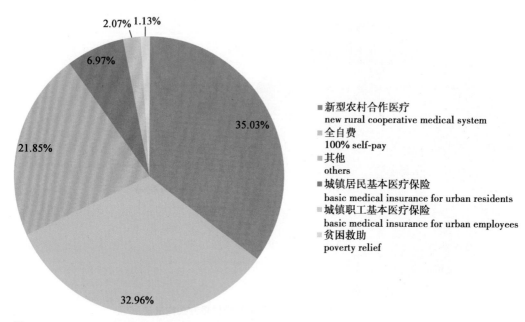

图 8-2-76　2017—2018 年甘肃淋巴瘤患儿住院费用医疗付费方式构成

Figure 8-2-76　Composition of medical payment methods for hospitalization expenses of children with lymphoma in Gansu in 2017-2018

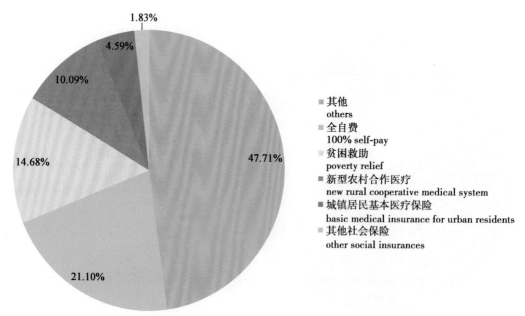

图 8-2-77　2017—2018 年青海淋巴瘤患儿住院费用医疗付费方式构成

Figure 8-2-77　Composition of medical payment methods for hospitalization expenses of children with lymphoma in Qinghai in 2017-2018

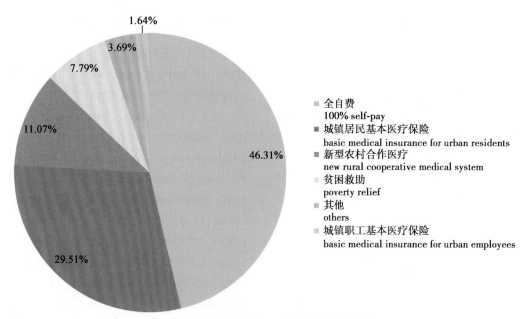

图 8-2-78　2017—2018 年宁夏淋巴瘤患儿住院费用医疗付费方式构成

Figure 8-2-78　Composition of medical payment methods for hospitalization expenses of children with lymphoma in Ningxia in 2017-2018

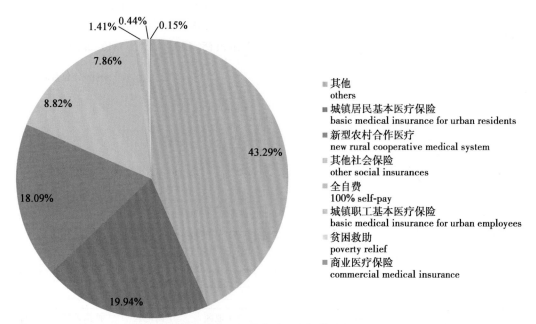

图 8-2-79　2017—2018 年新疆淋巴瘤患儿住院费用医疗付费方式构成

Figure 8-2-79　Composition of medical payment methods for hospitalization expenses of children with lymphoma in Xinjiang in 2017-2018

2.5 全国儿童肿瘤监测机构淋巴瘤患儿住院费用分析

2.5.1 全国儿童肿瘤监测机构淋巴瘤患儿次均住院费用情况

2.5.1.1 全国及六大区淋巴瘤患儿次均住院费用情况 全国淋巴瘤患儿次均住院费用(中位数)为 7 354.26 元。高于全国中位数水平的地区分别为中南地区(12 132.02 元)、西南地区(9 296.85元)、东北地区(8 206.09 元)和华东地区(7 858.60元),低于全国中位数水平的地区分别为华北地区(3 727.02 元)和西北地区(5 735.08 元)(图 8-2-80)。

2.5.1.2 各省份淋巴瘤患儿次均住院费用情况 根据淋巴瘤患儿次均住院费用(中位数),前 3 位的省份分别为天津(25 581.86 元)、广东(17 815.92 元)和河北(17 560.44 元),后 3 位分别为北京(3 158.88 元)、宁夏(3 243.49 元)和福建(5 429.24 元)(图 8-2-81)。

2.5 Analysis of hospitalization expenses of children with lymphoma in pediatric cancer surveillance sites in China

2.5.1 Expenses per hospitalization of children with lymphoma in pediatric cancer surveillance sites in China

2.5.1.1 Expenses per hospitalization of children with lymphoma in the six regions and the whole country Nationally, the median expenses per hospitalization was 7, 354.26 CNY. The regions above the national median were Central and Southern China (12, 132.02 CNY), Southwest China (9, 296.85 CNY), Northeast China (8, 260.09 CNY) and East China (7, 858.60 CNY), while those below the national median were North China (3, 727.02 CNY), and Northwest China (5, 735.08 CNY) (Figure 8-2-80).

2.5.1.2 Expenses per hospitalization of children with lymphoma in each provincial-level region In terms of the median expenses of each child with lymphoma per hospitalization, the top three provincial-level regions were Tianjin (25, 581.86 CNY), Guangdong (17, 815.92 CNY) and Hebei (17, 560.44 CNY), while the last three were Beijing (3, 158.88 CNY), Ningxia (3, 243.49 CNY) and Fujian (5, 429.24 CNY) (Figure 8-2-81).

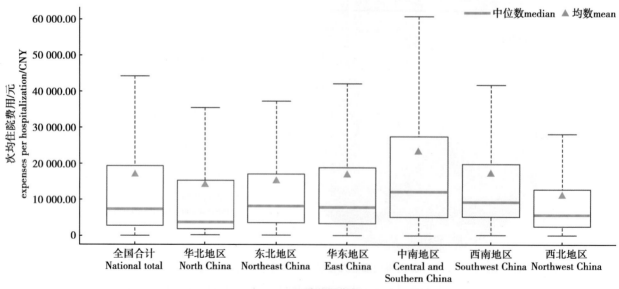

图 8-2-80 2017—2018 年全国及六大区淋巴瘤患儿次均住院费用

Figure 8-2-80 Expenses per hospitalization of children with lymphoma in the six regions and the whole country in 2017-2018

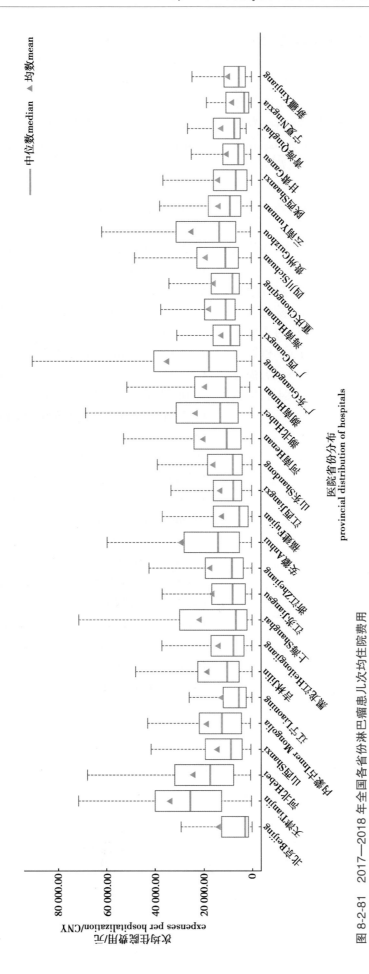

图 8-2-81　2017—2018 年全国各省份淋巴瘤患儿次均住院费用

Figure 8-2-81　Expenses per hospitalization of children with lymphoma in each provincial-level region in 2017-2018

2.5.2　全国儿童肿瘤监测机构淋巴瘤患儿次均住院分项费用情况

2.5.2.1　全国及六大区淋巴瘤患儿次均住院分项费用情况　根据全国淋巴瘤患儿次均住院分项费用(中位数),前 3 位分别为诊断类费用(1 824.36 元)、西药类费用(1 609.90 元)和综合医疗服务类费用(913.00 元)。六大区分项费用中位数的顺位与全国相比略有不同。如中南地区,次均住院分项费用(中位数)前 3 位分别为西药类费用(3 187.17 元)、诊断类费用(1 950.45 元)和综合医疗服务类费用(1 362.00 元)(图 8-2-82)。按均数统计的结果详见图 8-2-83。

2.5.2.2　各省份淋巴瘤患儿次均住院分项费用情况　根据各省份淋巴瘤患儿次均住院分项费用(中位数),以西药类费用为例,前 3 位的省份依次为河北(4 345.48 元)、湖北(4 249.70 元)和贵州(3 907.98 元),后 3 位依次为北京(405.35 元)、福建(707.22 元)和上海(1 078.70 元)(图 8-2-84)。按均数统计的结果详见图 8-2-85。

2.5.2　Expenses of each item per hospitalization of children with lymphoma in pediatric cancer surveillance sites in China

2.5.2.1　Expenses of each item per hospitalization of children with lymphoma in the six regions and the whole country　In terms of the median expenses of each item per hospitalization of children with lymphoma, the top three items were diagnostic expenses (1 824.36 CNY), western medication expenses (1 609.90 CNY) and comprehensive medical services expenses (913.00 CNY). The rank of the median expenses of each item in the six regions was slightly different from the national median. For example, in Central and Southern China, the top three median expenses of each item per hospitalization were western medication expenses (3 187.17 CNY), diagnostic expenses (1, 950.45 CNY) and comprehensive medical services expenses (1, 362.00 CNY)(Figure 8-2-82). Data by the mean expenses in Figure 8-2-83.

2.5.2.2　Expenses of each item per hospitalization of children with lymphoma in each provincial-level region　In terms of the median expenses of each item per hospitalization of children with lymphoma in each provincial-level region, taking western medication expenses as an example, the top three provincial-level regions were Hebei (4, 345.48 CNY), Hubei (4, 249.70 CNY) and Guizhou (3, 907.98 CNY). The last three were Beijing (405.35 CNY), Fujian (707.22 CNY) and Shanghai (1, 078.70 CNY)(Figure 8-2-84). Data by the mean expenses in Figure 8-2-85.

分项费用/元
expenses of each item/CNY

医院地区分布 regional distribution of hospitals	综合医疗服务类费用 comprehensive medical service expenses	诊断类费用 diagnostic expenses	治疗类费用 treatment expenses	康复类费用 rehabilitation expenses	中医类费用 traditional chinese medicine service expenses	西药类费用 western medication expenses	中药类费用 traditional chinese medication expenses	血液和血液制品类费用 blood and blood product expenses	耗材类费用 medical consumable expenses	其他类费用 others
全国合计 National total	913.00	1 824.36	0	0	0	1 609.90	0	0	334.56	0
华北地区 North China	299.00	1 681.00	0	0	0	578.76	0	0	325.02	0
东北地区 Northeast China	946.10	1 603.25	42.90	0	0	2 007.13	0	0	515.52	45.00
华东地区 East China	1 032.00	1 864.36	78.00	0	0	1 930.17	0	0	325.19	8.00
中南地区 Central and Southern China	1 362.00	1 950.45	83.00	0	0	3 187.17	0	0	562.02	6.00
西南地区 Southwest China	1 620.50	2 528.00	90.00	0	0	3 305.53	0	0	382.98	2.97
西北地区 Northwest China	661.00	1 676.00	50.00	0	0	1 373.80	0	0	109.86	6.00

图 8-2-82　2017—2018 年全国及六大区淋巴瘤患儿次均住院分项费用 (按中位数计)

Figure 8-2-82　Expenses of each item per hospitalization of children with lymphoma in the six regions and the whole country in 2017-2018 (by the median)

分项费用/元
expenses of each item/CNY

医院地区分布 regional distribution of hospitals	综合医疗服务类费用 comprehensive medical service expenses	诊断类费用 diagnostic expenses	治疗类费用 treatment expenses	康复类费用 rehabilitation expenses	中医类费用 traditional chinese medicine service expenses	西药类费用 western medication expenses	中药类费用 traditional chinese medication expenses	血液和血液制品类费用 blood and blood product expenses	耗材类费用 medical consumable expenses	其他类费用 others
全国合计 National total	2 238.22	4 016.92	657.38	10.53	21.44	5 342.60	131.22	917.37	1 407.59	604.13
华北地区 North China	2 024.89	3 839.44	194.92	1.46	4.89	4 304.42	41.18	949.78	1 645.59	311.42
东北地区 Northeast China	1 864.86	3 465.65	992.38	0.97	0.07	4 690.47	558.80	892.63	1 401.68	1 084.72
华东地区 East China	2 266.84	3 926.39	803.70	18.92	8.65	5 936.26	124.62	895.12	1 201.81	643.38
中南地区 Central and Southern China	2 674.93	4 899.66	1 221.62	11.77	85.86	8 006.56	268.24	1 085.58	1 882.57	1 618.83
西南地区 Southwest China	2 947.08	4 402.26	741.64	36.93	26.45	5 661.80	146.05	1 066.55	1 109.44	202.42
西北地区 Northwest China	1 513.58	3 078.33	1 000.93	3.14	19.63	3 765.25	57.28	369.85	579.15	264.28

图 8-2-83　2017—2018 年全国及六大区淋巴瘤患儿次均住院分项费用 (按均数计)

Figure 8-2-83　Expenses of each item per hospitalization of children with lymphoma in the six regions and the whole country in 2017-2018 (by the mean)

省份分布 provincial distribution of hospitals	综合医疗服务类费用 comprehensive medical service expenses	分项费用/元 expenses of each item/CNY								
		诊断类费用 diagnostic expenses	治疗类费用 treatment expenses	康复类费用 rehabilitation expenses	中医类费用 traditional chinese medicine service expenses	西药类费用 western medication expenses	中药类费用 traditional chinese medication expenses	血液和血液制品类费用 blood and blood product expenses	耗材类费用 medical consumable expenses	其他类费用 others
北京Beijing	247.65	1 601.00	0	0	0	405.35	0	0	303.94	0
天津Tianjin	3 779.00	8 801.00	200.00	0	0	3 466.85	0	35.55	1 978.35	0
河北Hebei	1 774.35	2 832.00	151.85	0	0	4 345.48	39.80	1 000.00	1 059.67	300.00
山西Shanxi	1 252.50	2 015.20	40.00	0	0	2 369.47	0	0	564.80	0
内蒙古Inner Mongolia	692.50	1 942.00	396.00	0	0	3 571.52	29.82	0	117.20	44.00
辽宁Liaoning	539.20	873.02	71.50	0	0	1 447.89	0	0	207.74	1 180.30
吉林Jilin	1 737.00	2 826.00	43.00	0	0	2 295.06	0	0	873.38	0
黑龙江Heilongjiang	921.00	1 343.00	140.00	0	0	2 834.47	0	0	795.20	52.00
上海Shanghai	1 363.00	2 607.50	0	0	0	1 078.70	0	0	512.22	0
江苏Jiangsu	1 028.00	1 569.00	235.40	6.00	0	2 195.94	53.00	62.50	534.28	240.00
浙江Zhejiang	715.00	2 326.00	94.00	22.00	0	2 116.20	0	0	299.08	16.00
安徽Anhui	1 333.25	3 096.75	90.00	0	0	2 794.21	40.15	0	301.13	107.78
福建Fujian	888.46	569.00	0	0	0	707.22	0	0	0	9.00
江西Jiangxi	1 043.00	1 998.00	72.00	0	0	2 933.20	142.14	10.00	384.71	49.50
山东Shandong	1 111.00	1 907.00	100.00	0	0	1 803.29	0	0	429.07	0
河南Henan	1 228.55	58.00	70.00	0	0	3 111.89	0	0	157.57	0
湖北Hubei	1 331.00	3 463.00	50.00	0	0	4 249.70	0	0	623.70	6.00
湖南Hunan	1 273.52	1 809.00	21.00	0	0	2 811.14	0	0	773.04	264.00
广东Guangdong	1 613.55	3 808.50	222.70	0	0	3 156.96	0	62.11	1 167.29	0
广西Guangxi	1 383.33	3 177.90	322.75	0	0	1 760.27	0	0	442.63	0
海南Hainan	1 550.60	2 059.91	222.00	0	0	3 285.53	79.64	0	715.60	6.00
重庆Chongqing	1 434.22	2 907.25	0	0	0	3 132.04	0	0	421.03	0
四川Sichuan	2 333.75	2 091.00	311.00	19.00	0	3 371.11	0	0	698.71	0
贵州Guizhou	1 721.06	3 043.50	278.40	0	0	3 907.98	0	0	525.45	70.80
云南Yunnan	1 510.00	2 478.00	120.00	0	0	3 289.44	69.00	0	114.62	0.05
陕西Shaanxi	994.00	1 041.25	100.00	0	0	1 664.72	0	0	117.48	0
甘肃Gansu	900.65	1 824.50	0	6.00	0	1 523.23	0	0	15.00	0
青海Qinghai	727.30	2 661.00	45.00	0	0	2 340.04	58.86	0	152.29	0
宁夏Ningxia	351.40	547.55	140.78	0	0	1 103.41	60.04	781.80	196.13	1.89
新疆Xinjiang	562.00	1 945.00	56.00	0	0	1 296.71	0	0	109.86	18.00

图 8-2-84　2017—2018 年全国各省份省级住院淋巴瘤患儿次均住院分项费用（按中位数计）

Figure 8-2-84　Expenses of each item per hospitalization of children with lymphoma in the six regions and the whole country in 2017-2018 (by the median)

医院省份分布 provincial distribution of hospitals	分项费用/元 expenses of each item/CNY								
	综合医疗服务类费用 comprehensive medical service expenses	诊断类费用 diagnostic expenses	治疗类费用 treatment expenses	康复类费用 rehabilitation expenses	中医类费用 traditional chinese medicine service expenses	西药类费用 western medication expenses	中药类费用 traditional chinese medication expenses	血液和血液制品类费用 blood and blood product expenses	耗材类费用 medical consumable expenses	其他类费用 others
北京Beijing	1 929.67	3 712.26	89.05	0.67	4.87	4 043.55	21.83	906.98	1 657.07	320.63
天津Tianjin	5 739.76	9 769.92	1 482.33	1.10	0	7 592.06	29.81	2 444.78	2 739.99	137.45
河北Hebei	2 945.25	5 187.87	981.05	0.88	12.80	7 556.61	159.43	2 639.38	2 066.80	729.14
山西Shanxi	2 157.47	3 679.20	650.90	15.45	3.74	4 870.51	301.91	582.29	1 102.13	20.24
内蒙古Inner Mongolia	1 377.11	3 119.66	2 592.42	0.66	11.85	7 879.22	170.03	1 164.21	573.62	229.10
辽宁Liaoning	1 266.22	2 220.46	1 468.89	0	0	4 235.90	151.19	880.63	742.29	2 584.50
吉林Jilin	2 599.73	5 267.46	762.59	1.67	0.12	4 632.09	850.75	1 074.12	1 855.43	424.79
黑龙江Heilongjiang	1 578.62	2 251.44	884.77	0	0	5 499.41	379.63	581.99	1 687.21	228.68
上海Shanghai	3 399.12	6 232.34	527.54	4.11	3.23	6 988.44	73.55	390.74	1 819.55	48.56
江苏Jiangsu	2 140.49	3 330.43	1 167.74	40.24	6.30	5 982.24	119.75	1 548.10	1 781.46	816.68
浙江Zhejiang	1 901.33	4 142.25	832.26	39.41	31.99	7 218.83	53.96	1 484.10	863.66	225.16
安徽Anhui	3 627.11	6 082.57	1 089.43	84.80	46.89	8 550.94	210.60	3 824.46	1 456.94	394.64
福建Fujian	2 026.15	1 675.64	226.94	0	0.02	4 386.06	4.74	182.62	107.97	874.57
江西Jiangxi	1 691.56	3 049.29	1 173.80	14.77	0.94	5 531.60	427.58	824.86	886.79	290.12
山东Shandong	2 139.94	4 024.59	766.53	11.71	1.72	5 042.16	137.62	661.19	1 241.29	1 212.88
河南Henan	2 285.92	1 810.84	1 007.83	6.20	58.71	6 691.14	122.11	582.03	545.86	697.92
湖北Hubei	2 621.85	6 753.07	840.35	17.36	2.04	8 890.89	257.61	284.18	1 672.26	328.19
湖南Hunan	2 799.84	3 940.24	634.62	13.68	453.44	5 308.27	921.11	1 044.48	1 633.38	1 159.06
广东Guangdong	3 293.90	8 194.73	1 953.26	11.02	3.58	10 144.82	61.07	2 333.46	3 144.63	3 953.29
广西Guangxi	2 334.89	4 013.84	1 047.96	1.76	10.70	2 806.50	22.78	264.20	1 212.72	118.91
海南Hainan	2 236.80	3 289.78	1 630.25	0	40.61	5 368.31	191.47	753.95	1 520.18	50.07
重庆Chongqing	2 919.27	5 066.53	506.59	36.45	23.03	4 313.49	75.23	974.28	1 165.16	28.98
四川Sichuan	3 793.01	3 793.46	1 196.53	48.21	44.77	5 680.81	87.86	1 163.35	1 416.40	378.43
贵州Guizhou	2 979.99	5 962.01	1 034.25	4.43	2.33	9 249.22	373.70	1 308.29	1 472.16	587.07
云南Yunnan	2 033.21	3 461.69	494.33	37.45	14.40	6 472.40	300.88	947.26	547.24	146.08
陕西Shaanxi	1 992.77	2 776.89	910.35	4.94	39.45	5 192.17	34.17	725.40	885.83	300.24
甘肃Gansu	1 635.15	3 309.42	423.78	16.94	75.40	2 831.90	221.64	371.96	941.63	348.43
青海Qinghai	1 062.03	3 597.12	2 800.93	0	0	4 837.60	192.09	71.39	337.63	78.98
宁夏Ningxia	787.70	2 331.18	639.62	4.92	0.37	2 618.50	86.39	1 825.97	854.83	13.34
新疆Xinjiang	1 328.61	3 189.82	1 112.55	0.20	4.90	3 395.95	32.14	188.66	357.14	248.95

图 8-2-85 2017—2018 年全国各省份淋巴瘤患儿次均住院分项费用(按均数计)

Figure 8-2-85 Expenses of each item per hospitalization of children with lymphoma in the six regions and the whole countryin 2017-2018(by the mean)

2.6　全国儿童肿瘤监测机构淋巴瘤患儿平均住院日分析

2.6.1　全国及六大区淋巴瘤患儿平均住院日情况

全国淋巴瘤患儿平均住院日的中位数为 6 天。高于全国中位数水平的地区为中南地区（8 天）和西南地区（8 天），与全国中位数水平相同的地区为东北地区（6 天）和西北地区（6 天），低于全国中位数水平的地区为华北地区（1 天）和华东地区（5 天）（图 8-2-86）。

2.6.2　各省份淋巴瘤患儿平均住院日情况

根据各省份淋巴瘤患儿平均住院日的中位数，淋巴瘤患儿平均住院日最长的省份是河北（17 天），其次是天津（15 天）、四川（11 天）、内蒙古（10.5 天）、山西（10 天）和贵州（10 天），最短的是北京（1 天）（图 8-2-87）。

2.6　Analysis of the average length of hospitalization of children with lymphoma in pediatric cancer surveillance sites in China

2.6.1　Average length of hospitalization of children with lymphoma in the six regions and the whole country

Nationally, the median of average length of hospitalization was 6 days. Central and Southern China (8 days), Southwest China (8 days) were above the national median. Northeast China (6 days) and Northwest China (6 days) were the same with the national median. North China (1 day) and East China (5 days) were below the national median (Figure 8-2-86).

2.6.2　Average length of hospitalization of children with lymphoma in each provincial-level region

In terms of the median of average length of hospitalization of children with lymphoma in each provincial-level region, the provincial-level regions with the longest average hospital stay was Hebei (17 days), followed by Tianjin (15 days), Sichuan (11 days), Inner Mongolia (10.5 days), Shanxi (10 days), and Guizhou (10 days), and the shortest was Beijing (1 day) (Figure 8-2-87).

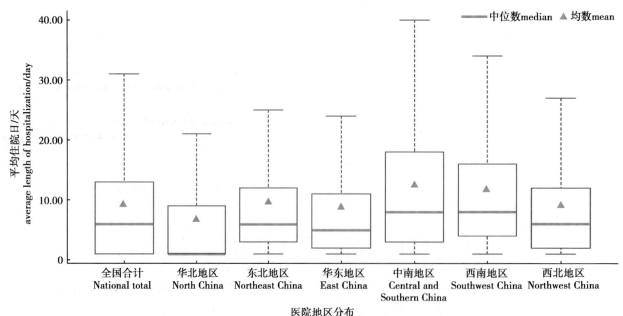

图 8-2-86　2017—2018 年全国及六大区淋巴瘤患儿平均住院日

Figure 8-2-86　Average length of hospitalization of children with lymphoma in the six regions and the whole country in 2017-2018

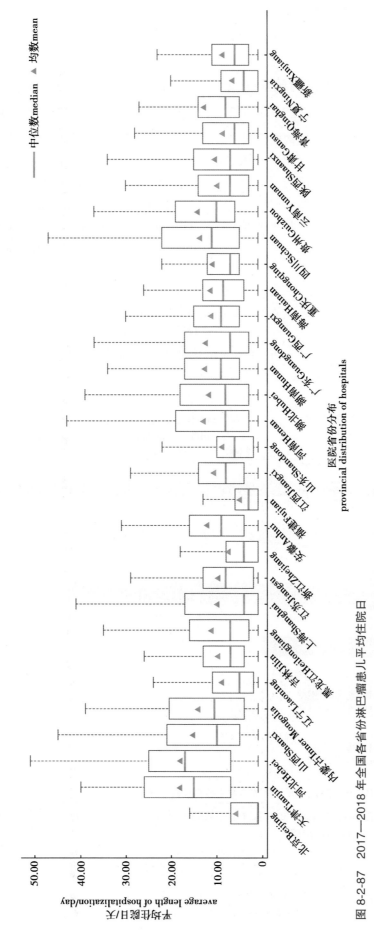

图 8-2-87　2017—2018 年全国各省份淋巴瘤患儿平均住院日

Figure8-2-87　Average length of hospitalization of children with lymphoma in each provincial-level region in 2017-2018

3 脑瘤

3.1 全国儿童肿瘤监测机构脑瘤患儿出院人次分析

3.1.1 六大区脑瘤患儿出院人次构成情况

在脑瘤患儿出院人次中,各大区出院人次占全部出院人次的比例由高到低依次为华北地区(32.40%)、华东地区(26.17%)、中南地区(23.64%)、西南地区(8.32%)、西北地区(5.07%)和东北地区(4.41%)(图8-3-1)。

3 Brain tumor

3.1 Analysis of discharges among children with brain tumor in pediatric cancer surveillance sites in China

3.1.1 Composition of discharges among children with brain tumor in the six regions

In terms of the discharges among children with brain tumor, the regions with the highest to the lowest proportion of discharges among children with brain tumor in all discharges were North China (32.40%), East China (26.17%), Central and Southern China (23.64%), Southwest China (8.32%), Northwest China (5.07%) and Northeast China (4.41%) (Figure 8-3-1).

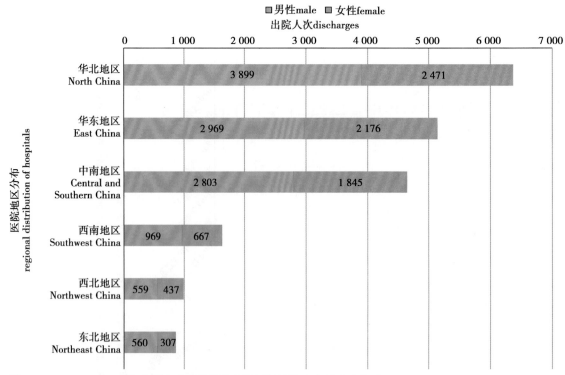

图 8-3-1 2017—2018 年全国六大区儿童肿瘤监测机构脑瘤出院人次构成

Figure 8-3-1 Composition of discharges among children with brain tumor in pediatric cancer surveillance sites in the six regions in 2017-2018

3.1.2　各省份脑瘤患儿出院人次构成情况

在所有省份中,脑瘤患儿出院人次占全部出院人次比例前 3 位的省份分别为北京(28.30%)、河南(10.18%)和山东(7.32%),后 3 位分别为西藏(0.04%)、青海(0.13%)和内蒙古(0.32%)(图 8-3-2,图 8-3-3)。

3.1.2　Composition of discharges among children with brain tumor in each provincial-level region

Among all provincial-level regions, Beijing (28.30%), Henan (10.18%) and Shandong (7.32%) were the three provincial-level regions with the highest proportions of discharges among children with brain tumor in all discharges, and Xizang (0.04%), Qinghai (0.13%) and Inner Mongolia (0.32%) had the lowest proportions of discharges among children with brain tumor (Figure 8-3-2~ Figure 8-3-3).

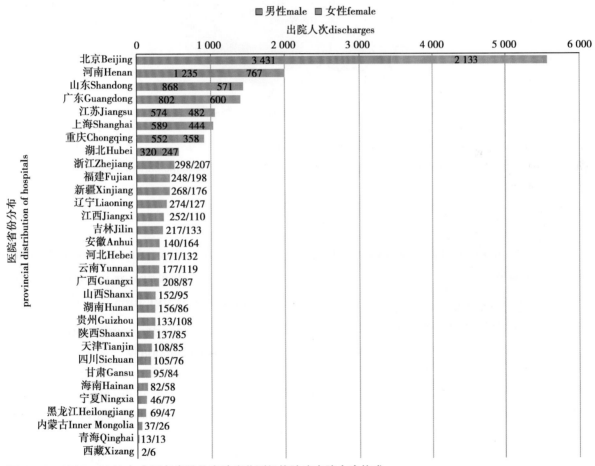

图 8-3-2　2017—2018 年全国各省份儿童肿瘤监测机构脑瘤出院人次构成

Figure 8-3-2　Composition of discharges among children with brain tumor in pediatric cancer surveillance sites in each provincial-level region in 2017-2018

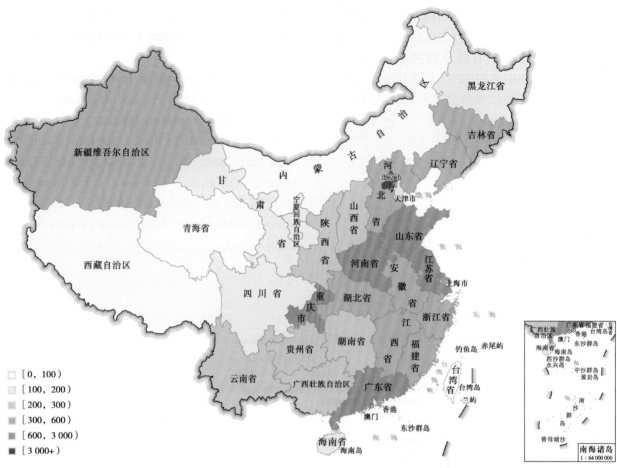

图 8-3-3　2017—2018 年全国各省份儿童肿瘤监测机构脑瘤出院人次分布

Figure 8-3-3　Distribution of discharges among children with brain tumor in pediatric cancer surveillance sites in each provincial-level region in 2017-2018

3.2　全国儿童肿瘤监测机构脑瘤患儿年龄/性别构成

3.2.1　全国脑瘤患儿年龄/性别构成情况

从性别分布来看,男性患儿占全部出院人次比例为 59.81%,女性患儿为 40.19%;男性患儿各年龄段的出院人次比例均高于女性患儿。从年龄分布来看,10 岁年龄组所占比例最高(7.43%),其次为11 岁(7.22%)和 13 岁(6.09%)年龄组(图 8-3-4)。

3.2　Age/gender composition of children with brain tumor in pediatric cancer surveillance sites in China

3.2.1　Age/gender composition of children with brain tumor nationally

In terms of gender distribution, male children accounted for 59.81% of all discharges, and female for 40.19%. The discharge proportions of male children at all ages were higher than those of female. In terms of age distribution, the 10-year age group accounted for the highest proportion (7.43%), followed by the 11-year age group (7.22%) and the 13-year age group (6.09%) (Figure 8-3-4).

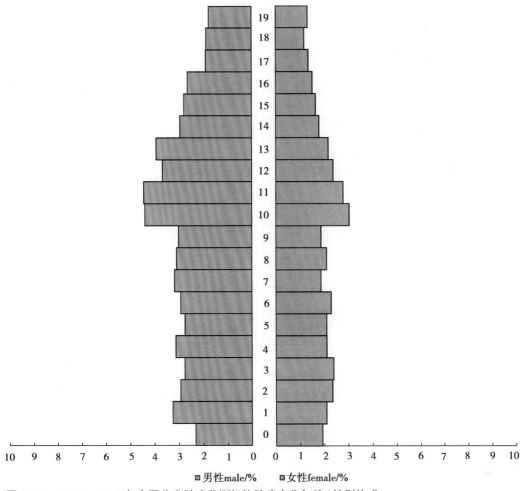

图 8-3-4　2017—2018 年全国儿童肿瘤监测机构脑瘤患儿年龄 / 性别构成

Figure 8-3-4　Age/gender composition of children with brain tumor in pediatric cancer surveillance sites in China in 2017-2018

3.2.2　六大区脑瘤患儿年龄 / 性别构成情况

从性别分布来看,六大区均显示男性患儿占全部出院人次比例高于女性患儿。从年龄分布来看,六大区的比例各有不同,其中华北地区的 10 岁年龄组所占比例最高;东北地区的 16 岁年龄组所占比例最高;华东地区的 2 岁年龄组所占比例最高;中南地区的 11 岁年龄组所占比例最高;西南地区的 4 岁年龄组所占比例最高;西北地区的 3 岁和 7 岁年龄组所占比例最高(图 8-3-5~ 图 8-3-10)。

3.2.2　Age/gender composition of children with brain tumor in the six regions

In terms of gender distribution, male children accounted for a higher proportion of all discharges than female in all the six regions. In terms of age distribution, the proportions of the six regions were different. The largest discharged age group for each region were as follows: 10-year age group in North China; 16-year age group in Northeast China; 2-year age group in East China; 11-year age group in Central and Southern China; 4-year age group in Southwest China; and both 3-year age group and 7-year age group in Northwest China (Figure 8-3-5~Figure 8-3-10).

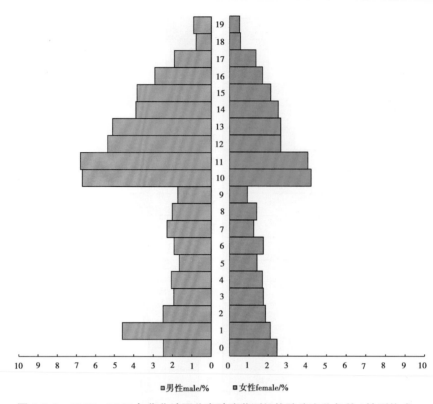

图 8-3-5　2017—2018 年华北地区儿童肿瘤监测机构脑瘤患儿年龄 / 性别构成

Figure 8-3-5　Age/gender composition of children with brain tumor in pediatric cancer surveillance sites in North China in 2017-2018

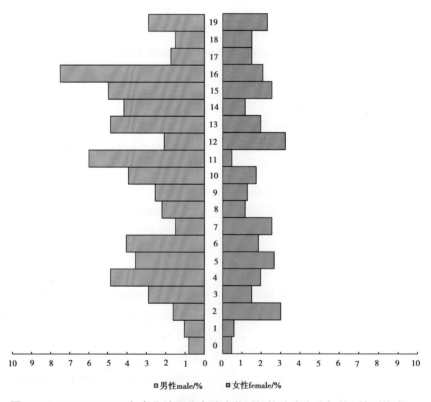

图 8-3-6　2017—2018 年东北地区儿童肿瘤监测机构脑瘤患儿年龄 / 性别构成

Figure 8-3-6　Age/gender composition of children with brain tumor in pediatric cancer surveillance sites in Northeast China in 2017-2018

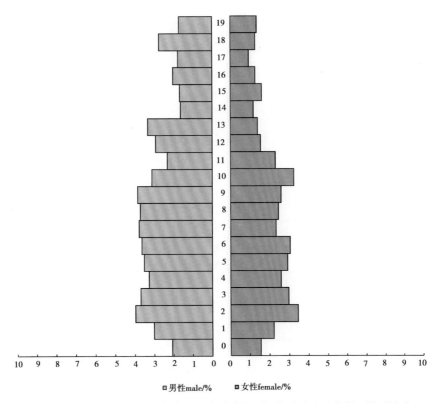

图 8-3-7　2017—2018 年华东地区儿童肿瘤监测机构脑瘤患儿年龄／性别构成

Figure 8-3-7　Age/gender composition of children with brain tumor in pediatric cancer surveillance sites in East China in 2017-2018

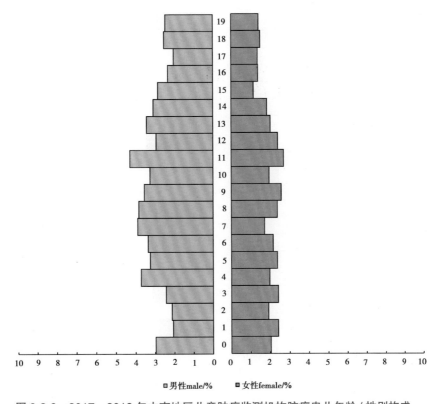

图 8-3-8　2017—2018 年中南地区儿童肿瘤监测机构脑瘤患儿年龄／性别构成

Figure 8-3-8　Age/gender composition of children with brain tumor in pediatric cancer surveillance sites in Central and Southern China in 2017-2018

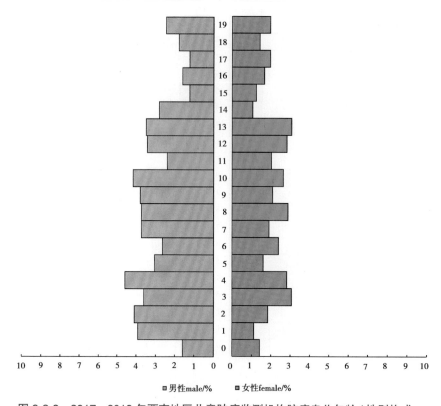

图 8-3-9 2017—2018 年西南地区儿童肿瘤监测机构脑瘤患儿年龄／性别构成

Figure 8-3-9 Age/gender composition of children with brain tumor in pediatric cancer surveillance sites in Southwest China in 2017-2018

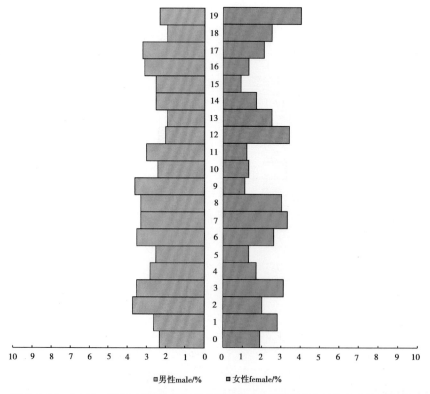

图 8-3-10 2017—2018 年西北地区儿童肿瘤监测机构脑瘤患儿年龄／性别构成

Figure 8-3-10 Age/gender composition of children with brain tumor in pediatric cancer surveillance sites in Northwest China in 2017-2018

3.2.3　各省份脑瘤患儿年龄/性别构成情况

从性别分布来看,除西藏外的其他30个省份出院患儿的性别分布均呈现男性比例高于女性;从年龄分布来看,各省份出院患儿的年龄分布各有不同。以山东为例,从性别分布来看,男性患儿占全部出院人次比例为60.32%,女性患儿为39.68%;从年龄分布来看,7岁年龄组所占比例最高(7.64%),其次为8岁(6.88%)和10岁(6.81%)年龄组(图8-3-11~图8-3-38)。

3.2.3　Age/gender composition of children with brain tumor in each provincial-level region

Apart from Xizang, the proportions of discharges among male children in other 30 provincial-level regions were higher than those of female. Age distribution differs across each provincial-level region. Taking Shandong as an example, in terms of gender distribution, male children and female children accounted for 60.32% and 39.68%, respectively. In terms of age distribution, the 7-year age group accounted for the highest proportion (7.64%), followed by the 8-year age group (6.88%) and the 10-year age group (6.81%) (Figure 8-3-11~Figure 8-3-38).

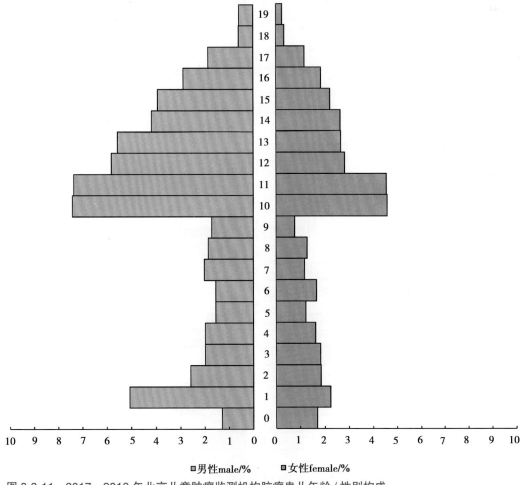

图 8-3-11　2017—2018 年北京儿童肿瘤监测机构脑瘤患儿年龄/性别构成

Figure 8-3-11　Age/gender composition of children with brain tumor in pediatric cancer surveillance sites in Beijing in 2017-2018

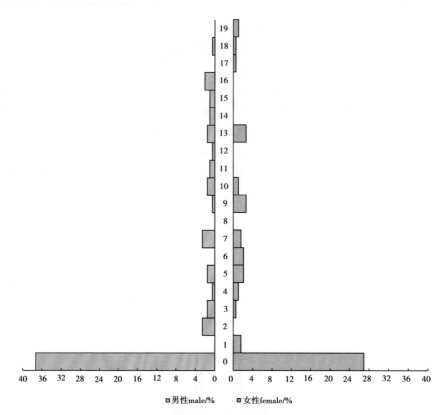

图 8-3-12 2017—2018 年天津儿童肿瘤监测机构脑瘤患儿年龄 / 性别构成

Figure 8-3-12 Age/gender composition of children with brain tumor in pediatric cancer surveillance sites in Tianjin in 2017-2018

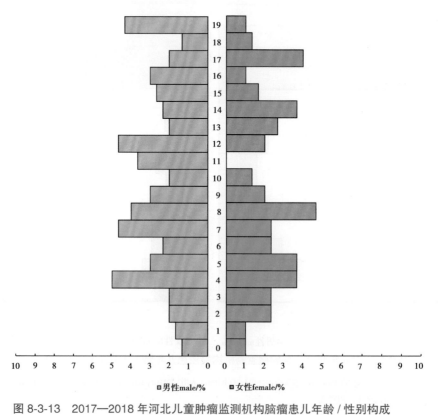

图 8-3-13 2017—2018 年河北儿童肿瘤监测机构脑瘤患儿年龄 / 性别构成

Figure 8-3-13 Age/gender composition of children with brain tumor in pediatric cancer surveillance sites in Hebei in 2017-2018

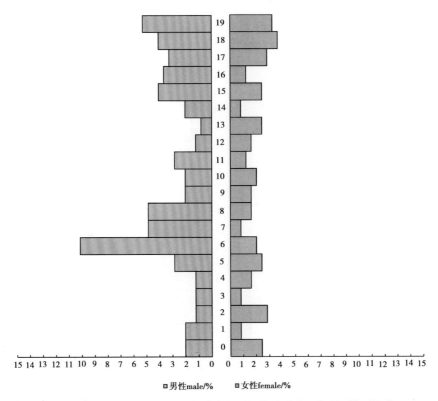

图 8-3-14　2017—2018 年山西儿童肿瘤监测机构脑瘤患儿年龄／性别构成

Figure 8-3-14　Age/gender composition of children with brain tumor in pediatric cancer surveillance sites in Shanxi in 2017-2018

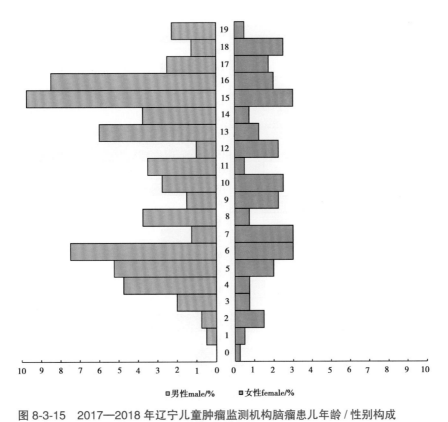

图 8-3-15　2017—2018 年辽宁儿童肿瘤监测机构脑瘤患儿年龄／性别构成

Figure 8-3-15　Age/gender composition of children with brain tumor in pediatric cancer surveillance sites in Liaoning in 2017-2018

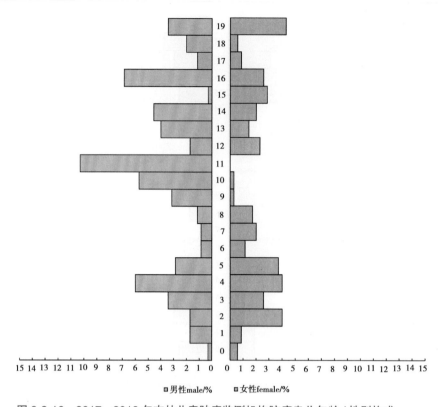

图 8-3-16　2017—2018 年吉林儿童肿瘤监测机构脑瘤患儿年龄 / 性别构成

Figure 8-3-16　Age/gender composition of children with brain tumor in pediatric cancer surveillance sites in Jilin in 2017-2018

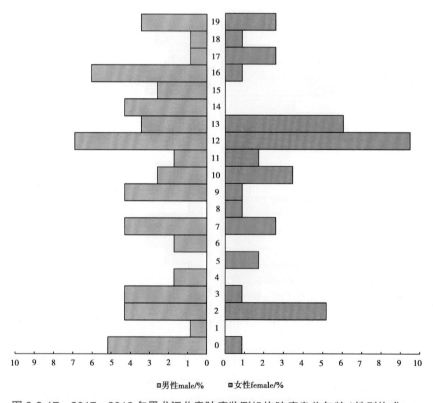

图 8-3-17　2017—2018 年黑龙江儿童肿瘤监测机构脑瘤患儿年龄 / 性别构成

Figure 8-3-17　Age/gender composition of children with brain tumor in pediatric cancer surveillance sites in Heilongjiang in 2017-2018

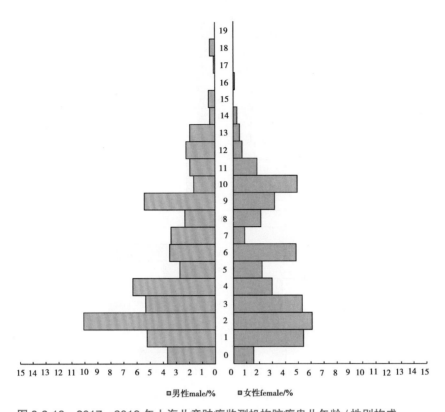

图 8-3-18　2017—2018 年上海儿童肿瘤监测机构脑瘤患儿年龄 / 性别构成

Figure 8-3-18　Age/gender composition of children with brain tumor in pediatric cancer surveillance sites in Shanghai in 2017-2018

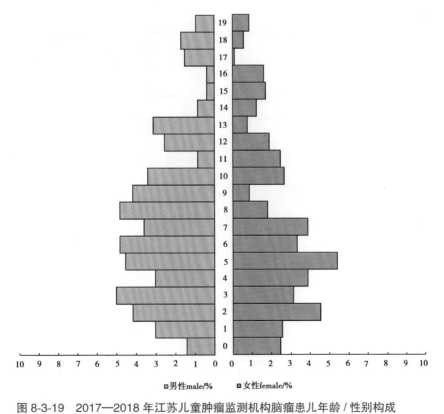

图 8-3-19　2017—2018 年江苏儿童肿瘤监测机构脑瘤患儿年龄 / 性别构成

Figure 8-3-19　Age/gender composition of children with brain tumor in pediatric cancer surveillance sites in Jiangsu in 2017-2018

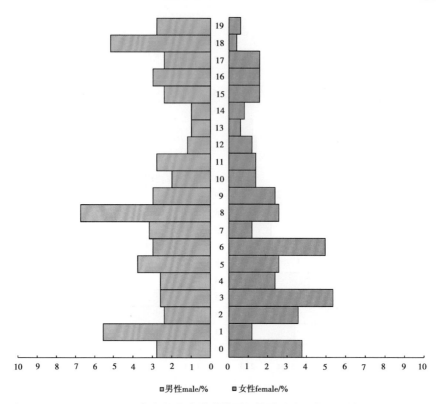

图 8-3-20　2017—2018 年浙江儿童肿瘤监测机构脑瘤患儿年龄／性别构成

Figure 8-3-20　Age/gender composition of children with brain tumor in pediatric cancer surveillance sites in Zhejiang in 2017-2018

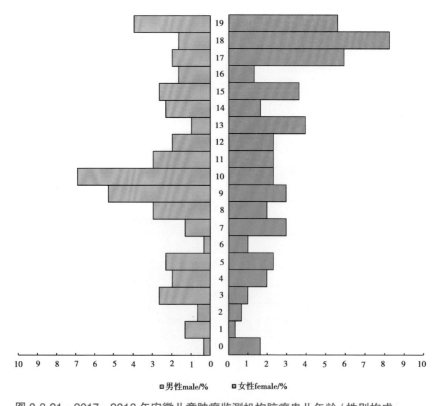

图 8-3-21　2017—2018 年安徽儿童肿瘤监测机构脑瘤患儿年龄／性别构成

Figure 8-3-21　Age/gender composition of children with brain tumor in pediatric cancer surveillance sites in Anhui in 2017-2018

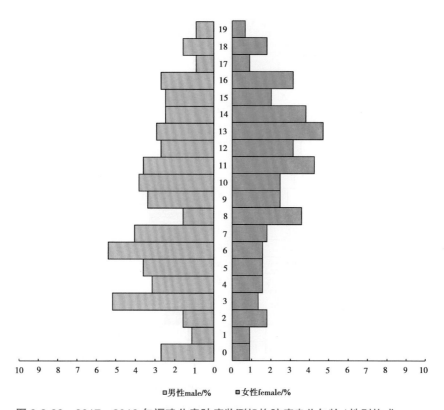

图 8-3-22　2017—2018 年福建儿童肿瘤监测机构脑瘤患儿年龄 / 性别构成

Figure 8-3-22　Age/gender composition of children with brain tumor in pediatric cancer surveillance sites in Fujian in 2017-2018

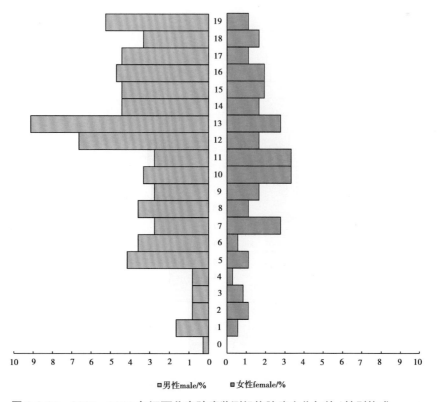

图 8-3-23　2017—2018 年江西儿童肿瘤监测机构脑瘤患儿年龄 / 性别构成

Figure 8-3-23　Age/gender composition of children with brain tumor in pediatric cancer surveillance sites in Jiangxi in 2017-2018

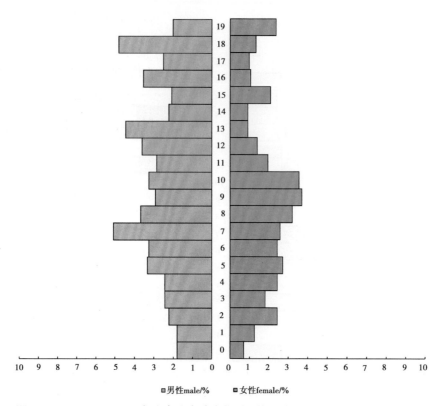

图 8-3-24 2017—2018 年山东儿童肿瘤监测机构脑瘤患儿年龄／性别构成

Figure 8-3-24 Age/gender composition of children with brain tumor in pediatric cancer surveillance sites in Shandong in 2017-2018

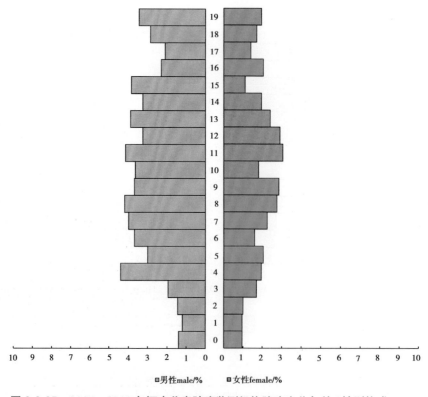

图 8-3-25 2017—2018 年河南儿童肿瘤监测机构脑瘤患儿年龄／性别构成

Figure 8-3-25 Age/gender composition of children with brain tumor in pediatric cancer surveillance sites in Henan in 2017-2018

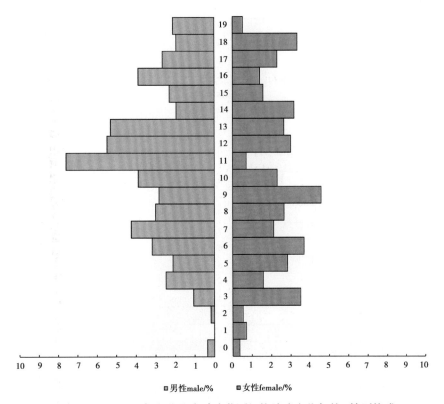

图 8-3-26　2017—2018 年湖北儿童肿瘤监测机构脑瘤患儿年龄 / 性别构成

Figure 8-3-26　Age/gender composition of children with brain tumor in pediatric cancer surveillance sites in Hubei in 2017-2018

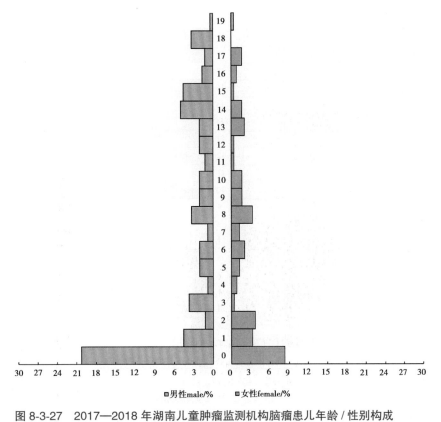

图 8-3-27　2017—2018 年湖南儿童肿瘤监测机构脑瘤患儿年龄 / 性别构成

Figure 8-3-27　Age/gender composition of children with brain tumor in pediatric cancer surveillance sites in Hunan in 2017-2018

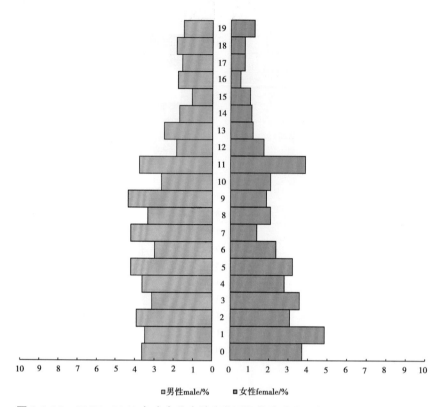

图 8-3-28　2017—2018 年广东儿童肿瘤监测机构脑瘤患儿年龄／性别构成

Figure 8-3-28　Age/gender composition of children with brain tumor in pediatric cancer surveillance sites in Guangdong in 2017-2018

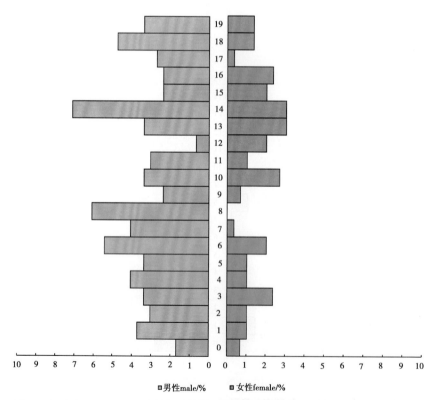

图 8-3-29　2017—2018 年广西儿童肿瘤监测机构脑瘤患儿年龄／性别构成

Figure 8-3-29　Age/gender composition of children with brain tumor in pediatric cancer surveillance sites in Guangxi in 2017-2018

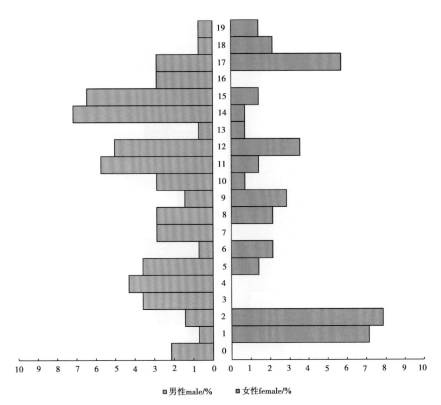

图 8-3-30　2017—2018 年海南儿童肿瘤监测机构脑瘤患儿年龄／性别构成

Figure 8-3-30　Age/gender composition of children with brain tumor in pediatric cancer surveillance sites in Hainan in 2017-2018

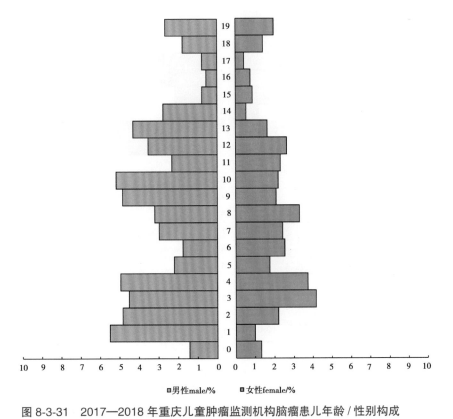

图 8-3-31　2017—2018 年重庆儿童肿瘤监测机构脑瘤患儿年龄／性别构成

Figure 8-3-31　Age/gender composition of children with brain tumor in pediatric cancer surveillance sites in Chongqing in 2017-2018

249

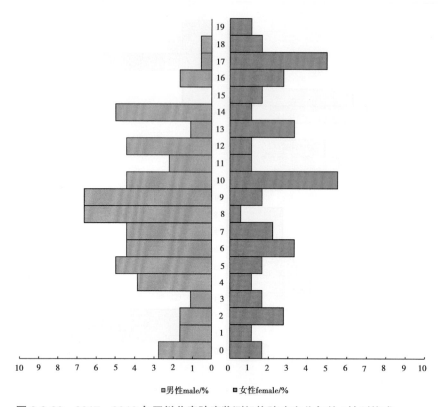

图 8-3-32　2017—2018 年四川儿童肿瘤监测机构脑瘤患儿年龄／性别构成

Figure 8-3-32　Age/gender composition of children with brain tumor in pediatric cancer surveillance sites in Sichuan in 2017-2018

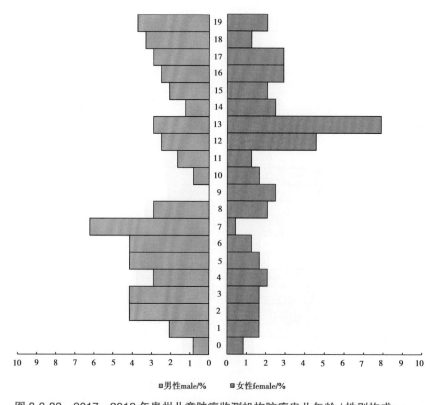

图 8-3-33　2017—2018 年贵州儿童肿瘤监测机构脑瘤患儿年龄／性别构成

Figure 8-3-33　Age/gender composition of children with brain tumor in pediatric cancer surveillance sites in Guizhou in 2017-2018

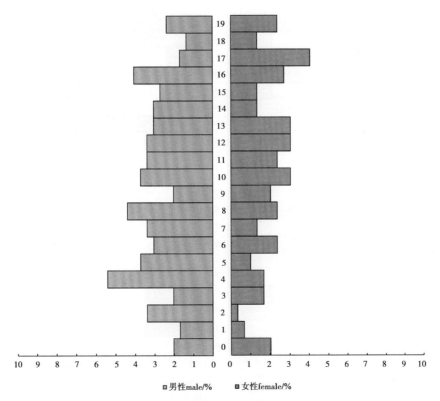

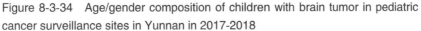

图 8-3-34　2017—2018 年云南儿童肿瘤监测机构脑瘤患儿年龄／性别构成

Figure 8-3-34　Age/gender composition of children with brain tumor in pediatric cancer surveillance sites in Yunnan in 2017-2018

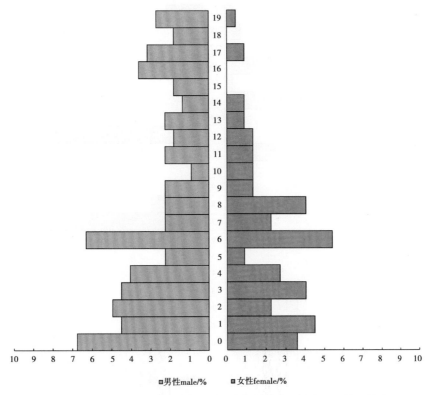

图 8-3-35　2017—2018 年陕西儿童肿瘤监测机构脑瘤患儿年龄／性别构成

Figure 8-3-35　Age/gender composition of children with brain tumor in pediatric cancer surveillance sites in Shaanxi in 2017-2018

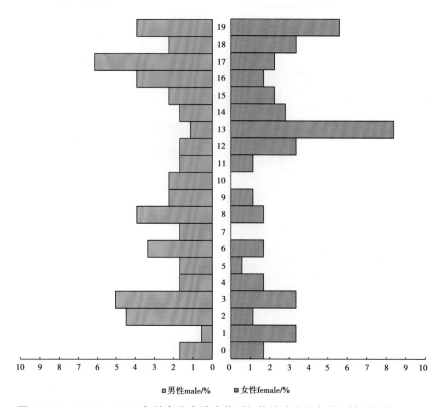

图 8-3-36　2017—2018 年甘肃儿童肿瘤监测机构脑瘤患儿年龄／性别构成

Figure 8-3-36　Age/gender composition of children with brain tumor in pediatric cancer surveillance sites in Gansu in 2017-2018

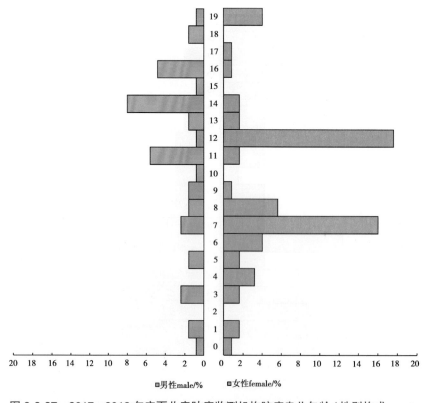

图 8-3-37　2017—2018 年宁夏儿童肿瘤监测机构脑瘤患儿年龄／性别构成

Figure 8-3-37　Age/gender composition of children with brain tumor in pediatric cancer surveillance sites in Ningxia in 2017-2018

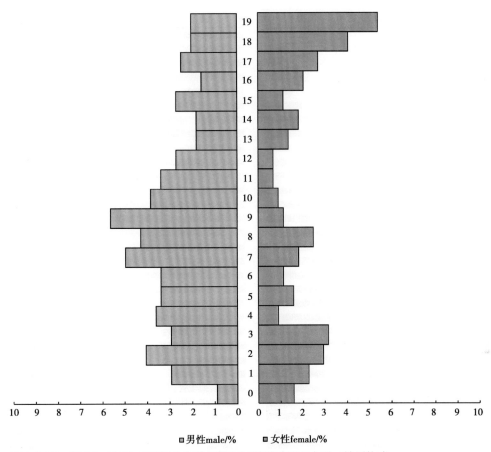

图 8-3-38　2017—2018 年新疆儿童肿瘤监测机构脑瘤患儿年龄／性别构成

Figure 8-3-38　Age/gender composition of children with brain tumor in pediatric cancer surveillance sites in Xinjiang in 2017-2018

3.3　全国儿童肿瘤监测机构脑瘤患儿就医省份分布

3.3.1　全国各省份脑瘤患儿本省就医与省外就医的分布情况

总体而言，脑瘤患儿本省就医的比例为59.24%。在所有省份中，本省就医比例前 3 位的省份分别为北京（98.65%）、广东（89.81%）和上海（89.58%）。省外就医比例前 3 位分别为内蒙古（81.50%）、河北（79.39%）和四川（75.87%）（图8-3-39）。

3.3　Distribution of provincial-level regions visited by children with brain tumor in pediatric cancer surveillance sites in China

3.3.1　Distribution of children with brain tumor receiving medical treatment in and out of their own provincial-level regions

In general, 59.24% of all children with brain tumor sought medical treatment in their own provincial-level regions. Beijing (98.65%), Guangdong (89.81%) and Shanghai (89.58%) were the top three provincial-level regions receiving out-province patients. Inner Mongolia (81.50%), Hebei (79.39%) and Sichuan (75.87%) were the top three provincial-level regions in terms of the proportion of patients going to other provincial-level regions for medical treatment (Figure 8-3-39).

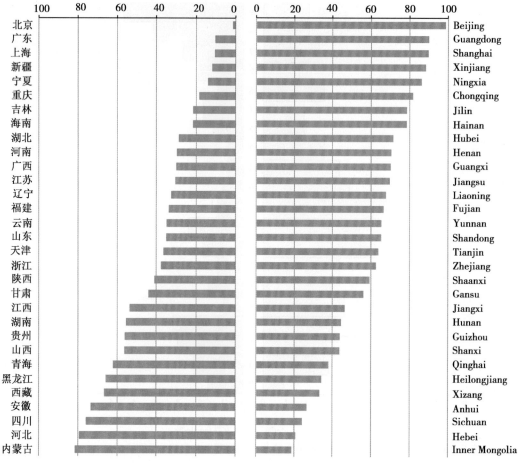

省外就医比例 proportion of patients receiving treatment out of their own provinces /%

本省就医比例 proportion of patients receiving treatment in their own provinces/%

图 8-3-39　2017—2018 年全国各省份脑瘤患儿本省就医与省外就医比例 /%

Figure 8-3-39　Proportion of children with brain tumor receiving medical treatment in and out of their own provincial-level regions in 2017-2018/%

3.3.2　全国各省份脑瘤患儿省外就医的去向省份分布情况

各省份脑瘤患儿选择省外就医的去向分布呈现明显的规律，主要的去向省份为北京、上海、重庆、广东和江苏。如户籍地为安徽的脑瘤患儿，选择省外就医的主要去向为北京、上海和江苏，分别占户籍地为安徽的脑瘤患儿选择省外就医总数的32.8%、29.6% 和 28.9%。再如户籍地为贵州的脑瘤患儿，选择省外就医的主要去向为重庆和北京，分别占户籍地为贵州的脑瘤患儿选择省外就医总数的54.7% 和 18.3%（图 8-3-40，按行方向查看）。

3.3.2　Distribution of provincial-level regions receiving pediatric brain tumor patients from other provincial-level regions

The distribution of provincial-level regions receiving children with brain tumor from outside the provincial-level regions showed obvious regularity. The main destinations were Beijing, Shanghai, Chongqing, Guangdong and Jiangsu. For Anhui children with brain tumor, the main destinations were Beijing, Shanghai and Jiangsu, accounting for 32.8%, 29.6% and 28.9%, respectively. For Guizhou children with brain tumor, Chongqing and Beijing were the main destinations, accounting for 54.7%, and 18.3%, respectively (Figure 8-3-40, view in rows).

收治省外就医肿瘤患儿的医院省份分布
provincial distribution of hospitals receiving children with cancer from outside the province

患儿户籍所在省份来源分布 distribution of the provinces of origin of children with cancer receiving treatment out of their own provinces	北京 Beijing	天津 Tianjin	河北 Hebei	山西 Shanxi	内蒙古 Inner Mongolia	辽宁 Liaoning	吉林 Jilin	黑龙江 Heilongjiang	上海 Shanghai	江苏 Jiangsu	浙江 Zhejiang	安徽 Anhui	福建 Fujian	江西 Jiangxi	山东 Shandong	河南 Henan	湖北 Hubei	湖南 Hunan	广东 Guangdong	广西 Guangxi	海南 Hainan	重庆 Chongqing	四川 Sichuan	贵州 Guizhou	云南 Yunnan	西藏 Xizang	陕西 Shaanxi	甘肃 Gansu	青海 Qinghai	宁夏 Ningxia	新疆 Xinjiang	合计 total
北京 Beijing	98.3	0	0	0	0	0	0	0	0	0	0	0	0	0	0	0	0	0	0	0	0	0	0	0	0	0	0	0	0	0	0	100
天津 Tianjin	50.0	50.0	0	0	0	0	0	0	0	0	0	0	0	0	0	0	0	0	0	0	0	0	0	0	1.7	0	0	0	0	0	0	100
河北 Hebei	93.8	4.8	0	0	0	0	0	0	0.1	0	0	0	0	0	0.4	0.1	0	0	0.3	0	0	0	0.3	0.6	0	0	0.3	0	0	0.3	0	100
山西 Shanxi	94.3	0.4	0	0	0	0	0	0	0.3	0.3	0	0	0.3	0	0	1.0	0	0.3	0.3	0	0	0.3	0.3	0	0	0	0.6	0	0	0.4	0	100
内蒙古 Inner Mongolia	80.0	1.5	0	0	0	4.6	9.6	3.1	0.4	0	0	0	0	0	0	0	0	0	0	0	0	0	0	0	0	0	0	0.4	0	0.4	0	100
辽宁 Liaoning	88.3	1.1	0	0.6	1.2	0	7.7	0	1.2	0	0	0	0	0	0	0	0	0	0	0	0	0	0	0	0	0	0	0	0	0	0	100
吉林 Jilin	90.4	0	0	0	0	4.8	0	0	0	0.5	0	0	0	0	0	1.4	0	0	1.0	0	1.2	0	0.5	0	0	0	1.0	0	0	0.5	0.5	100
黑龙江 Heilongjiang	88.9	1.4	0	1.4	1.2	1.4	0	0	1.0	0.5	0.6	0	0	0	0.9	0	0	0	0.9	0.3	0.5	0	0	0	0.5	0	0	0	0	0.5	0	100
上海 Shanghai	50.0	0	0	0	0	0	0	0	0	15.0	0	0	0	0	0	0	15.0	0	15.0	0	0.5	0	0	0	0	0	0	0	0	0	0	100
江苏 Jiangsu	41.8	0	0	0	0	0	0	0	54.9	0	0.6	0	0.4	0.6	0.9	1.3	0	0	0.9	0.3	0	0.1	0	0	0	0	0	0	0	0	0	100
浙江 Zhejiang	57.0	1.7	0.1	0.1	0	0.1	0.1	0	36.6	1.3	0	0	0.5	0	0.9	1.3	0	0.1	0.4	0.3	1.3	0.1	0	0	0	0	0	0.1	0	0	0	100
安徽 Anhui	32.9	0.4	0	0	0.1	0	0	0	29.6	28.9	4.5	0	0.5	0	0.4	0.4	0.7	0.1	0.9	0	0	0.1	0	0.1	0	0	0	0	0	0.2	0	100
福建 Fujian	63.5	1.9	0	0.5	0	0	0	0	21.6	0.5	1.9	0	0	0.5	0	0	0	0	9.1	0.2	0	1.4	0	0.1	0	0	0	0	0	0	0.1	100
江西 Jiangxi	41.6	0	0	0	0	0	0	0	27.9	1.0	4.3	0.2	0.2	0	0	0.7	1.0	1.0	20.3	0	0.1	0	0	0	0.1	0	0	0	0	0	0	100
山东 Shandong	89.9	0.4	0.5	0.1	0	0.3	0	0	4.3	1.3	1.3	1.2	0	0	0	1.5	0	0	0.3	0	0.1	0.4	0	0	0	0	0.5	0.1	0	0.1	0.5	100
河南 Henan	84.6	0.7	0.6	0	0	0.1	0.2	0	5.5	0.9	1.3	0	1.0	0.1	0.5	0	2.3	0	1.8	0	0.1	0.4	0	0	0	0	0.5	0	0	0.1	0	100
湖北 Hubei	88.8	0	0	0	0	0	0	0	4.7	1.0	0	0	1.0	0	0.5	1.0	0	0	11.0	0	0.5	9.1	0	0	0.5	0	0.5	0	0	0	0	100
湖南 Hunan	58.8	0	0	0	0	0	0	0	1.7	2.4	4.8	0	0.3	0	3.8	0.3	2.7	0	24.6	0	0.3	0	0	0	0.3	0	0	0	0	0	0	100
广东 Guangdong	81.1	0	0.9	0	0	0	0.9	0	2.7	7.2	0	0.8	0.9	0	0	0.8	0.9	0	0	2.7	0.9	0	0	0.8	0.3	0	0.9	0	0	0.9	0	100
广西 Guangxi	32.8	0.7	0	0	0	0.1	0	0	2.5	1.6	0.8	0.8	0	0	0	0.8	0.8	0	56.6	0	0	2.5	0	0.8	0	0	0	0	0.1	0	0	100
海南 Hainan	5.9	0	0	0	0	0	0	0	0	0	0	0	0	0	0	0	0	2.9	91.2	0	0	0	0	0	0	0	0	0	0	0	0	100
重庆 Chongqing	68.4	0	0	0	0	0	0	0	13.0	0	0	0.2	1.1	0	0	3.3	1.1	0	10.9	0	0.2	0	1.1	0.8	0	0	1.1	0	0	0	0.8	100
四川 Sichuan	19.4	0.6	0.2	0	0	0	0	0	6.3	0.6	0	0	2.7	0	2.9	0.3	0.8	0	8.4	0	0.7	56.3	0	0.2	0.4	0	0	0	0	0	0	100
贵州 Guizhou	18.4	0	0	0	0	0	0	0	3.3	0.3	3.0	0	1.7	0	0	0.3	0	0	9.7	1.3	0.7	54.7	0.3	0	6.3	0	0	0	0	0	0	100
云南 Yunnan	65.4	0	0	0	0	0	0	0	11.1	4.9	11.1	0	0.7	0	0	0	0	0	1.4	0	0	3.5	1.4	0.7	6.3	0	0	0	0	0	0	100
西藏 Xizang	25.0	0	0	0	0	0	0	0	3.1	43.7	0	0	6.3	0	0	0.8	0	0	0.8	0	0	12.5	12.5	0	0	0	0	0	0	0	0	100
陕西 Shaanxi	84.3	2.2	0	0	1.6	0	1.6	0	4.4	0.7	1.6	0	0	0	0	0.8	0	0	0.8	0	0	0	0	0.7	0	0	12.5	0	0	0.8	0.8	100
甘肃 Gansu	64.1	0.7	0.8	0	0	0	0	0	4.4	0	1.5	0	0	0	2.4	6.6	0	0	0.7	0	0	0	4.4	0	0	0	0	0	0	0	3.7	100
青海 Qinghai	78.1	0	0	0	0	0	0	0	0	7.4	0	0	0	0	0	0	0	0	4.9	0	0	0	2.4	0	0	0	0	2.4	0	0	2.4	100
宁夏 Ningxia	68.3	0	0	0	0	0	0	0	0	7.4	0	0	0	0	2.4	5.3	0	0	4.9	0	0	0	2.4	0	0	0	21.1	2.4	0	0	0	100
新疆 Xinjiang	56.0	0	0	0	0	0	0	0	21.0	5.3	0	0	0	0	5.3	8.8	0	0	1.8	0	0	1.8	0	0	0	0	1.8	5.3	0	0	0	100

图 8-3-40　2017—2018 年全国各省份户籍地脑瘤患儿选择省外就医的省份分布/%

Figure 8-3-40　Distribution of provincial-level regions receiving children with brain tumor from other provincial-level regions in 2017-2018/%

255

3.3.3　全国各省份收治脑瘤患儿来源的省份分布情况

各省份儿童肿瘤监测机构收治的省外就医脑瘤患儿来源分布略有差异,多数省份收治的脑瘤患儿来源以其相邻省份为主。如辽宁,其收治的省外就医脑瘤患儿主要来源于内蒙古、吉林和黑龙江,分别占辽宁收治的省外就医脑瘤患儿总数的52.2%、17.4%和13.0%。再如陕西,其收治的省外就医脑瘤患儿主要来源于甘肃、宁夏和河南,分别占陕西收治的省外就医脑瘤患儿总数的45.9%、10.8%和10.8%(图8-3-41,按列方向查看)。

3.4　全国儿童肿瘤监测机构脑瘤患儿住院费用医疗付费方式构成

3.4.1　全国脑瘤患儿住院费用医疗付费方式构成情况

全国脑瘤患儿住院费用的医疗付费方式中,占比最高的前3种类型分别为全自费(26.64%)、新型农村合作医疗(25.36%)和其他(16.30%)(图8-3-42)。

3.4.2　六大区脑瘤患儿住院费用医疗付费方式构成情况

六大区的医疗付费方式所占比例各不相同,西南地区和华东地区均以全自费占比最高,分别为37.20%和32.87%。而中南地区、西北地区、东北地区和华北地区则以新型农村合作医疗占比最高,分别为40.23%、31.27%、28.98%和21.99%(图8-3-43~图8-3-48)。

3.3.3　Distribution of the provincial-level regions of origin of children with brain tumor receiving treatment out of their own provincial-level regions

There was a slight difference in the distribution of the provincial-level regions of origin of children with brain tumor admitted to surveillance sites across the provincial-level regions, and most of the children were from their neighboring provincial-level regions. For example, in Liaoning, the children hospitalized from other provincial-level regions were mainly from Inner Mongolia, Jilin and Heilongjiang, accounting for 52.2%, 17.4% and 13.0%, respectively. In Shaanxi, children hospitalized from other provincial-level regions were mainly from Gansu, Ningxia and Henan, accounting for 45.9%, 10.8% and 10.8%, respectively (Figure 8-3-41, view in lines).

3.4　Composition of medical payment methods for hospitalization expenses of children with brain tumor in pediatric cancer surveillance sites in China

3.4.1　Composition of medical payment methods for hospitalization expenses of children with brain tumor nationally

Among the medical payment methods of children with brain tumor nationally, the top three methods were 100% self-pay (26.64%), new rural cooperative medical system (25.36%), and through other payment methods (16.30%) (Figure 8-3-42).

3.4.2　Composition of medical payment methods for hospitalization expenses of children with brain tumor in the six regions

The proportions of medical payment methods in the six regions were different, and the proportion of 100% self-pay was the highest in Southwest China and East China, accounting for 37.2% and 32.87%, respectively. In Central and Southern China, Northwest China, Northeast China and North China, new rural cooperative medical system was the highest, accounting for 40.23%, 31.27%, 28.98% and 21.99%, respectively (Figure 8-3-43~Figure 8-3-48).

图 8-3-41　2017—2018 年全国各省份儿童肿瘤监测机构省外就医脑瘤患儿来源分布 /%

Figure 8-3-41　Distribution of provincial-level regions of origin of children with brain tumor receiving treatment out of their own provincial-level regions in 2017-2018/%

收治省外级医院肿瘤患儿的医院省份分布

provincial distribution of hospitals receiving children with cancer from outside the province

患儿来源分布 / distribution of the provinces of origin of children receiving treatment out of their own provinces

来源 Origin	北京 Beijing	天津 Tianjin	河北 Hebei	山西 Shanxi	内蒙古 Inner Mongolia	辽宁 Liaoning	吉林 Jilin	黑龙江 Heilongjiang	上海 Shanghai	江苏 Jiangsu	浙江 Zhejiang	安徽 Anhui	福建 Fujian	江西 Jiangxi	山东 Shandong	河南 Henan	湖北 Hubei	湖南 Hunan	广东 Guangdong	广西 Guangxi	海南 Hainan	重庆 Chongqing	四川 Sichuan	贵州 Guizhou	云南 Yunnan	西藏 Xizang	陕西 Shaanxi	甘肃 Gansu	青海 Qinghai	宁夏 Ningxia	新疆 Xinjiang
北京 Beijing	1.1	2.2							0.2															14.2							0
天津 Tianjin	19.9	59.3							0.1						10.7						23.4	0.2			4.0		8.2				0
河北 Hebei	5.6	1.1	0			0	0	0	0.1	0.3			2.8	20.0		5.8			0.7		23.4	0.2	6.6				5.4			14.2	0
山西 Shanxi	3.9	4.4		16.6		52.3	55.7		0.1				2.8		4.3	5.8											5.4	16.6		14.3	0
内蒙古 Inner Mongolia	3.0	2.2			0		31.1	100.0													5.9	0.2		14.3				16.6			0
辽宁 Liaoning	1.4	0	0	16.6	25.0	17.4			0.1						4.3	5.8			0.5		5.9		6.7				0			14.3	0
吉林 Jilin	3.5	3.3	0	50.0		13.0			0.2	0.3					2.1		6.5		0.7	11.2	5.9	0.2					5.4				0
黑龙江 Heilongjiang	0.2	0							20.9	1.0	1.7			40.0	6.4				0.7		17.6			14.3			0				6.2
上海 Shanghai	2.6	4.4							9.9		30.5		2.8		6.4	5.9	12.8	14.3	0.2			0.2		14.3			2.7			14.3	0
江苏 Jiangsu	2.5	4.4	7.6	16.7		4.3	2.2		27.6	76.4	3.4		11.4					14.3	1.7			0.2									6.2
浙江 Zhejiang	5.0	3.3			25.0				5.2	0.3	15.3	7.7	2.9	20.0		5.9	8.5	57.1	4.5	11.1		1.2							100.0		25.0
安徽 Anhui	2.5	4.4							13.4	1.3	9.3	69.2			0	21.6			19.8		5.9	0.6			4.0		10.8	16.7		14.3	0
福建 Fujian	3.3	0							3.7	2.3	2.5		0	20.0	2.1		40.4		0.5			3.8					2.7				0
江西 Jiangxi	12.7	2.2					4.4		5.2	0.7	11.9	7.7	5.7		2.1	3.9			3.5		5.9	0	4.0	14.3				2.7			25.0
山东 Shandong	13.1	5.5							1.2	2.3	2.5		2.8		23.4	2.0	17.0		5.4		5.9		4.0				2.7			14.3	0
河南 Henan	2.7	0							0.6	0.7	11.9		2.9						17.0	33.3											0
湖北 Hubei	3.3	0									0.8	7.7				2.0	2.1	14.3	16.3			0.6					2.7			14.3	0
湖南 Hunan	1.7	3.3							1.4				2.9			5.9	2.1		7.3												25.0
广东 Guangdong	0.8	0							3.8	1.0	7.6		40.0		31.9		8.5		10.4	44.4	5.9	58.7	6.7	14.3	8.0						0
广西 Guangxi	0.1	0	7.7				2.2		1.2	2.3	13.6		14.3			2.0			6.8		11.8	32.7	6.7	14.3	76.0			16.7			0
海南 Hainan	1.2	0							1.9	2.3			2.9				2.1	14.3	0.5			1.0	13.3								0
重庆 Chongqing	1.9	3.3		50.0		8.7			0.5		1.7	7.7			2.1	2.0	2.1		0.2			0.4	13.3				45.9			14.3	6.2
四川 Sichuan	1.0	1.1		16.7		4.3	4.4		0.7	0.3	1.7					17.6			0.2				40.0	14.3							31.3
贵州 Guizhou	1.8	0							0										0				6.7					16.7			6.3
云南 Yunnan	0.1	0							0.5										0								10.8				0
西藏 Xizang	2.0	3.3			50.0				0.7	0.3	1.7					2.0			0.2			0.2					2.7	50.0			0
陕西 Shaanxi	1.7	1.1													2.1				0.5											0	0
甘肃 Gansu	0.6	0								0.3						2.0		14.3													0
青海 Qinghai	0.2	0														9.8															0
宁夏 Ningxia	0.6	0							1.4	0.3					6.4																0
新疆 Xinjiang	0.6	0																													0
合计 Total	100	100	100	100	100	100	100	100	100	100	100	100	100	100	100	100	100	100	100	100	100	100	100	100	100	100	100	100	100	100	100

257

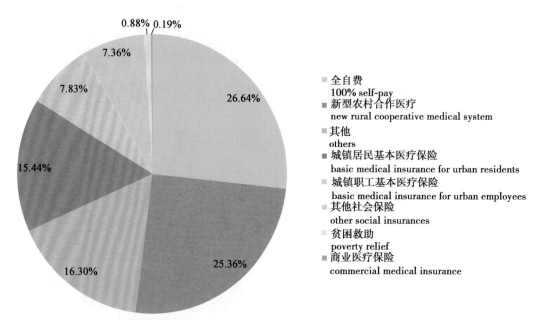

图 8-3-42　2017—2018 年全国脑瘤患儿住院费用医疗付费方式构成

Figure 8-3-42　Composition of medical payment methods for hospitalization expenses of children with brain tumor nationally in 2017-2018

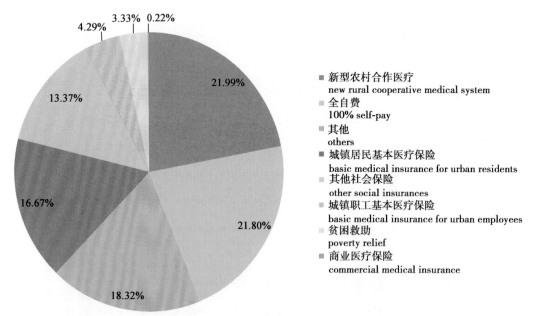

图 8-3-43　2017—2018 年华北地区脑瘤患儿住院费用医疗付费方式构成

Figure 8-3-43　Composition of medical payment methods for hospitalization expenses of children with brain tumor in North China in 2017-2018

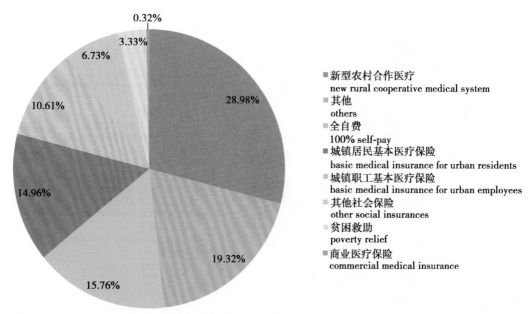

图 8-3-44 2017—2018 年东北地区脑瘤患儿住院费用医疗付费方式构成

Figure 8-3-44 Composition of medical payment methods for hospitalization expenses of children with brain tumor in Northeast China in 2017-2018

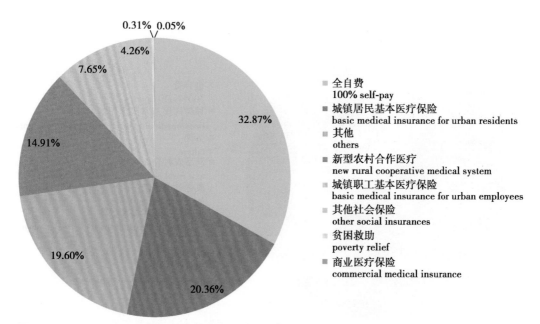

图 8-3-45 2017—2018 年华东地区脑瘤患儿住院费用医疗付费方式构成

Figure 8-3-45 Composition of medical payment methods for hospitalization expenses of children with brain tumor in East China in 2017-2018

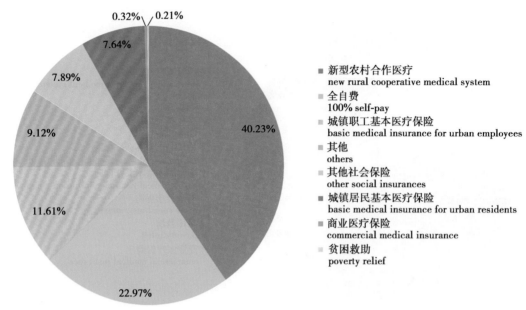

图 8-3-46　2017—2018 年中南地区脑瘤患儿住院费用医疗付费方式构成

Figure 8-3-46　Composition of medical payment methods for hospitalization expenses of children with brain tumor in Central and Southern China in 2017-2018

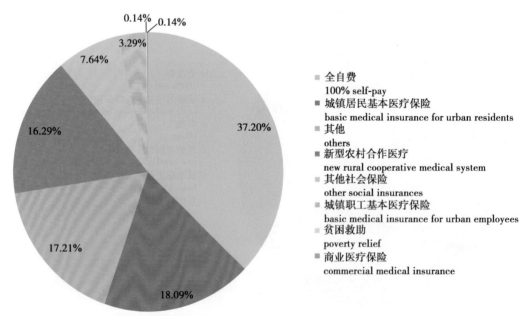

图 8-3-47　2017—2018 年西南地区脑瘤患儿住院费用医疗付费方式构成

Figure 8-3-47　Composition of medical payment methods for hospitalization expenses of children with brain tumor in Southwest China in 2017-2018

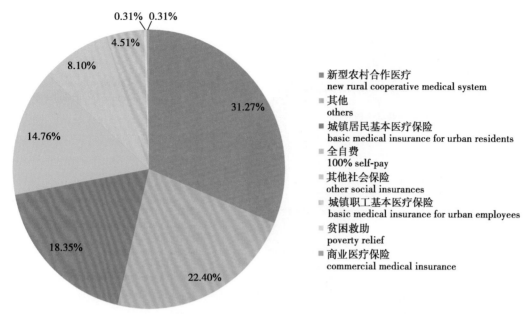

0.31% 0.31%
4.51%
8.10%
14.76%
18.35%
22.40%
31.27%

- 新型农村合作医疗
  new rural cooperative medical system
- 其他
  others
- 城镇居民基本医疗保险
  basic medical insurance for urban residents
- 全自费
  100% self-pay
- 其他社会保险
  other social insurances
- 城镇职工基本医疗保险
  basic medical insurance for urban employees
- 贫困救助
  poverty relief
- 商业医疗保险
  commercial medical insurance

图 8-3-48　2017—2018 年西北地区脑瘤患儿住院费用医疗付费方式构成

Figure 8-3-48　Composition of medical payment methods for hospitalization expenses of children with brain tumor in Northwest China in 2017-2018

3.4.3　各省份脑瘤患儿住院费用医疗付费方式构成情况

河北、内蒙古、黑龙江、江苏、安徽、江西、湖南、广东、四川、贵州、西藏和宁夏 12 个省份均以全自费所占比例最高。山西、吉林、福建、河南、广西、海南、陕西和新疆 8 个省份的新型农村合作医疗占比最高。北京、上海、山东和重庆 4 个省份的城镇居民基本医疗保险占比最高（图 8-3-49~ 图 8-3-79）。

3.4.3　Composition of medical payment methods for hospitalization expenses of children with brain tumor in each provincial-level region

The proportion of 100% self-pay was the highest in the following 12 provincial-level regions: Hebei, Inner Mongolia, Heilongjiang, Jiangsu, Anhui, Jiangxi, Hunan, Guangdong, Sichuan, Guizhou, Xizang and Ningxia. Payment by new rural cooperative medical system was the highest for Shanxi, Jilin, Fujian, Henan, Guangxi, Hainan, Shaanxi and Xinjiang. The following four provincial-level regions—Beijing, Shanghai, Shandong and Chongqing—had the highest proportions of payment by basic medical insurance for urban residents (Figure 8-3-49~Figure 8-3-79).

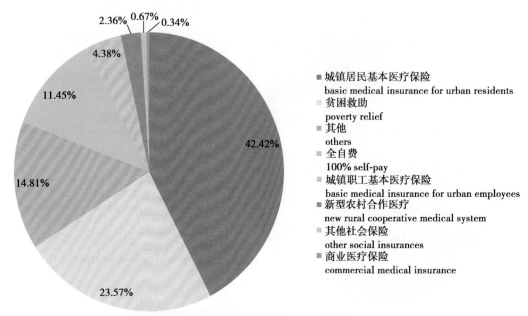

图 8-3-49　2017—2018 年北京脑瘤患儿住院费用医疗付费方式构成

Figure 8-3-49　Composition of medical payment methods for hospitalization expenses of children with brain tumor in Beijing in 2017-2018

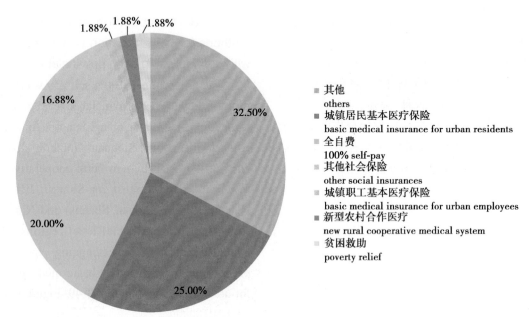

图 8-3-50　2017—2018 年天津脑瘤患儿住院费用医疗付费方式构成

Figure 8-3-50　Composition of medical payment methods for hospitalization expenses of children with brain tumor in Tianjin in 2017-2018

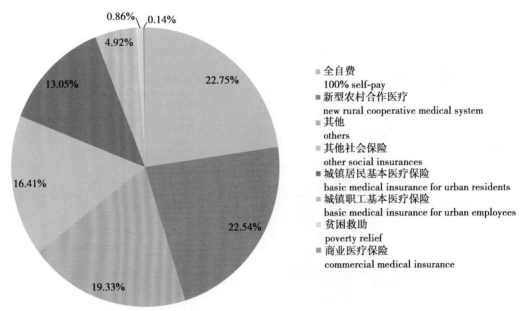

图 8-3-51　2017—2018 年河北脑瘤患儿住院费用医疗付费方式构成

Figure 8-3-51　Composition of medical payment methods for hospitalization expenses of children with brain tumor in Hebei in 2017-2018

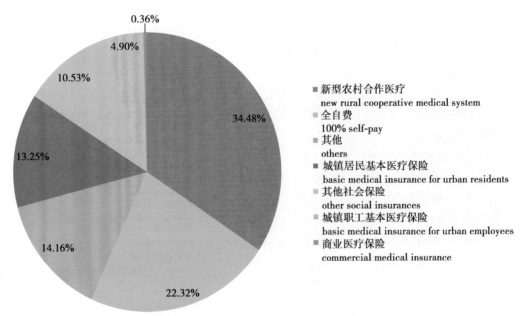

图 8-3-52　2017—2018 年山西脑瘤患儿住院费用医疗付费方式构成

Figure 8-3-52　Composition of medical payment methods for hospitalization expenses of children with brain tumor in Shanxi in 2017-2018

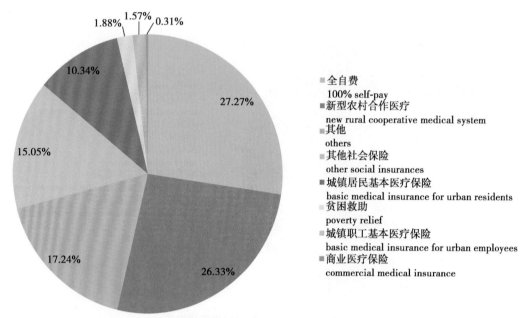

图 8-3-53　2017—2018 年内蒙古脑瘤患儿住院费用医疗付费方式构成

Figure 8-3-53　Composition of medical payment methods for hospitalization expenses of children with brain tumor in Inner Mongolia in 2017-2018

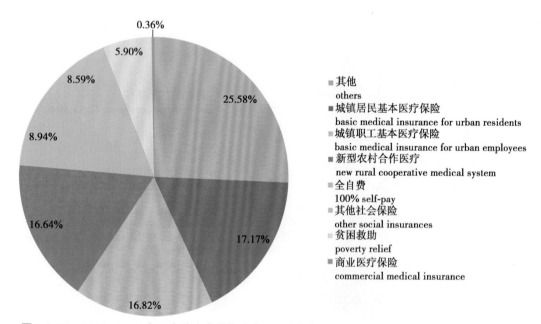

图 8-3-54　2017—2018 年辽宁脑瘤患儿住院费用医疗付费方式构成

Figure 8-3-54　Composition of medical payment methods for hospitalization expenses of children with brain tumor in Liaoning in 2017-2018

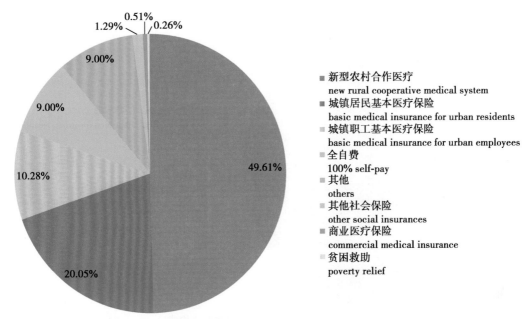

图 8-3-55　2017—2018 年吉林脑瘤患儿住院费用医疗付费方式构成

Figure 8-3-55　Composition of medical payment methods for hospitalization expenses of children with brain tumor in Jilin in 2017-2018

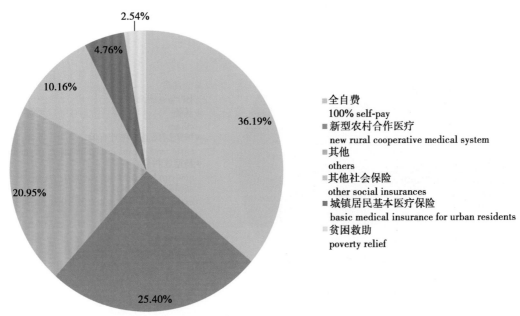

图 8-3-56　2017—2018 年黑龙江脑瘤患儿住院费用医疗付费方式构成

Figure 8-3-56　Composition of medical payment methods for hospitalization expenses of children with brain tumor in Heilongjiang in 2017-2018

265

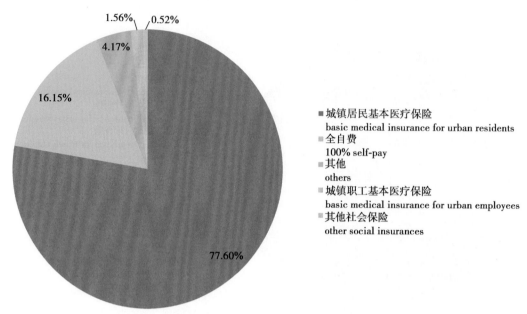

图 8-3-57 2017—2018 年上海脑瘤患儿住院费用医疗付费方式构成

Figure 8-3-57 Composition of medical payment methods for hospitalization expenses of children with brain tumor in Shanghai in 2017-2018

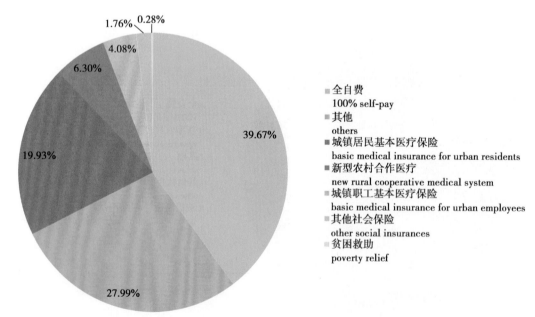

图 8-3-58 2017—2018 年江苏脑瘤患儿住院费用医疗付费方式构成

Figure 8-3-58 Composition of medical payment methods for hospitalization expenses of children with brain tumor in Jiangsu in 2017-2018

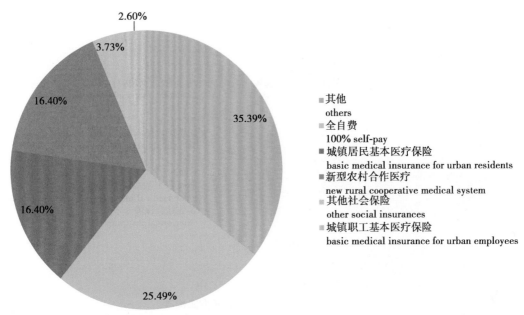

图 8-3-59　2017—2018 年浙江脑瘤患儿住院费用医疗付费方式构成

Figure 8-3-59　Composition of medical payment methods for hospitalization expenses of children with brain tumor in Zhejiang in 2017-2018

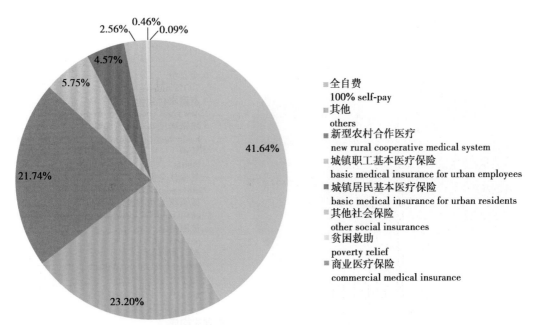

图 8-3-60　2017—2018 年安徽脑瘤患儿住院费用医疗付费方式构成

Figure 8-3-60　Composition of medical payment methods for hospitalization expenses of children with brain tumor in Anhui in 2017-2018

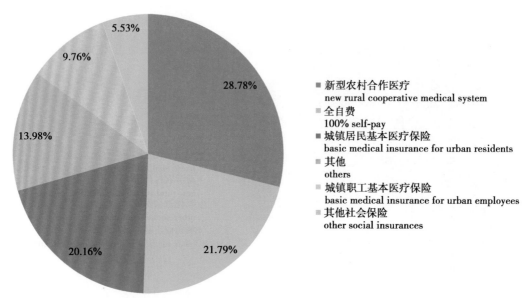

图 8-3-61　2017—2018 年福建脑瘤患儿住院费用医疗付费方式构成

Figure 8-3-61　Composition of medical payment methods for hospitalization expenses of children with brain tumor in Fujian in 2017-2018

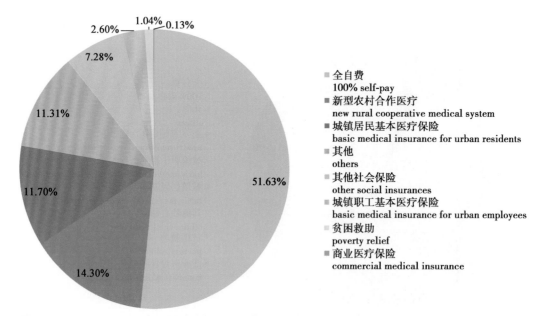

图 8-3-62　2017—2018 年江西脑瘤患儿住院费用医疗付费方式构成

Figure 8-3-62　Composition of medical payment methods for hospitalization expenses of children with brain tumor in Jiangxi in 2017-2018

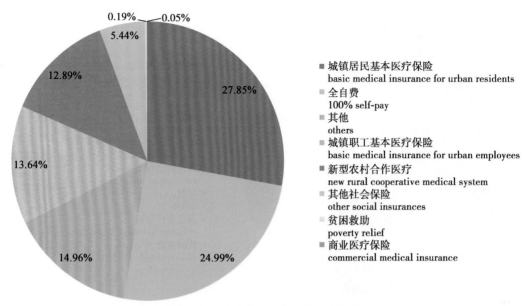

图 8-3-63　2017—2018 年山东脑瘤患儿住院费用医疗付费方式构成

Figure 8-3-63　Composition of medical payment methods for hospitalization expenses of children with brain tumor in Shandong in 2017-2018

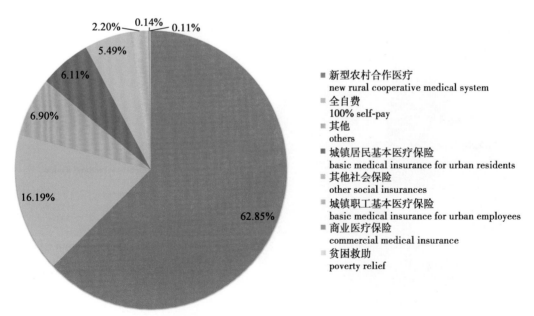

图 8-3-64　2017—2018 年河南脑瘤患儿住院费用医疗付费方式构成

Figure 8-3-64　Composition of medical payment methods for hospitalization expenses of children with brain tumor in Henan in 2017-2018

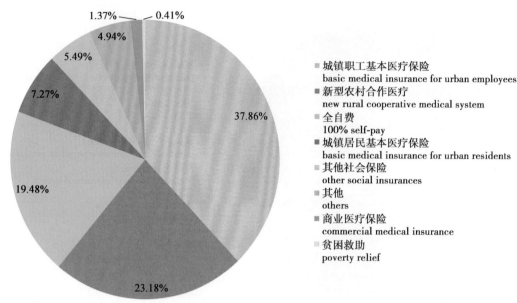

图 8-3-65　2017—2018 年湖北脑瘤患儿住院费用医疗付费方式构成

Figure 8-3-65　Composition of medical payment methods for hospitalization expenses of children with brain tumor in Hubei in 2017-2018

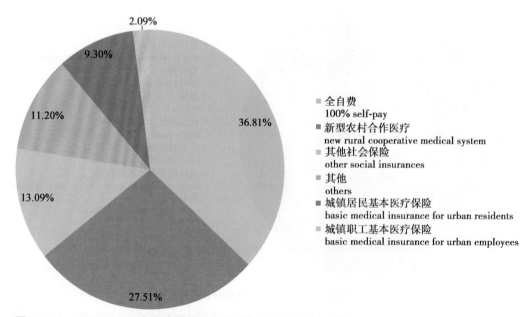

图 8-3-66　2017—2018 年湖南脑瘤患儿住院费用医疗付费方式构成

Figure 8-3-66　Composition of medical payment methods for hospitalization expenses of children with brain tumor in Hunan in 2017-2018

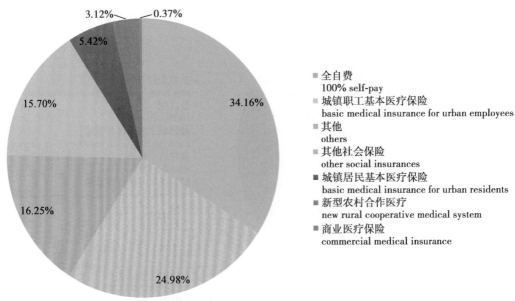

图 8-3-67　2017—2018 年广东脑瘤患儿住院费用医疗付费方式构成

Figure 8-3-67　Composition of medical payment methods for hospitalization expenses of children with brain tumor in Guangdong in 2017-2018

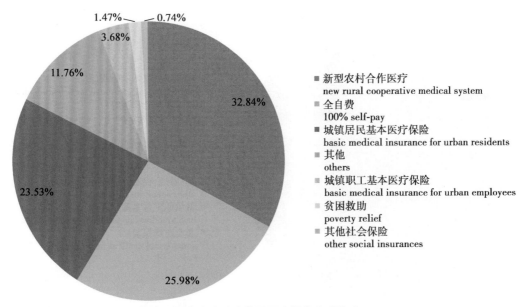

图 8-3-68　2017—2018 年广西脑瘤患儿住院费用医疗付费方式构成

Figure 8-3-68　Composition of medical payment methods for hospitalization expenses of children with brain tumor in Guangxi in 2017-2018

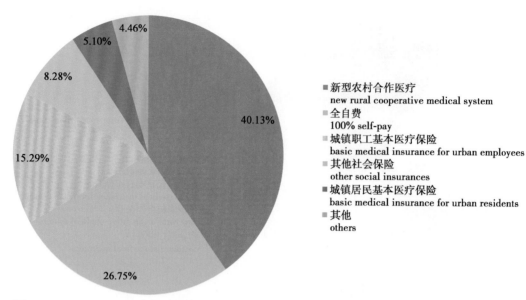

图 8-3-69　2017—2018 年海南脑瘤患儿住院费用医疗付费方式构成

Figure 8-3-69　Composition of medical payment methods for hospitalization expenses of children with brain tumor in Hainan in 2017-2018

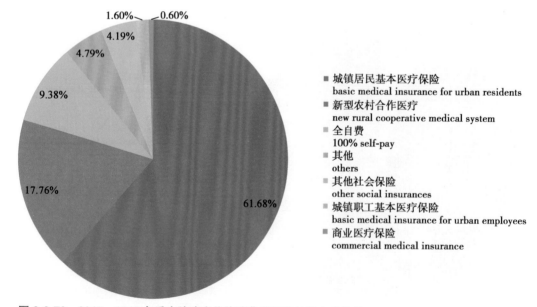

图 8-3-70　2017—2018 年重庆脑瘤患儿住院费用医疗付费方式构成

Figure 8-3-70　Composition of medical payment methods for hospitalization expenses of children with brain tumor in Chongqing in 2017-2018

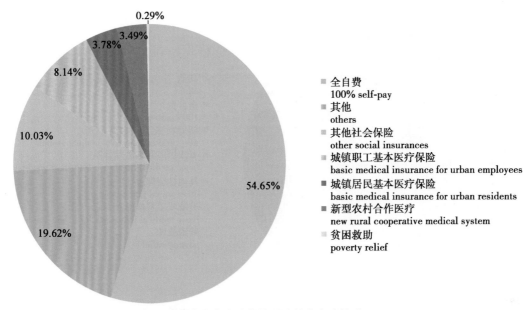

图 8-3-71　2017—2018 年四川脑瘤患儿住院费用医疗付费方式构成

Figure 8-3-71　Composition of medical payment methods for hospitalization expenses of children with brain tumor in Sichuan in 2017-2018

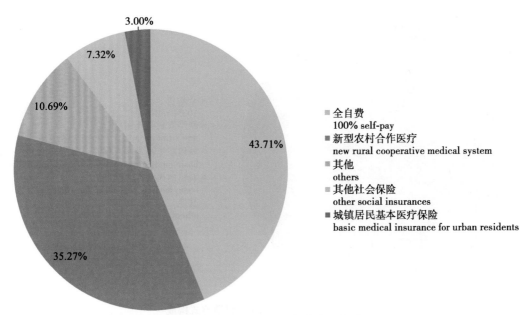

图 8-3-72　2017—2018 年贵州脑瘤患儿住院费用医疗付费方式构成

Figure 8-3-72　Composition of medical payment methods for hospitalization expenses of children with brain tumor in Guizhou in 2017-2018

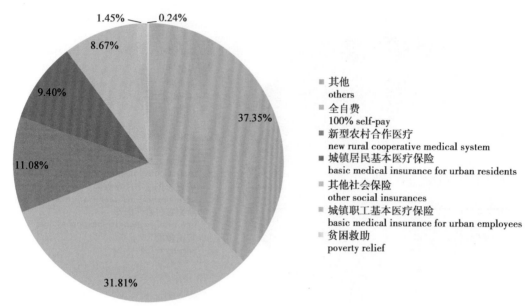

图 8-3-73　2017—2018 年云南脑瘤患儿住院费用医疗付费方式构成

Figure 8-3-73　Composition of medical payment methods for hospitalization expenses of children with brain tumor in Yunnan in 2017-2018

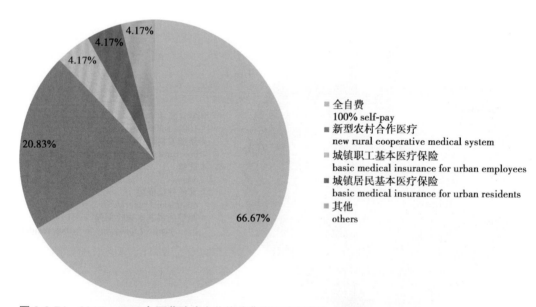

图 8-3-74　2017—2018 年西藏脑瘤患儿住院费用医疗付费方式构成

Figure 8-3-74　Composition of medical payment methods for hospitalization expenses of children with brain tumor in Xizang in 2017-2018

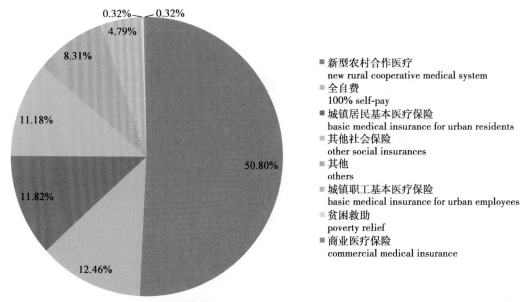

图 8-3-75   2017—2018 年陕西脑瘤患儿住院费用医疗付费方式构成

Figure 8-3-75   Composition of medical payment methods for hospitalization expenses of children with brain tumor in Shaanxi in 2017-2018

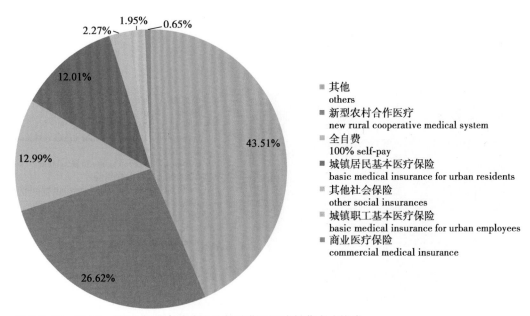

图 8-3-76   2017—2018 年甘肃脑瘤患儿住院费用医疗付费方式构成

Figure 8-3-76   Composition of medical payment methods for hospitalization expenses of children with brain tumor in Gansu in 2017-2018

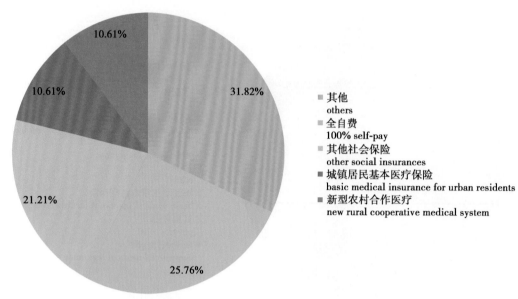

图 8-3-77　2017—2018 年青海脑瘤患儿住院费用医疗付费方式构成

Figure 8-3-77　Composition of medical payment methods for hospitalization expenses of children with brain tumor in Qinghai in 2017-2018

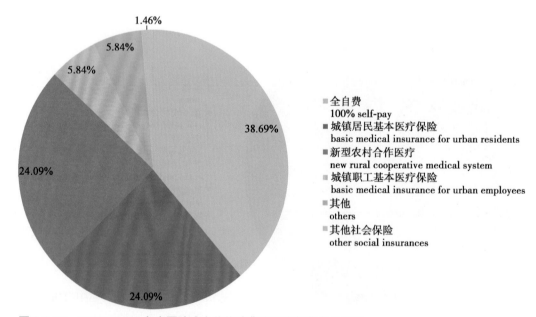

图 8-3-78　2017—2018 年宁夏脑瘤患儿住院费用医疗付费方式构成

Figure 8-3-78　Composition of medical payment methods for hospitalization expenses of children with brain tumor in Ningxia in 2017-2018

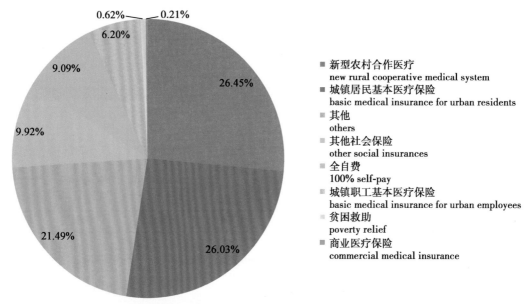

新型农村合作医疗
new rural cooperative medical system
城镇居民基本医疗保险
basic medical insurance for urban residents
其他
others
其他社会保险
other social insurances
全自费
100% self-pay
城镇职工基本医疗保险
basic medical insurance for urban employees
贫困救助
poverty relief
商业医疗保险
commercial medical insurance

图 8-3-79　2017—2018 年新疆脑瘤患儿住院费用医疗付费方式构成

Figure 8-3-79　Composition of medical payment methods for hospitalization expenses of children with brain tumor in Xinjiang in 2017-2018

3.5　全国儿童肿瘤监测机构脑瘤患儿住院费用分析

3.5.1　全国儿童肿瘤监测机构脑瘤患儿次均住院费用情况

3.5.1.1　全国及六大区脑瘤患儿次均住院费用情况　全国脑瘤患儿次均住院费用（中位数）为 12 721.42 元。高于全国中位数水平的地区分别为西北地区（16 631.01 元）、西南地区（15 346.08 元）、中南地区（14 440.74 元）和东北地区（13 603.92 元），低于全国中位数水平的地区分别为华北地区（11 360.16 元）和华东地区（11 867.26 元）（图 8-3-80）。

3.5　Analysis of hospitalization expenses of children with brain tumor in pediatric cancer surveillance sites in China

3.5.1　Expenses per hospitalization of children with brain tumor in pediatric cancer surveillance sites in China

3.5.1.1　Expenses per hospitalization of children with brain tumor in the six regions and the whole country　Nationally, the median expenses per hospitalization was 12, 721.42 CNY. The regions above the national median were Northwest China (16, 631.01 CNY), Southwest China (15, 346.08 CNY), Central and Southern China (14, 440.74 CNY) and Northeast China (13, 603.92 CNY), while those below the national median were North China (11, 360.16 CNY) and East China (11, 867.26 CNY) (Figure 8-3-80).

277

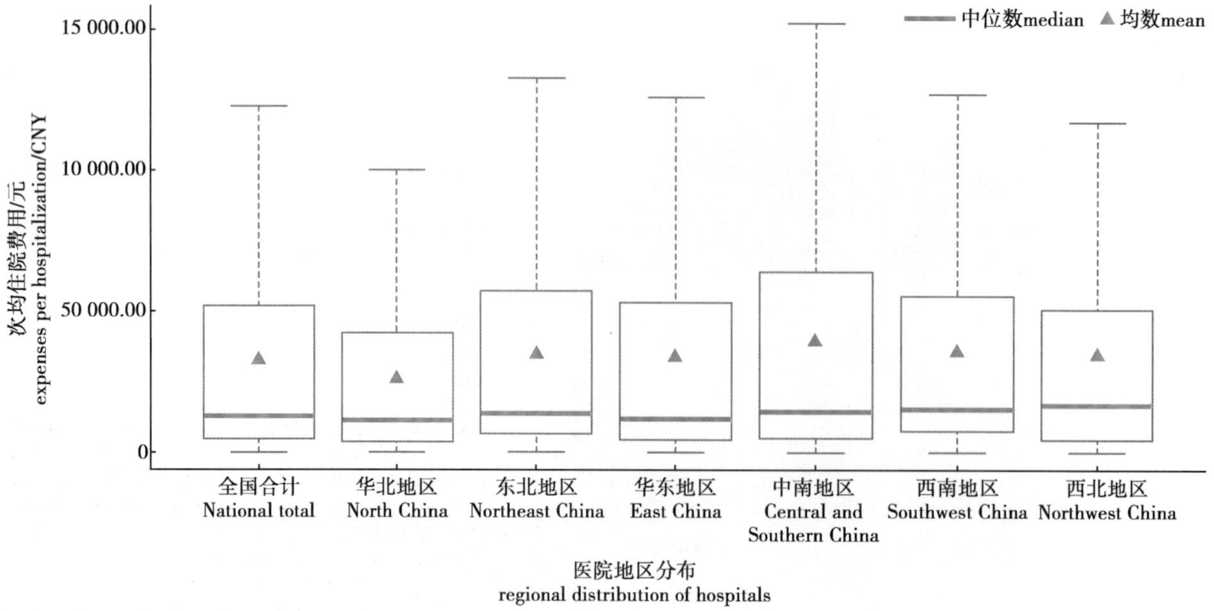

图 8-3-80　2017—2018 年全国及六大区脑瘤患儿次均住院费用

Figure 8-3-80　Expenses per hospitalization of children with brain tumor in the six regions and the whole country in 2017-2018

3.5.1.2　各省份脑瘤患儿次均住院费用情况　根据脑瘤患儿次均住院费用(中位数),前 3 位的省份分别为河北(38 942.96 元)、云南(34 004.78 元)和陕西(31 032.51 元),后 3 位分别为宁夏(4 384.53 元)、西藏(7 354.55 元)和江苏(7 781.26 元)(图 8-3-81)。

3.5.2　全国儿童肿瘤监测机构脑瘤患儿次均住院分项费用情况

3.5.2.1　全国及六大区脑瘤患儿次均住院分项费用情况　根据全国脑瘤患儿次均住院分项费用(中位数),前 3 位分别为诊断类费用(2 156.00 元)、西药类费用(2 059.35 元)和综合医疗服务类费用(1 517.95 元)。六大区分项费用中位数的顺位与全国相比略有不同。如西北地区,次均住院分项费用(中位数)前 3 位分别为治疗类费用(4 761.62 元)、诊断类费用(3 908.95 元)和西药类费用(1 830.78 元)(图 8-3-82)。按均数统计的结果详见图 8-3-83。

3.5.1.2　Expenses per hospitalization of children with brain tumor in each provincial-level region　In terms of the median expenses per hospitalization of children with brain tumor, the top three provincial-level regions were Hebei (38, 942.96 CNY), Yunnan (34, 004.78 CNY) and Shaanxi (31, 032.51 CNY), while the last three were Ningxia (4, 384.53 CNY), Xizang (7, 354.55 CNY) and Jiangsu (7, 781.26 CNY) (Figure 8-3-81).

3.5.2　Expenses of each item per hospitalization of children with brain tumor in pediatric cancer surveillance sites in China

3.5.2.1　Expenses of each item per hospitalization of children with brain tumor in the six regions and the whole country　The top three expenses of each item per hospitalization were for diagnostic expenses (2, 156.00 CNY), western medication expenses (2, 059.35 CNY) and comprehensive medical services expenses (1, 517.95 CNY). The order of regional median for itemized expenses of each item differed slightly from that of the national. For example, in Northwest China, the top three median itemized expenses for each hospitalization were treatment expenses (4, 761.62 CNY), diagnostic expenses (3, 908.95 CNY) and western medication expenses (1, 830.78 CNY)(Figure 8-3-82). Data by the mean expenses in Figure 8-3-83.

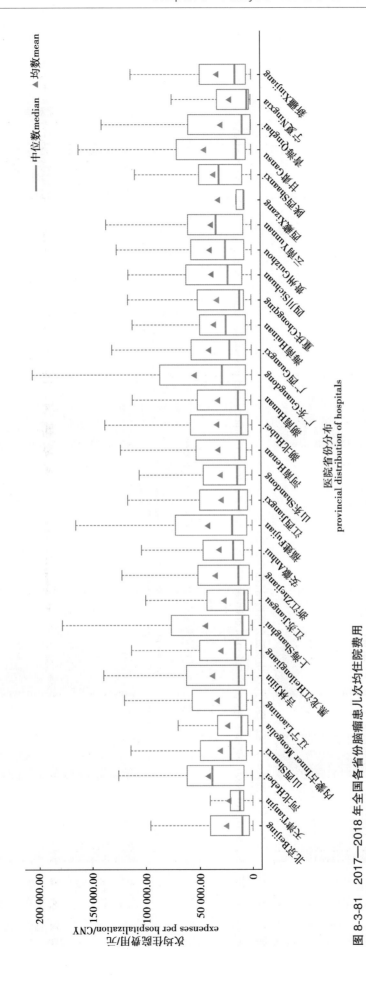

图 8-3-81　2017—2018 年全国各省份脑瘤患儿次均住院费用

Figure 8-3-81　Expenses per hospitalization of children with brain tumor in each provincial-level region in 2017-2018

分项费用/元 expenses of each item/CNY

图像分区分布 regional distribution of hospitals	综合医疗服务类费用 comprehensive medical service expenses	诊断类费用 diagnostic expenses	治疗类费用 treatment expenses	康复类费用 rehabilitation expenses	中医类费用 traditional chinese medicine service expenses	西药类费用 western medication expenses	中药类费用 traditional chinese medication expenses	血液和血液制品类费用 blood and blood product expenses	耗材类费用 medical consumable expenses	其他类费用 others
全国合计 National total	1 517.95	2 156.00	200.00	0	0	2 059.35	0	0	604.27	0
华北地区 North China	1 224.80	1 450.00	0	0	0	1 735.41	0	0	665.53	0
东北地区 Northeast China	1 670.50	2 475.00	464.00	0	0	3 321.12	0	135.00	718.37	36.60
华东地区 East China	1 376.20	2 321.95	394.50	0	0	1 606.21	0	0	491.04	108.00
中南地区 Central and Southern China	1 791.50	3 445.30	815.10	0	0	2 536.07	0	0	864.86	0
西南地区 Southwest China	2 388.41	4 158.11	600.00	0	0	4 084.01	0	0	471.72	9.00
西北地区 Northwest China	1 706.00	3 908.95	4 761.62	0	0	1 830.78	0	0	385.05	8.00

图 8-3-82 2017—2018 年全国及六大区脑瘤患儿次均住院分项费用（按中位数计）

Figure 8-3-82 Expenses of each item per hospitalization of children with brain tumor in the six regions and the whole country in 2017-2018 (by the median)

分项费用/元 expenses of each item/CNY

图像分区分布 regional distribution of hospitals	综合医疗服务类费用 comprehensive medical service expenses	诊断类费用 diagnostic expenses	治疗类费用 treatment expenses	康复类费用 rehabilitation expenses	中医类费用 traditional chinese medicine service expenses	西药类费用 western medication expenses	中药类费用 traditional chinese medication expenses	血液和血液制品类费用 blood and blood product expenses	耗材类费用 medical consumable expenses	其他类费用 others
全国合计 National total	3 727.85	4 440.71	6 053.00	68.91	44.85	5 458.63	225.83	505.45	9 127.45	1 780.57
华北地区 North China	3 129.37	2 604.52	4 776.43	4.04	5.53	4 223.29	243.80	507.90	9 257.46	325.21
东北地区 Northeast China	3 125.13	4 383.72	8 679.11	66.98	8.58	7 280.29	733.84	796.05	8 320.91	1 704.86
华东地区 East China	4 081.13	4 456.82	6 078.97	140.64	72.42	5 300.82	86.50	442.04	9 865.27	2 489.12
中南地区 Central and Southern China	4 119.04	6 559.40	8 184.58	67.46	107.35	6 787.36	331.15	516.87	9 297.31	4 204.53
西南地区 Southwest China	4 538.08	6 567.34	5 081.76	152.70	41.76	7 123.58	171.15	604.68	7 042.16	1 366.86
西北地区 Northwest China	3 761.54	5 925.97	7 288.78	72.31	31.84	6 130.28	191.93	400.79	7 806.76	1 416.08

图 8-3-83 2017—2018 年全国及六大区脑瘤患儿次均住院分项费用（按均数计）

Figure 8-3-83 Expenses of each item per hospitalization of children with brain tumor in the six regions and the whole country in 2017-2018 (by the mean)

3.5.2.2　各省份脑瘤患儿次均住院分项费用情况　根据各省份脑瘤患儿次均住院分项费用(中位数),以诊断类费用为例,前3位的省份依次为广东(6 251.73元)、四川(5 819.00元)和云南(5 632.63元),后3位依次为河南(849.90元)、北京(1 247.00元)和宁夏(1 261.50元)(图8-3-84)。按均数统计的结果详见图8-3-85。

3.6　全国儿童肿瘤监测机构脑瘤患儿平均住院日分析

3.6.1　全国及六大区脑瘤患儿平均住院日情况

全国脑瘤患儿平均住院日的中位数为8天。高于全国中位数水平的地区分别为西北地区(14天)、西南地区(11天)、东北地区(10天)、中南地区(10天)和华东地区(9天),低于全国中位数水平的地区为华北地区(5天)(图8-3-86)。

3.5.2.2　Expenses of each item per hospitalization of children with brain tumor in each provincial-level region　In terms of the median expenses of each item per hospitalization of children with brain tumor in each provincial-level region, taking diagnostic expenses as an example, the top three provincial-level regions were Guangdong (6, 251.73 CNY), Sichuan (5, 819.00 CNY) and Yunnan (5, 632.63 CNY). The last three were Henan (849.90 CNY), Beijing (1, 247.00 CNY) and Ningxia (1, 261.50 CNY) (Figure 8-3-84). Data by the mean expenses in Figure 8-3-85.

3.6　Analysis of the average length of hospitalization of children with brain tumor in pediatric cancer surveillance sites in China

3.6.1　Average length of hospitalization of children with brain tumor in the six regions and the whole country

Nationally, the median of average length of hospitalization was 8 days. Northwest China (14 days), Southwest China (11 days), Northeast China (10 days), Central and Southern China (10 days) and East China (9 days) were above the national median, and North China (5 days) was below the national median (Figure 8-3-86).

医院省份分布 provincial distribution of hospitals	综合医疗服务类费用 comprehensive medical service expenses	诊断类费用 diagnostic expenses	治疗类费用 treatment expenses	康复类费用 rehabilitation expenses	中医类费用 traditional chinese medicine service expenses	西药类费用 western medication expenses	中药类费用 traditional chinese medication expenses	血液和血液制品类费用 blood and blood product expenses	耗材类费用 medical consumable expenses	其他类费用 others
北京Beijing	1 120.50	1 247.00		0	0	1 664.85	27.93	0	642.59	0
天津Tianjin	4 142.50	4 698.50	464.00	0	0	644.45	0	29.00	630.13	544.04
河北Hebei	2 903.60	4 207.00	3 249.20	0	0	4 603.85	0	159.00	1 693.33	425.96
山西Shanxi	2 472.40	3 498.20	3 469.50	0	0	3 028.34	0	0	1 229.10	9.50
内蒙古Inner Mongolia	665.00	1 719.00	20.00	0	0	2 183.71	0	0	101.26	185.00
辽宁Liaoning	1 396.90	1 916.20	6 965.48	0	0	3 429.94	0	245.00	314.64	1 390.40
吉林Jilin	2 008.50	3 111.50	163.00	0	0	3 093.09	0	125.00	915.05	0
黑龙江Heilongjiang	1 620.40	1 556.50	60.00	0	0	4 418.46	0	0	936.95	136.00
上海Shanghai	2 126.00	2 057.00	100.00	0	0	1 475.10	0	0	1 154.04	0
江苏Jiangsu	838.00	2 204.50	544.70	9.00	0	1 530.42	0	115.00	479.00	168.00
浙江Zhejiang	1 581.35	2 195.01	542.50	22.00	0	1 790.15	0	0	638.66	0
安徽Anhui	1 661.00	2 520.20	283.50	0	0	4 482.36	0	0	152.90	153.30
福建Fujian	3 639.00	4 903.00	4 609.00	0	0	2 499.64	0	0	209.24	0
江西Jiangxi	1 437.00	2 297.00	2 645.50	0	0	3 519.08	0	0	376.62	120.00
山东Shandong	1 219.00	2 161.00	90.00	0	0	831.60	0	0	450.06	488.15
河南Henan	1 186.90	849.90	110.00	0	0	3 516.73	0	0	185.57	0
湖北Hubei	1 138.50	2 749.25	134.00	0	0	2 811.66	0	0	267.92	0
湖南Hunan	2 047.74	3 732.00	299.50	0	0	1 172.41	0	0	751.43	115.78
广东Guangdong	2 593.15	6 251.73	6 720.98	0	0	2 355.18	0	0	2 592.64	0
广西Guangxi	2 235.40	4 032.50	4 451.90	0	0	3 844.11	0	0	1 227.81	0
海南Hainan	2 333.40	3 661.76	5 720.00	0	0	1 987.21	0	0	1 472.90	0
重庆Chongqing	2 125.15	3 239.70	0	24.00	0	4 293.26	0	0	364.91	9.00
四川Sichuan	2 687.10	5 819.00	1 800.00	0	0	1 667.83	0	0	1 007.76	6.00
贵州Guizhou	2 525.53	4 420.50	3 048.00	0	0	3 131.74	0	95.00	157.56	65.20
云南Yunnan	4 157.03	5 632.63	4 480.00	120.00	0	5 795.88	0	230.00	5 979.48	0.05
西藏Xizang	2 426.00	1 389.50	–	100.00	–	3 217.22	0	–	–	270.02
陕西Shaanxi	3 666.90	5 147.50	7 695.00	0	0	5 364.27	0	0	2 456.96	0
甘肃Gansu	1 596.00	4 525.50	915.00	0	0	1 764.38	0	0	878.40	0
青海Qinghai	645.00	1 642.00	4 589.45	0	0	902.95	41.80	0	64.63	0
宁夏Ningxia	836.30	1 261.50	1 057.70	8.00	0	688.50	0	306.70	340.45	15.75
新疆Xinjiang	1 628.75	3 589.50	3 623.88	0	0	1 889.76	0	0	173.92	44.00

分项费用/元 expenses of each item/CNY

图 8-3-84 2017—2018 年全国各省份脑瘤患儿次均住院分项费用（按中位数计）

Figure 8-3-84 Expenses of each item per hospitalization of children with brain tumor in each provincial-level region in 2017-2018 (by the median)

provincial distribution of hospitals	综合医疗服务费用 comprehensive medical service expenses	诊断类费用 diagnostic expenses	治疗类费用 treatment expenses	康复类费用 rehabilitation expenses	中医类费用 traditional chinese medicine service expenses	西药类费用 western medication expenses	中药类费用 traditional chinese medication expenses	血液和血液制品类费用 blood and blood product expenses	耗材类费用 medical consumable expenses	其他类费用 others
北京Beijing	2 913.16	2 201.01	4 637.67	1.98	0.19	3 927.71	227.90	494.75	9 714.68	171.54
天津Tianjin	6 295.66	5 514.58	2 490.46	0	1.45	2 374.59	261.14	320.95	2 858.39	779.03
河北Hebei	4 595.34	6 164.45	6 193.12	14.00	55.39	8 998.09	36.84	1 044.72	9 504.85	3 142.52
山西Shanxi	3 798.03	4 961.96	8 373.00	42.27	41.00	6 230.88	196.00	468.94	5 672.63	380.01
内蒙古Inner Mongolia	2 794.04	2 854.27	4 073.89	38.40	284.25	5 077.28	186.52	412.69	1 472.33	1 131.24
辽宁Liaoning	2 596.03	4 002.12	11 508.57	178.12	4.31	6 119.08	40.52	697.22	8 055.04	3 792.91
吉林Jilin	3 792.08	5 273.52	6 871.20	42.07	11.97	8 715.41	111.59	938.11	9 038.56	373.30
黑龙江Heilongjiang	2 923.54	2 932.60	7 572.99	0	0	6 804.22	120.43	459.66	7 040.29	706.65
上海Shanghai	5 787.04	6 047.05	4 131.50	266.20	188.25	6 331.65	122.94	211.45	17 787.71	1 318.67
江苏Jiangsu	2 102.54	3 847.76	5 076.33	232.92	51.10	4 174.12	228.86	787.97	9 022.85	1 371.68
浙江Zhejiang	3 724.83	4 677.74	8 385.32	74.04	42.08	5 492.78	517.63	873.88	9 265.05	833.63
安徽Anhui	3 106.28	4 257.29	5 038.38	243.72	84.10	7 387.77	374.06	974.84	5 877.56	498.52
福建Fujian	11 731.50	6 570.32	8 564.94	39.87	33.54	6 132.42	1 616.04	317.14	7 510.68	1 078.47
江西Jiangxi	3 080.24	3 261.33	8 571.81	297.93	53.08	7 709.89	1 036.87	212.01	5 701.34	549.94
山东Shandong	2 871.87	3 464.62	6 362.73	13.70	11.18	4 046.74	70.30	301.41	7 406.65	5 652.93
河南Henan	2 735.53	2 784.87	4 562.72	68.86	533.95	7 209.06	540.95	279.89	4 918.04	1 052.97
湖北Hubei	2 604.80	5 769.08	7 063.25	6.23	7.89	6 851.46	124.50	392.12	5 269.50	2 761.40
湖南Hunan	4 932.76	6 005.97	3 945.01	79.22	36.31	4 200.15	328.38	151.73	9 797.30	1 006.06
广东Guangdong	5 289.78	8 922.06	10 248.44	100.33	28.09	6 800.51	52.48	769.76	12 152.97	7 132.98
广西Guangxi	4 153.67	6 846.10	7 833.91	38.18	38.65	8 338.37	11.97	247.16	9 014.01	184.69
海南Hainan	3 825.63	4 857.66	9 536.20	0	602.86	6 480.05	69.53	287.57	7 654.76	1 890.74
重庆Chongqing	4 435.94	6 484.39	4 126.95	102.91	47.69	6 704.28	105.00	458.20	5 635.33	46.79
四川Sichuan	4 787.57	7 593.94	8 409.43	175.81	12.28	5 228.42	10.72	945.25	8 570.26	145.15
贵州Guizhou	4 119.41	6 429.42	5 391.73	23.38	19.64	7 031.03	14.37	742.61	5 856.24	6 789.62
云南Yunnan	4 844.49	6 241.07	5 311.89	545.11	76.87	9 325.14	61.34	737.02	10 709.10	376.45
西藏Xizang	9 807.25	7 395.44	-	291.25	-	10 427.97	11.40	-	-	2 839.32
陕西Shaanxi	4 655.10	6 472.65	6 984.65	20.28	42.17	7 056.51	281.95	269.79	9 378.41	40.60
甘肃Gansu	5 365.57	7 551.74	6 442.11	113.21	3.89	8 166.91	797.31	797.31	10 435.51	372.15
青海Qinghai	2 073.88	4 861.86	7 854.12	25.56		8 515.07	691.75	339.33	8 316.17	256.61
宁夏Ningxia	1 966.86	3 879.46	6 651.60	637.92	142.09	2 736.27	24.14	1 300.63	5 960.96	25.45
新疆Xinjiang	3 268.28	5 649.12	7 891.89	29.42	34.45	5 687.72	72.97	157.05	6 454.97	2 631.15

图 8-3-85　2017—2018 年全国各省份协脑瘤患儿次均住院分项费用（按均数计）

Figure 8-3-85　Expenses of each item per hospitalization of children with brain tumor in each provincial-level region in 2017-2018 (by the mean)

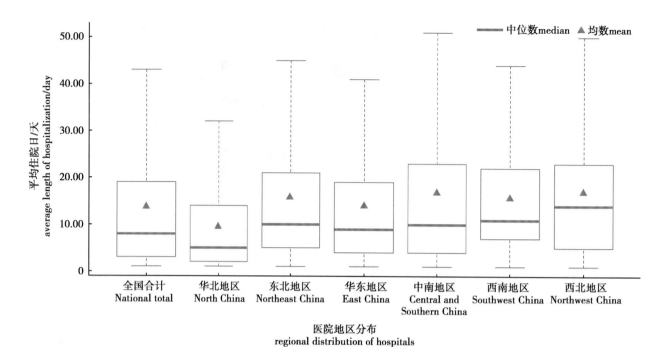

图 8-3-86　2017—2018 年全国及六大区脑瘤患儿平均住院日

Figure 8-3-86　Average length of hospitalization of children with brain tumor in the six regions and the whole countryin 2017-2018

3.6.2　各省份脑瘤患儿平均住院日情况

根据各省份脑瘤患儿平均住院日的中位数,脑瘤患儿平均住院日最长的省份是云南(20 天),其次是河北(19 天)、陕西(18 天)和四川(16 天),最短的是北京(4 天)(图 8-3-87)。

3.6.2　Average length of hospitalization of children with brain tumor in each provincial-level region

In terms of the median of average length of hospitalization of children with brain tumor in each provincial-level region, the provincial-level region with the longest average hospital stay was Yunnan (20 days), followed by Hebei (19 days), Shaanxi (18 days) and Sichuan (16 days), and the shortest was Beijing (4 days) (Figure 8-3-87).

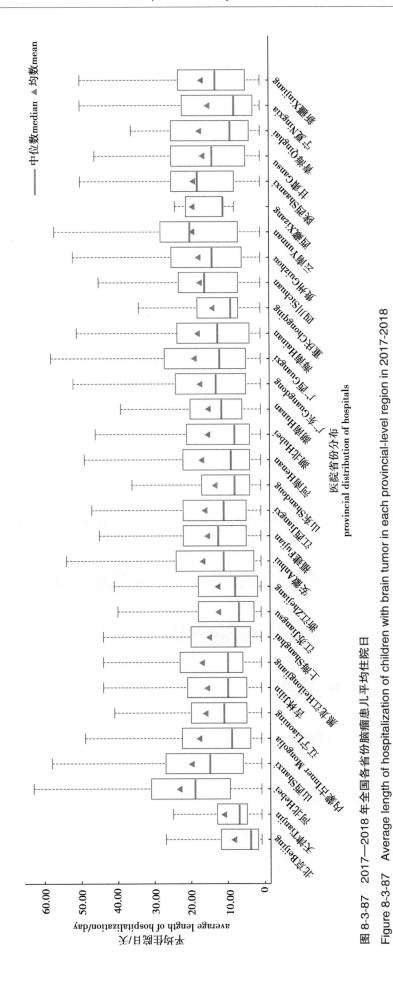

图 8-3-87   2017—2018 年全国各省份脑瘤患儿平均住院日

Figure 8-3-87   Average length of hospitalization of children with brain tumor in each provincial-level region in 2017-2018

4 骨肿瘤

4.1 全国儿童肿瘤监测机构骨肿瘤患儿出院人次分析

4.1.1 六大区骨肿瘤患儿出院人次构成情况

在骨肿瘤患儿出院人次中,各大区出院人次占全部出院人次的比例由高到低依次为华北地区(35.65%)、中南地区(28.64%)、华东地区(17.15%)、东北地区(7.16%)、西南地区(6.46%)和西北地区(4.94%)(图 8-4-1)。

4 Bone cancer

4.1 Analysis of discharges among children with bone cancer in pediatric cancer surveillance sites in China

4.1.1 Composition of discharges among children with bone cancer in the six regions

In terms of the discharges among children with bone cancer, the regions with the highest to the lowest proportions of discharges among children with bone cancer in all discharges were North China (35.65%), Central and Southern China (28.64%), East China (17.15%), Northeast China (7.16%), Southwest China (6.46%) and Northwest China (4.94%) (Figure 8-4-1).

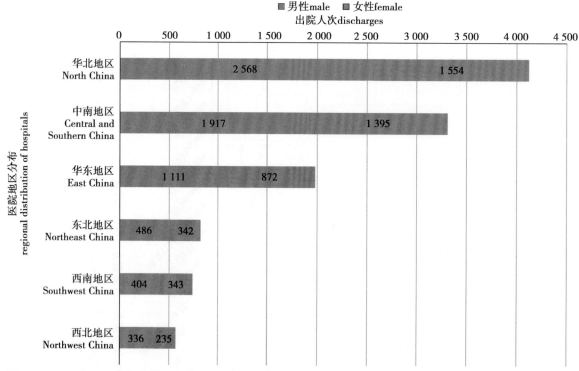

图 8-4-1　2017—2018 年全国六大区儿童肿瘤监测机构骨肿瘤出院人次构成

Figure 8-4-1　Composition of discharges among children with bone cancer in pediatric cancer surveillance sites in the six regions in 2017-2018

4.1.2　各省份骨肿瘤患儿出院人次构成情况

在所有省份中,骨肿瘤患儿出院人次占全部出院人次比例前 3 位的省份分别为北京(29.93%)、河南(12.17%)和山东(7.13%),后 3 位分别为西藏(0.05%)、青海(0.20%)和海南(0.22%)(图 8-4-2,图 8-4-3)。

4.1.2　Composition of discharges among children with bone cancer in each provincial-level region

Among all provincial-level regions, Beijing (29.93%), Henan (12.17%) and Shandong (7.13%) were the three provincial-level regions with the highest proportions of discharges among children with bone cancer in all discharges, and Xizang (0.05%), Qinghai (0.20%) and Hainan (0.22%) had the lowest proportions of discharges among children with bone cancer (Figure 8-4-2~Figure 8-4-3).

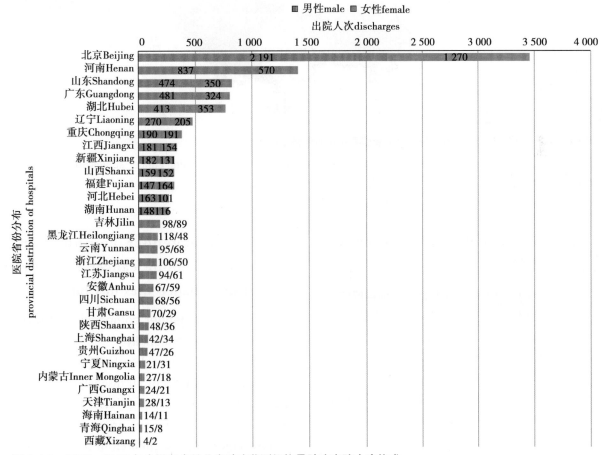

图 8-4-2　2017—2018 年全国各省份儿童肿瘤监测机构骨肿瘤出院人次构成

Figure 8-4-2　Composition of discharges among children with bone cancer in pediatric cancer surveillance sites in each provincial-level region in 2017-2018

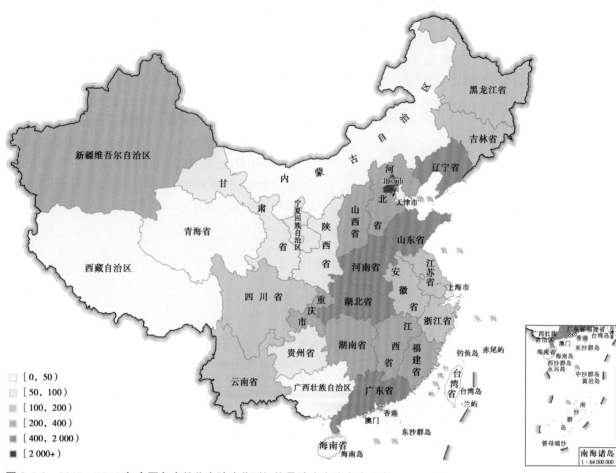

图 8-4-3 2017—2018 年全国各省份儿童肿瘤监测机构骨肿瘤出院人次分布

Figure 8-4-3 Distribution of discharges among children with bone cancer in pediatric cancer surveillance sites in each provincial-level region in 2017-2018

4.2　全国儿童肿瘤监测机构骨肿瘤患儿年龄/性别构成

4.2.1　全国骨肿瘤患儿年龄/性别构成情况

从性别分布来看,男性患儿占全部出院人次比例为 59.00%,女性患儿为 41.00%;除 3 岁、8 岁和 11 岁年龄组外,其他年龄段的男性患儿出院人次比例均高于女性患儿。从年龄分布来看,15 岁年龄组所占比例最高(9.61%),其次为 14 岁(9.39%)和 13 岁(8.83%)年龄组(图 8-4-4)。

4.2　Age/gender composition of children with bone cancer in pediatric cancer surveillance sites in China

4.2.1　Age/gender composition of children with bone cancer nationally

In terms of gender distribution, male children accounted for 59.00% of all discharges, and female for 41.00%; Except for the 3-year age group, 8-year age group, and 11-year age group, the proportions of discharges of male children in other age groups were higher than those of females. In terms of age distribution, the 15-year age group had the highest proportion (9.61%), followed by the 14-year age group (9.39%) and 13-year age group (8.83%)(Figure 8-4-4).

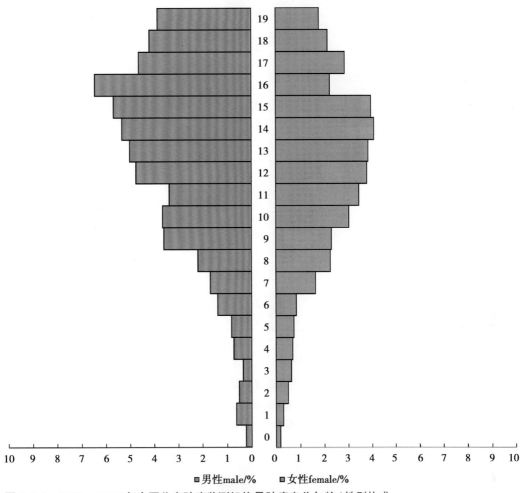

图 8-4-4　2017—2018 年全国儿童肿瘤监测机构骨肿瘤患儿年龄 / 性别构成

Figure 8-4-4　Age/gender composition of children with bone cancer in pediatric cancer surveillance sites in China in 2017-2018

4.2.2　六大区骨肿瘤患儿年龄 / 性别构成情况

从性别分布来看,六大区均显示男性患儿占全部出院人次比例高于女性患儿。从年龄分布来看,六大区的比例各有不同,其中华北地区、中南地区和西北地区的 15 岁年龄组所占比例最高;东北地区的 12 岁年龄组所占比例最高;华东地区的 16 岁年龄组所占比例最高;西南地区的 14 岁年龄组所占比例最高(图 8-4-5~ 图 8-4-10)。

4.2.2　Age/gender composition of children with bone cancer in the six regions

In terms of gender distribution, male children accounted for a higher proportion of all discharges than female in all the six regions. In terms of age distribution, the proportions of the six regions were different, among which the proportions of the 15-year age group in North China, Central and Southern China and Northwest China were the highest. The proportions of 12-year age group in Northeast were the highest. The proportions of 16-year age group in East China were the highest. The proportions of 14-year age group in Southwest China were the highest (Figure 8-4-5~Figure 8-4-10).

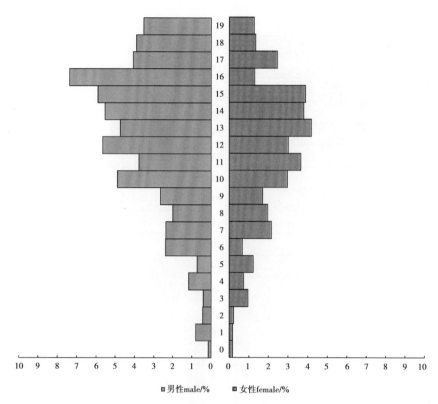

图 8-4-5 2017—2018 年华北地区儿童肿瘤监测机构骨肿瘤患儿年龄／性别构成

Figure 8-4-5 Age/gender composition of children with bone cancer in pediatric cancer surveillance sites in North China in 2017-2018

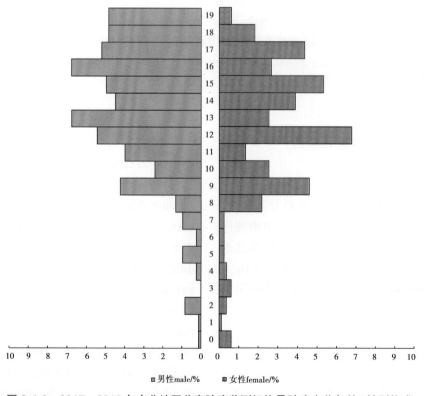

图 8-4-6 2017—2018 年东北地区儿童肿瘤监测机构骨肿瘤患儿年龄／性别构成

Figure 8-4-6 Age/gender composition of children with bone cancer in pediatric cancer surveillance sites in Northeast China in 2017-2018

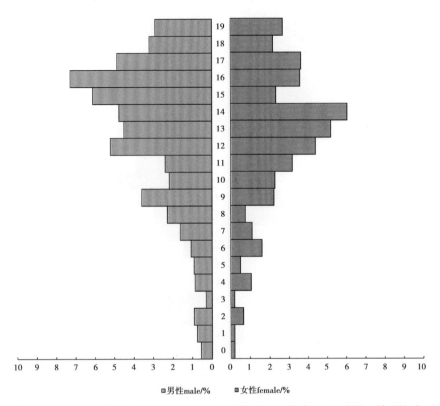

图 8-4-7　2017—2018 年华东地区儿童肿瘤监测机构骨肿瘤患儿年龄 / 性别构成

Figure 8-4-7　Age/gender composition of children with bone cancer in pediatric cancer surveillance sites in East China in 2017-2018

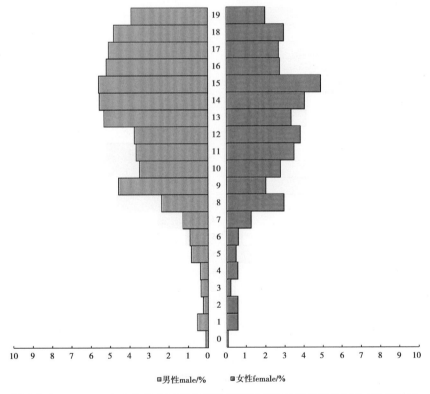

图 8-4-8　2017—2018 年中南地区儿童肿瘤监测机构骨肿瘤患儿年龄 / 性别构成

Figure 8-4-8　Age/gender composition of children with bone cancer in pediatric cancer surveillance sites in Central and Southern China in 2017-2018

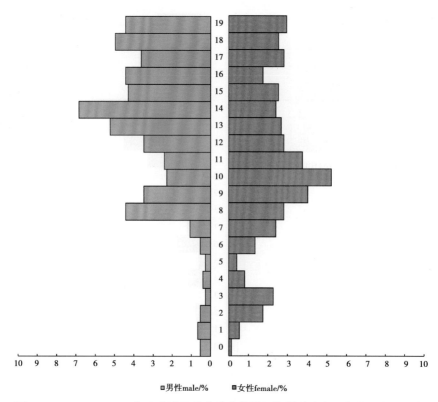

图 8-4-9　2017—2018 年西南地区儿童肿瘤监测机构骨肿瘤患儿年龄／性别构成

Figure 8-4-9　Age/gender composition of children with bone cancer in pediatric cancer surveillance sites in Southwest China in 2017-2018

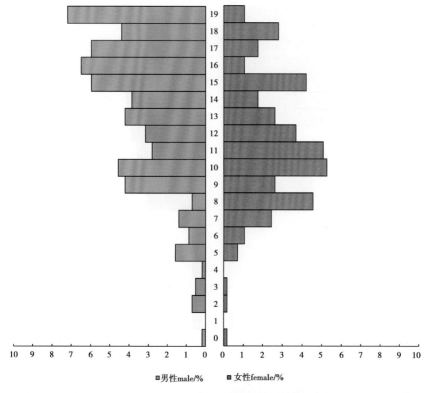

图 8-4-10　2017—2018 年西北地区儿童肿瘤监测机构骨肿瘤患儿年龄／性别构成

Figure 8-4-10　Age/gender composition of children with bone cancer in pediatric cancer surveillance sites in Northwest China in 2017-2018

4.2.3　各省份骨肿瘤患儿年龄/性别构成情况

从性别分布来看,除福建、宁夏、重庆外的其他28个省份出院患儿的性别分布均呈现男性比例高于女性;从年龄分布来看,各省份出院患儿的年龄分布各有不同。以广东为例,从性别分布来看,男性患儿占全部出院人次比例为59.75%,女性为40.25%;从年龄分布来看,15岁年龄组所占比例最高(9.44%),其次为12岁(9.32%)、17岁(8.94%)和18岁(8.94%)年龄组(图8-4-11~图8-4-30)。

4.2.3　Age/gender composition of children with bone cancer in each provincial-level region

In terms of gender distribution, the proportions of discharges among male children were higher than those of female in 28 provincial-level regions except Fujian, Ningxia, and Chongqing. From the perspective of age distribution, each provincial-level region had different distribution for discharges. Taking Guangdong as an example, from the perspective of gender distribution, male children accounted for 59.75% of all discharges, and female accounted for 40.25%. As for age distribution, the 15-year age group had accounted for the highest proportion (9.44%), followed by the 12-year age group (9.32%), 17-year age group (8.94%) and 18-year age group (8.94%)(Figure 8-4-11~Figure 8-4-30).

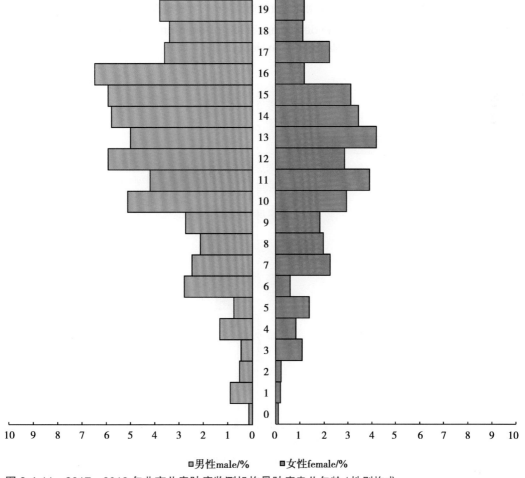

■男性male/%　　■女性female/%

图8-4-11　2017—2018年北京儿童肿瘤监测机构骨肿瘤患儿年龄/性别构成

Figure 8-4-11　Age/gender composition of children with bone cancer in pediatric cancer surveillance sites in Beijing in 2017-2018

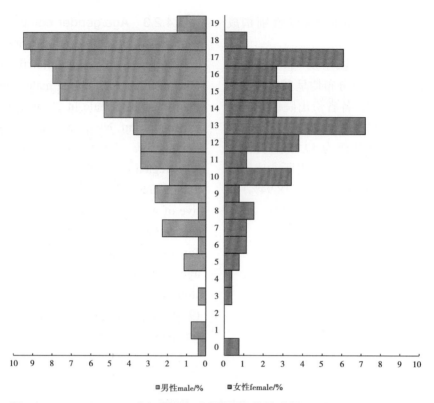

图 8-4-12 2017—2018 年河北儿童肿瘤监测机构骨肿瘤患儿年龄 / 性别构成

Figure 8-4-12 Age/gender composition of children with bone cancer in pediatric cancer surveillance sites in Hebei in 2017-2018

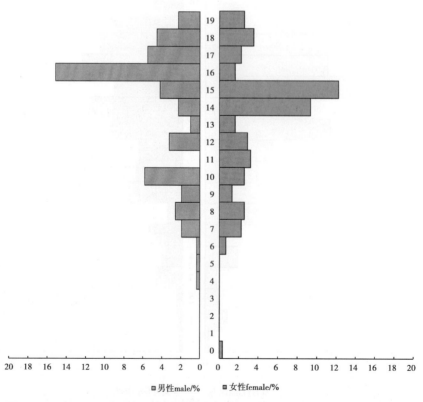

图 8-4-13 2017—2018 年山西儿童肿瘤监测机构骨肿瘤患儿年龄 / 性别构成

Figure 8-4-13 Age/gender composition of children with bone cancer in pediatric cancer surveillance sites in Shanxi in 2017-2018

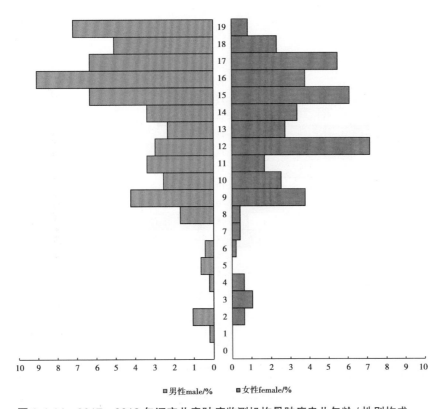

图 8-4-14　2017—2018 年辽宁儿童肿瘤监测机构骨肿瘤患儿年龄／性别构成

Figure 8-4-14　Age/gender composition of children with bone cancer in pediatric cancer surveillance sites in Liaoning in 2017-2018

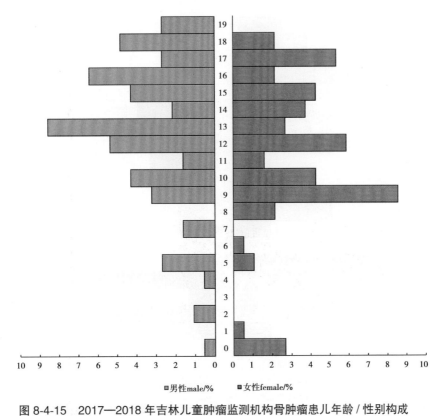

图 8-4-15　2017—2018 年吉林儿童肿瘤监测机构骨肿瘤患儿年龄／性别构成

Figure 8-4-15　Age/gender composition of children with bone cancer in pediatric cancer surveillance sites in Jilin in 2017-2018

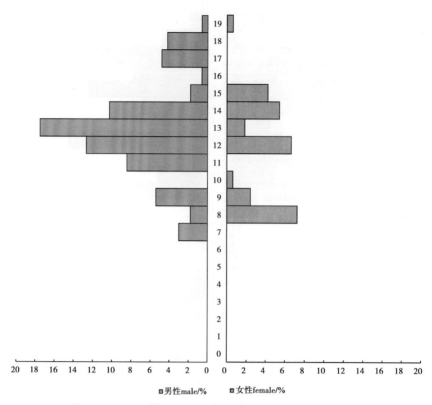

图 8-4-16　2017—2018 年黑龙江儿童肿瘤监测机构骨肿瘤患儿年龄／性别构成

Figure 8-4-16　Age/gender composition of children with bone cancer in pediatric cancer surveillance sites in Heilongjiang in 2017-2018

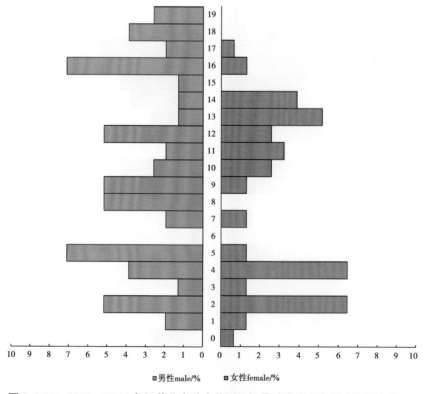

图 8-4-17　2017—2018 年江苏儿童肿瘤监测机构骨肿瘤患儿年龄／性别构成

Figure 8-4-17　Age/gender composition of children with bone cancer in pediatric cancer surveillance sites in Jiangsu in 2017-2018

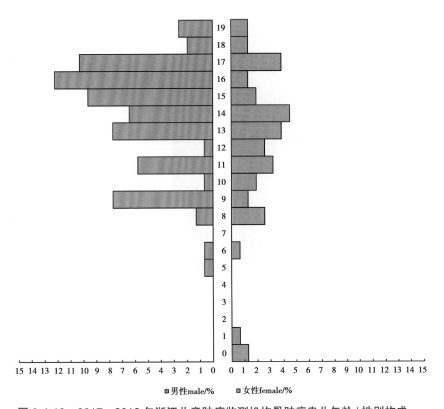

图 8-4-18　2017—2018 年浙江儿童肿瘤监测机构骨肿瘤患儿年龄 / 性别构成

Figure 8-4-18　Age/gender composition of children with bone cancer in pediatric cancer surveillance sites in Zhejiang in 2017-2018

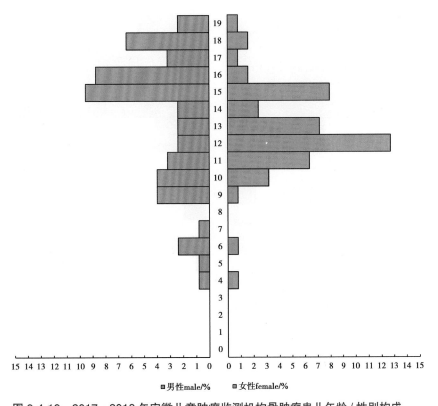

图 8-4-19　2017—2018 年安徽儿童肿瘤监测机构骨肿瘤患儿年龄 / 性别构成

Figure 8-4-19　Age/gender composition of children with bone cancer in pediatric cancer surveillance sites in Anhui in 2017-2018

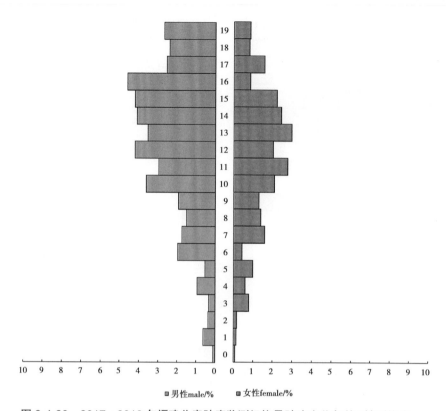

图 8-4-20　2017—2018 年福建儿童肿瘤监测机构骨肿瘤患儿年龄 / 性别构成

Figure 8-4-20　Age/gender composition of children with bone cancer in pediatric cancer surveillance sites in Fujian in 2017-2018

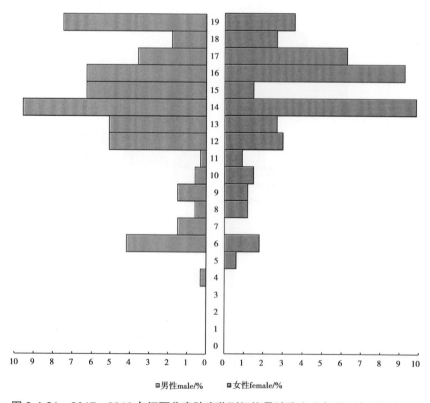

图 8-4-21　2017—2018 年江西儿童肿瘤监测机构骨肿瘤患儿年龄 / 性别构成

Figure 8-4-21　Age/gender composition of children with bone cancer in pediatric cancer surveillance sites in Jiangxi in 2017-2018

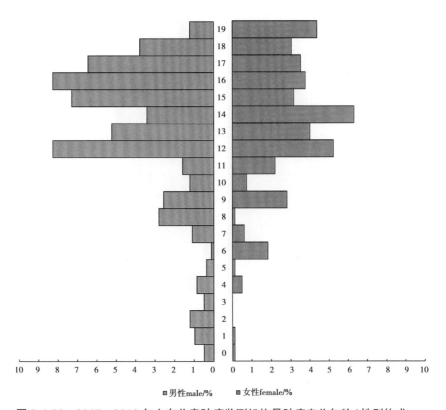

图 8-4-22 2017—2018 年山东儿童肿瘤监测机构骨肿瘤患儿年龄 / 性别构成

Figure 8-4-22 Age/gender composition of children with bone cancer in pediatric cancer surveillance sites in Shandong in 2017-2018

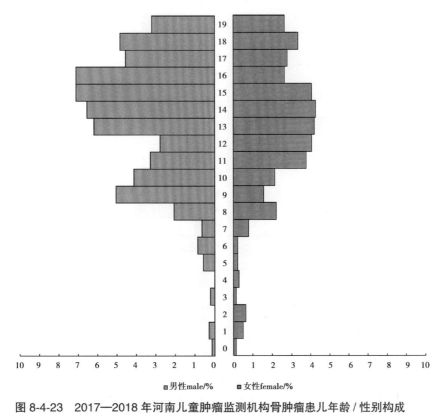

图 8-4-23 2017—2018 年河南儿童肿瘤监测机构骨肿瘤患儿年龄 / 性别构成

Figure 8-4-23 Age/gender composition of children with bone cancer in pediatric cancer surveillance sites in Henan in 2017-2018

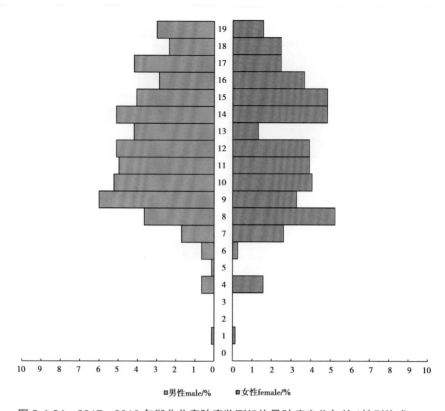

图 8-4-24　2017—2018 年湖北儿童肿瘤监测机构骨肿瘤患儿年龄／性别构成

Figure 8-4-24　Age/gender composition of children with bone cancer in pediatric cancer surveillance sites in Hubei in 2017-2018

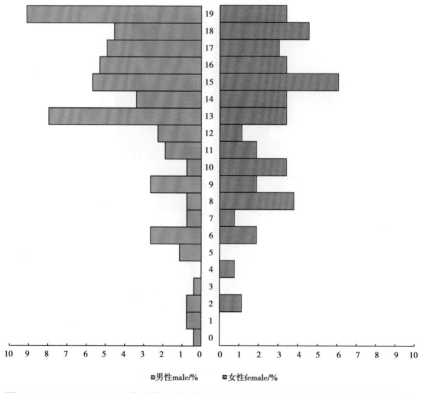

图 8-4-25　2017—2018 年湖南儿童肿瘤监测机构骨肿瘤患儿年龄／性别构成

Figure 8-4-25　Age/gender composition of children with bone cancer in pediatric cancer surveillance sites in Hunan in 2017-2018

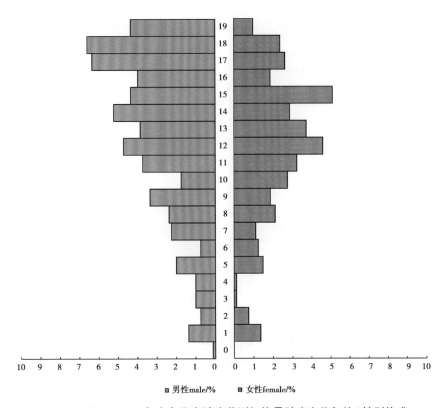

图 8-4-26　2017—2018 年广东儿童肿瘤监测机构骨肿瘤患儿年龄／性别构成

Figure 8-4-26　Age/gender composition of children with bone cancer in pediatric cancer surveillance sites in Guangdong in 2017-2018

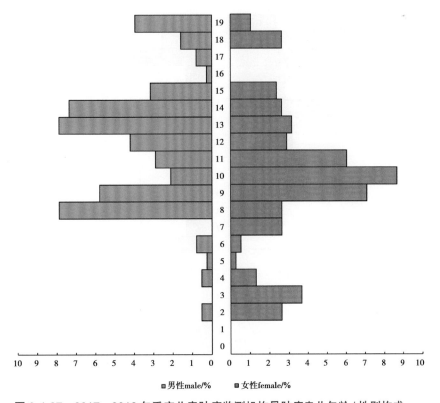

图 8-4-27　2017—2018 年重庆儿童肿瘤监测机构骨肿瘤患儿年龄／性别构成

Figure 8-4-27　Age/gender composition of children with bone cancer in pediatric cancer surveillance sites in Chongqing in 2017-2018

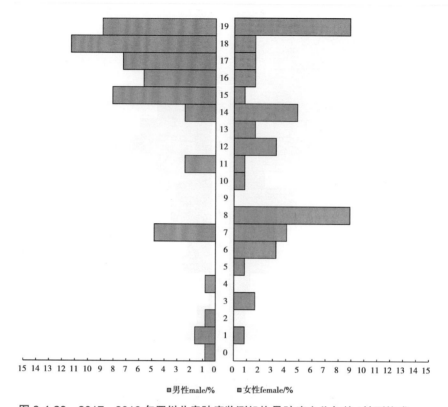

图 8-4-28　2017—2018 年四川儿童肿瘤监测机构骨肿瘤患儿年龄 / 性别构成

Figure 8-4-28　Age/gender composition of children with bone cancer in pediatric cancer surveillance sites in Sichuan in 2017-2018

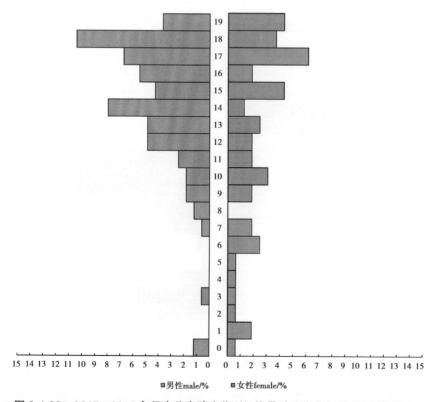

图 8-4-29　2017—2018 年云南儿童肿瘤监测机构骨肿瘤患儿年龄 / 性别构成

Figure 8-4-29　Age/gender composition of children with bone cancer in pediatric cancer surveillance sites in Yunnan in 2017-2018

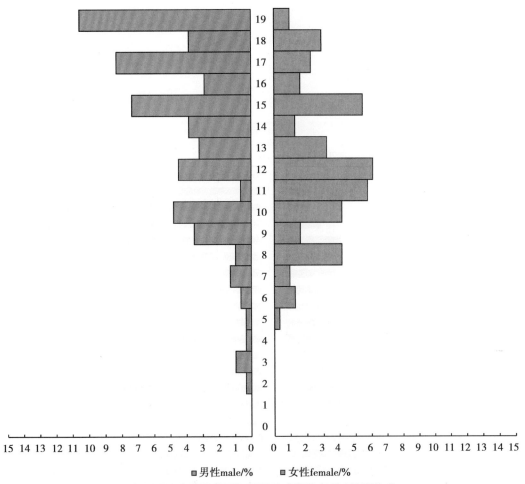

图 8-4-30　2017—2018 年新疆儿童肿瘤监测机构骨肿瘤患儿年龄 / 性别构成

Figure 8-4-30　Age/gender composition of children with bone cancer in pediatric cancer surveillance sites in Xinjiang in 2017-2018

4.3　全国儿童肿瘤监测机构骨肿瘤患儿就医省份分布

4.3.1　全国各省份骨肿瘤患儿本省就医与省外就医的分布情况

总体而言，骨肿瘤患儿本省就医的比例为 62.66%。在所有省份中，本省就医比例前 3 位的省份分别为北京（99.25%）、广东（91.12%）和新疆（89.80%）。省外就医比例前 3 位分别为内蒙古（85.95%）、贵州（70.78%）和安徽（67.54%）（图 8-4-31）。

4.3　Distribution of provincial-level regions visited by children with bone cancer in pediatric cancer surveillance sites in China

4.3.1　Distribution of children with bone cancer receiving medical treatment in and out of their own provincial-level regions

In general, 62.66% of all children with bone cancer sought medical treatment in their own provincial-level regions. Beijing (99.25%), Guangdong (91.12%) and Xinjiang (89.80%) were the top three recipients of patients from other provincial-level regions. Inner Mongolia (85.95%), Guizhou (70.78%) and Anhui (67.54%) were the top three provincial-level regions in terms of the proportion of patients going to other provincial-level regions for medical treatment (Figure 8-4-31).

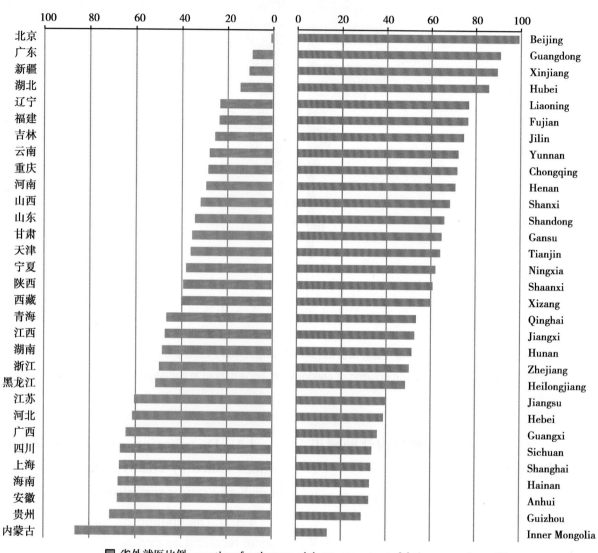

图 8-4-31　2017—2018 年全国各省份骨肿瘤患儿本省就医与省外就医比例 /%

Figure 8-4-31　Proportion of children with bone cancer receiving medical treatment in and out of their own provincial-level regions in 2017-2018/%

4.3.2　全国各省份骨肿瘤患儿省外就医的去向省份分布情况

各省份骨肿瘤患儿选择省外就医的去向分布呈现明显的规律，主要的去向省份为北京、广东、重庆、湖北和上海。如户籍地为河南的骨肿瘤患儿，选择省外就医的主要去向为北京和湖北，分别占户籍地为河南的骨肿瘤患儿选择省外就医总数的75.3%和19.1%。再如户籍地为贵州的骨肿瘤患儿，选择省外就医的主要去向为北京、重庆和广东，分别占户籍地为贵州的骨肿瘤患儿选择省外就医总数的47.1%、26.2%和12.8%（图8-4-32，按行方向查看）。

4.3.3　全国各省份收治骨肿瘤患儿来源的省份分布情况

各省份儿童肿瘤监测机构收治的省外就医骨肿瘤患儿来源分布略有差异，多数省份收治的骨肿瘤患儿来源以其相邻省份为主。如北京，其收治的省外就医骨肿瘤患儿主要来源于河南、山东和河北，分别占北京收治的省外就医骨肿瘤患儿总数的12.4%、11.9%和11.4%。再如江苏，其收治的省外就医骨肿瘤患儿主要来源于安徽，占江苏收治的省外就医骨肿瘤患儿的69.2%（图8-4-33，按列方向查看）。

4.3.2　Distribution of provincial-level regions receiving children with bone cancer from outside the provincial-level regions

The distribution of provincial-level regions receiving children with bone cancer from outside the provincial-level regions showed obvious regularity. The main destinations provincial-level regions were Beijing, Guangdong, Chongqing, Hubei and Shanghai. For example, for children with bone cancer in Henan, major destinations for medical treatment outside their own provincial-level regions were Beijing and Hubei, accounting for 75.3% and 19.1%, respectively. Another example is the children with bone cancer from Guizhou. Their main destinations were Beijing, Chongqing and Guangdong, accounting for 47.1%, 26.2% and 12.8%, respectively (Figure 8-4-32, view in rows).

4.3.3　Distribution of the provincial-level regions of origin of children with bone cancer receiving treatment out of their own provincial-level regions

There was a slight difference in the distribution of the provincial-level regions of origin of children with bone cancer admitted to surveillance sites in different provincial-level regions, and most of the children were mainly from their neighboring provincial-level regions. For example, in Beijing, the children with bone cancer admitted to hospitals out of their provincial-level regions were mainly from Henan, Shandong and Hebei, accounting for 12.4%, 11.9% and 11.4% of the total number of children with bone cancer admitted to Beijing out of their own provincial-level regions, respectively. Another example is Jiangsu. Children hospitalized from other provincial-level regions were mainly from Anhui, accounting for 69.2% (Figure 8-4-33, view in lines).

收治省外级医院肿瘤患儿的医院省份分布

provincial distribution of hospitals receiving children with cancer from outside the province

户籍地 distribution of the provinces of origin of children with cancer out of their own provinces	北京 Beijing	天津 Tianjin	河北 Hebei	山西 Shanxi	内蒙古 Inner Mongolia	辽宁 Liaoning	吉林 Jilin	黑龙江 Heilongjiang	上海 Shanghai	江苏 Jiangsu	浙江 Zhejiang	安徽 Anhui	福建 Fujian	江西 Jiangxi	山东 Shandong	河南 Henan	湖北 Hubei	湖南 Hunan	广东 Guangdong	广西 Guangxi	海南 Hainan	重庆 Chongqing	四川 Sichuan	贵州 Guizhou	云南 Yunnan	西藏 Xizang	陕西 Shaanxi	甘肃 Gansu	青海 Qinghai	宁夏 Ningxia	新疆 Xinjiang	合计 total
北京Beijing	90.0	0	0	0	0	0	0	0	0	0	0	0	0	0	0	0	0	0	0	0	0	0	0	0	0	0	0	0	0	0	0	100
天津Tianjin	95.6	0	0	0	0	0	0	0	0	0	0	0	0	0	0	0	0	0	0	0	0	0	0	0	0	0	0	0	0	0	0	100
河北Hebei	97.1	0	0	0	0	0	0	0	0	0	0	0	0	0	0	0	0	0	0	0	0	0	0.5	0	0	0	0	0	0	0	0.3	100
山西Shanxi	0	1.0	0	0	0.8	0	0	0	0	0	0	0	0	0	0.9	2.2	0	10.0	0	0	0	0	0	0	0	0	0	0	0	0	0	100
内蒙古Inner Mongolia	82.8	0.4	0	0	0	5.1	11.7	0	0	0	0	0	0	0	0	0	0	0	0	0	0	0	0	0	0	0	0	0	0	0	0	100
辽宁Liaoning	98.4	0.8	0	0	0	0	0	0	0	0	0	0	0	0	0	0	0	0	0	0	0	0	0	0	0	0	0	0	0	0	0	100
吉林Jilin	94.1	0	0	0	0	5.9	0	0	0	0	0	0	0	0	0	0	0	0	0	0	0	0	0	0	0	0	0	0	0	0	0	100
黑龙江Heilongjiang	89.2	1.7	0	0	0	5.7	2.3	0	0	0	0	0	0	0	0	0	0	0	0	0	0	0	0	0	0	0	0	0	0	0	0	100
上海Shanghai	100.0	0	0	0	0	0	0	0	0	0	0	0	0	0	0	0	0	0	0	0	0	0	0	0	0	0	0	0	0	0	0	100
江苏Jiangsu	75.6	2.0	0	0	0	0	0	0	19.9	0	0	0	0	0	0	0	0	0	1.0	0	0	0	0	0	0	0	0	0	0	0	0	100
浙江Zhejiang	94.6	0	0	0	0	0	0	0	0	0.9	0	0	0	0	0	0	0.9	0	0	0	0	0	0	0	0	0	0	0.4	0	0	0	100
安徽Anhui	76.0	0.3	0.4	3.1	0	0	0	0	2.7	7.0	1.6	0	0	0	0	5.4	2.7	0	0.8	0	0	0	0	0	0	0	0	0	0	0	0	100
福建Fujian	78.4	0	0	0	0	0	0	0	2.3	0	2.2	0	0	1.0	0	0	0	0	5.4	0	0	0	0	0	0	0	0	0	0	0	0	100
江西Jiangxi	68.4	0	0	0	0	0	0	0	14.0	0	9.1	0.5	0	0	0	0	0.7	0.7	17.8	0	0.3	0	0	0	0	0	0	0	0	0	0	100
山东Shandong	94.6	1.0	1.0	0.9	0	1.2	0	0	2.0	0.4	0	0	0	0	0	1.0	0.5	0	0.5	0	0	0	0	0	0	0	0	0	0	0	0	100
河南Henan	75.2	0.4	0.5	0	0	0	0	0	0.2	0	0	0.2	0	0	0	0	19.1	0	1.1	0	0	0	0	0	0	0	0.2	0	0	0	0.5	100
湖北Hubei	91.2	0	0	0	0	0	0	0	0.2	0	1.0	0	2.9	0	0	0	0	0.2	2.9	0	0	0	0	0	0	0	0	0	0	0	0	100
湖南Hunan	74.1	0	0	0	0	0.4	0	0	0	0	0	0	0	0	0	0.4	0	0	23.5	0	0	0	0	0.8	0.9	0	0	0	0	0	0	100
广东Guangdong	90.5	1.9	0	0	0	0	0	0	0	3.8	0	0	0	0	0	0	1.9	0	0	1.9	0	0	0	0	0	0	0	0	0	0	0	100
广西Guangxi	23.7	0	0	0	0	1.3	1.3	0	0	0	0	0	0	0	0	0	1.9	1.3	63.2	0	1.3	7.9	0	0.5	0	0	0	0	0	0	0	100
海南Hainan	0	0	7.4	0	0	0	0	0	0	0	0	0	0	0	0	0	0	1.2	90.2	1.3	0	0	0	0	0	0	0	0	0	0	0	100
重庆Chongqing	90.7	0	0	0	0	0	0	0	0	0	0	0	0	0	0	2.4	5.8	0	3.5	0	0	0	0	0	0	0	0	0	0	0	0	100
四川Sichuan	35.2	0	0	0	0	0	0	0	0	0	0	0	0	0	0	0.5	5.5	0	6.9	0	0	48.6	0	2.3	0.5	0	0	0	0	0	0	100
贵州Guizhou	47.1	0	0	0	0	0	0	0	0	0.5	0.9	0	0	0	0	1.7	0	0	12.8	0	0	26.2	0	0	9.3	0	0	0	0	0	0	100
云南Yunnan	72.8	0	0	0	0	0	0	0	0	1.8	5.5	0	0	0	0	0	1.8	0	3.6	0	0	7.3	0	0	0	0	0	0	0	0	0	100
西藏Xizang	25.0	0	0	0	0	0	0	0	0	0	0	0	0	0	0	0	0	0	0	0	0	0	75.0	0	0	0	0	0	0	0	0	100
陕西Shaanxi	91.6	0	0	0	0	0	0	0	0	0	0	0	0	0	0	0	0	0	0	0	0	0	0	0	2.8	0	0	0	0	0	0	100
甘肃Gansu	11.6	0	0	0	0	0	0	0	0	0	0	0	0	0	0	30.8	0	0	2.8	0	0	0	0	0	0	0	51.9	0	0	2.8	0	100
青海Qinghai	15.0	0	0	0	0	0	0	0	0	0	0	0	0	0	0	85.0	0	0	3.8	0	0	0	0	0	0	0	0	0	0	0	1.9	100
宁夏Ningxia	96.8	0	0	0	0	0	0	0	0	0	0	0	0	0	0	0	0	0	0	0	0	3.2	0	0	0	0	0	0	0	0	0	100
新疆Xinjiang	71.4	0	0	0	0	0	2.9	0	0	0	0	0	0	0	0	5.7	0	0	2.9	0	0	3.2	11.4	0	0	0	0	5.7	0	0	0	100

图 8-4-32 2017—2018年全国各省份户籍地骨肿瘤患儿选择省外就医的省份分布 /%

Figure 8-4-32 Distribution of provincial-level regions receiving children with bone cancer from outside the provincial-level regions in 2017-2018

表示肿瘤患儿的来源省份分布 / distribution of the provinces of origin of children with cancer receiving treatment out of their own provinces

收治省外就医肿瘤患儿的医院所在省份分布 / provincial distribution of hospitals receiving children with cancer from outside the province

来源 Origin \ 医院 Hospital	北京 Beijing	天津 Tianjin	河北 Hebei	山西 Shanxi	内蒙古 Inner Mongolia	辽宁 Liaoning	吉林 Jilin	黑龙江 Heilongjiang	上海 Shanghai	江苏 Jiangsu	浙江 Zhejiang	安徽 Anhui	福建 Fujian	江西 Jiangxi	山东 Shandong	河南 Henan	湖北 Hubei	湖南 Hunan	广东 Guangdong	广西 Guangxi	海南 Hainan	重庆 Chongqing	四川 Sichuan	贵州 Guizhou	云南 Yunnan	西藏 Xizang	陕西 Shaanxi	甘肃 Gansu	青海 Qinghai	宁夏 Ningxia	新疆 Xinjiang
北京 Beijing	0.4	0	0	0	0	0	0	0	0	0	0	0	0	0	11.2	0	0	0	0	0	0	0	0	0	0	0	0	0	0	0	0
天津 Tianjin	11.5	26.2	0	0	0	0	0	0	0	0	0	0	0	0	0	0	0	20.0	0	0	0	0	0	0	0	0	0	0	0	0	20.0
河北 Hebei	3.9	0	0	23.5	100.0	2.5	0	0	0	0	0	0	0	0	0	0	0	0	0	0	0	0	15.3	0	0	0	0	0	0	0	0
山西 Shanxi	6.4	0	0	0	0	33.3	0	0	0	0	0	0	0	0	0	4.9	0	0	0	0	0	0	0	50.0	0	0	0	0	0	0	0
内蒙古 Inner Mongolia	3.9	4.4	0	0	0	0	83.3	0	0	0	0	0	0	0	0	0	0	0	0	0	0	0	0	0	0	0	0	0	0	0	0
辽宁 Liaoning	1.4	4.3	0	0	0	0	0	0	0	0	2.4	0	0	0	0	0	0	0	0	0	0	0	0	0	0	0	0	0	0	0	0
吉林 Jilin	4.7	0	0	0	0	7.7	0	0	0	0	0	0	0	0	0	0	0	0	0	0	0	0	0	0	0	0	0	0	0	0	0
黑龙江 Heilongjiang	0.3	13.0	0	0	0	25.6	11.1	0	0	0	0	0	0	0	22.2	0	0	0	0	0	0	0	0	0	0	0	0	0	0	0	0
上海 Shanghai	4.4	0	0	0	0	0	0	0	54.9	0	0	50.0	0	0	0	0	0	0	0	0	0	0	0	0	0	0	0	0	0	0	0
江苏 Jiangsu	3.2	17.4	0	0	0	0	0	0	4.2	3.9	0	0	0	0	0	0	0.8	0	0	0	0	0	0	0	0	0	0	0	0	0	0
浙江 Zhejiang	5.9	4.3	0	0	0	0	0	0	8.5	69.3	0	0	0	0	0	0	5.1	0	0	0	0	0	0	0	5.2	0	0	0	0	0	0
安徽 Anhui	2.2	0	9.0	47.1	0	0	0	0	18.3	0	9.8	0	0	0	0	22.6	0	0	0	0	0	0	0	50.0	0	0	0	33.3	0	0	0
福建 Fujian	6.1	0	0	0	0	0	0	0	8.5	0	4.9	0	0	0	0	0	0	0	0	0	0	0	0	0	0	0	0	0	0	0	0
江西 Jiangxi	11.9	17.4	0	0	0	0	0	0	0	0	65.9	0	50.0	0	0	6.5	1.5	40.0	20.3	0	20.0	0	0	0	0	0	0	0	0	0	0
山东 Shandong	12.4	8.7	36.4	0	0	12.8	0	0	1.4	0	0	0	0	0	0	0	1.5	0	0.8	0	0	0	0	0	0	0	0	0	0	0	60.0
河南 Henan	2.8	0	27.3	29.4	0	10.3	0	0	1.4	0	0	50.0	0	0	11.1	0	76.6	20.0	2.3	0	0	0	0	0	0	0	3.6	0	0	0	0
湖北 Hubei	5.4	0	0	0	0	0	0	0	1.4	3.8	2.4	0	50.0	0	0	1.6	0	0	1.1	0	0	0	0	0	0	0	0	0	0	0	0
湖南 Hunan	1.4	0	0	0	0	2.6	2.8	0	0	7.7	2.4	0	0	0	0	0	0.7	0	1.6	0	0	0	0	0	0	0	0	0	0	0	0
广东 Guangdong	0.5	4.3	0	0	0	0	0	0	0	0	0	0	0	100.0	0	0	0.7	0	21.8	50.0	60.0	0	0	0	0	0	0	0	0	0	0
广西 Guangxi	0	0	27.3	0	0	2.6	0	0	0	0	0	0	0	0	0	1.6	0	20.0	18.4	0	0	3.7	0	0	0	0	0	0	0	0	0
海南 Hainan	0	0	0	0	0	0	0	0	0	7.7	0	0	0	0	0	0	0	0	14.2	0	0	0	0	0	0	0	0	0	0	0	0
重庆 Chongqing	2.3	0	0	0	0	0	0	0	0	3.8	4.9	0	0	0	22.2	1.6	3.6	0	1.1	0	0	65.4	0	0	5.3	0	0	0	0	0	0
四川 Sichuan	2.3	0	0	0	0	0	0	0	0	0	0	0	0	0	0	0	0	0	5.7	0	0	27.8	30.8	0	0	0	0	0	0	0	0
贵州 Guizhou	2.4	0	0	0	0	0	0	0	0	0	0	0	0	0	0	4.8	8.8	0	8.4	50.0	0	2.5	0	0	84.2	0	0	0	0	0	0
云南 Yunnan	1.2	0	0	0	0	2.6	0	0	1.4	3.8	7.3	0	0	0	22.2	0	0.7	0	0.8	0	0	0	0	0	0	0	0	0	0	0	0
西藏 Xizang	0.1	0	0	0	0	0	0	0	0	0	0	0	0	0	0	0	0	0	0	0	0	0	23.1	0	0	0	0	0	0	0	0
陕西 Shaanxi	1.0	0	0	0	0	0	0	0	0	0	0	0	0	0	0	25.8	0	0	0.4	0	0	0	0	0	5.3	0	96.4	0	0	100.0	0
甘肃 Gansu	0.2	0	0	0	0	0	0	0	0	0	0	0	0	0	0	27.4	0	0	0.8	0	0	0	0	0	0	0	0	66.7	0	0	20.0
青海 Qinghai	0.1	0	0	0	0	0	0	0	0	0	0	0	0	0	0	0	0	0	0	0	0	0	0	0	0	0	0	0	0	0	0
宁夏 Ningxia	0.9	0	0	0	0	0	0	0	0	0	0	0	0	0	0	0	0	0	0	0	0	0	0	0	0	0	0	0	0	0	0
新疆 Xinjiang	0.8	0	0	0	0	0	2.8	0	0	0	0	0	0	0	0	3.2	0	0	0	0	0	0.6	30.8	0	0	0	0	0	0	0	0
合计 total	100	100	100	100	100	100	100	100	100	100	100	100	100	100	100	100	100	100	100	100	100	100	100	100	100	100	100	100	100	100	100

图 8-4-33　2017—2018 年全国各省份儿童肿瘤监测机构省外就医骨肿瘤患儿来源分布 /%

Figure 8-4-33　Distribution of the provincial-level regions of origin of children with bone cancer receiving treatment out of their own provincial-level regions in 2017-2018

4.4 全国儿童肿瘤监测机构骨肿瘤患儿住院费用医疗付费方式构成

4.4.1 全国骨肿瘤患儿住院费用医疗付费方式构成情况

全国骨肿瘤患儿住院费用的医疗付费方式中，占比最高的前 3 种类型分别为城镇居民基本医疗保险 (27.54%)、新型农村合作医疗 (26.07%) 和全自费 (21.56%)(图 8-4-34)。

4.4.2 六大区骨肿瘤患儿住院费用医疗付费方式构成情况

六大区的医疗付费方式所占比例各不相同，中南地区、东北地区和西北地区均以新型农村合作医疗占比最高，分别为 40.45%、32.46% 和 31.78%；华北地区、西南地区和华东地区均以城镇居民医疗保险占比最高，分别为 35.26%、34.71% 和 33.28%(图 8-4-35~ 图 8-4-40)。

4.4 Composition of medical payment methods for hospitalization expenses of children with bone cancer in pediatric cancer surveillance sites in China

4.4.1 Composition of medical payment methods for hospitalization expenses of children with bone cancer nationally

Among the medical payment methods of children with bone cancer nationally, the top three methods were basic medical insurance for urban residents (27.54%), new rural cooperative medical system (26.07%), and 100% self-pay (21.56%)(Figure 8-4-34).

4.4.2 Composition of medical payment methods for hospitalization expenses of children with bone cancer in the six regions

The proportions of different payment methods in the six regions were different. Central and Southern China, Northeast and Northwest China had the highest proportions of new rural cooperative medical system, which were 40.45%, 32.46% and 31.78%, respectively. As for North China, Southwest China and East China, basic medical insurance for urban residents accounted for the highest proportions, which were 35.26%, 34.71% and 33.28%, respectively (Figure 8-4-35~Figure 8-4-40).

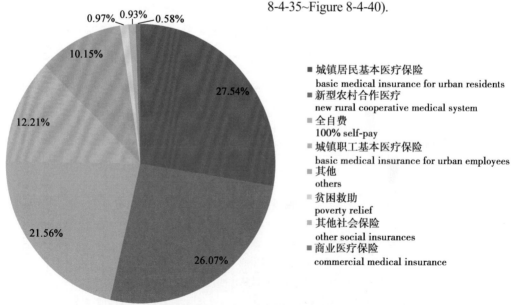

■ 城镇居民基本医疗保险
basic medical insurance for urban residents
■ 新型农村合作医疗
new rural cooperative medical system
■ 全自费
100% self-pay
■ 城镇职工基本医疗保险
basic medical insurance for urban employees
■ 其他
others
■ 贫困救助
poverty relief
■ 其他社会保险
other social insurances
■ 商业医疗保险
commercial medical insurance

图 8-4-34 2017—2018 年全国骨肿瘤患儿住院费用医疗付费方式构成

Figure 8-4-34 Composition of medical payment methods for hospitalization expenses of children with bone cancer nationally in 2017-2018

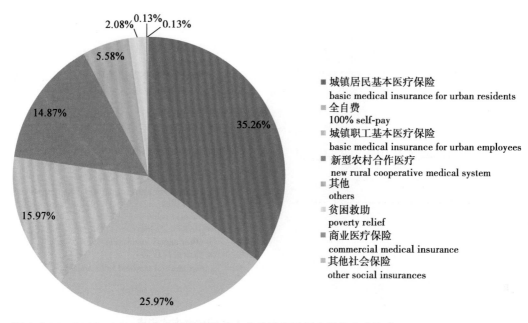

图 8-4-35   2017—2018 年华北地区骨肿瘤患儿住院费用医疗付费方式构成

Figure 8-4-35   Composition of medical payment methods for hospitalization expenses of children with bone cancer in North China in 2017-2018

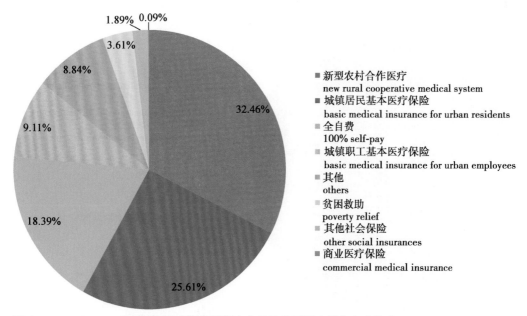

图 8-4-36   2017—2018 年东北地区骨肿瘤患儿住院费用医疗付费方式构成

Figure 8-4-36   Composition of medical payment methods for hospitalization expenses of children with bone cancer in Northeast China in 2017-2018

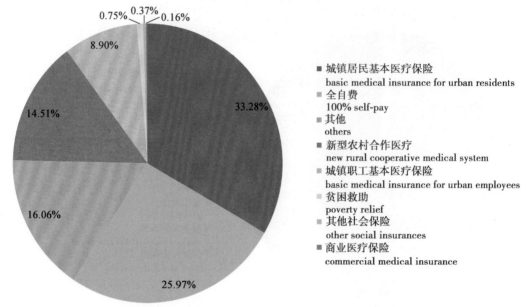

图 8-4-37　2017—2018 年华东地区骨肿瘤患儿住院费用医疗付费方式构成

Figure 8-4-37　Composition of medical payment methods for hospitalization expenses of children with bone cancer in East China in 2017-2018

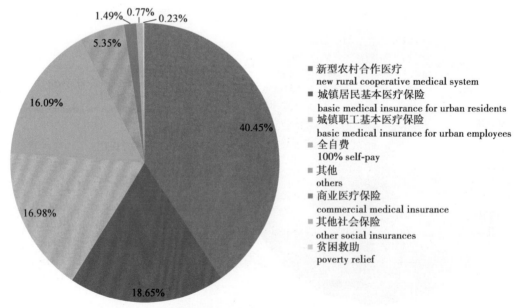

图 8-4-38　2017—2018 年中南地区骨肿瘤患儿住院费用医疗付费方式构成

Figure 8-4-38　Composition of medical payment methods for hospitalization expenses of children with bone cancer in Central and Southern China in 2017-2018

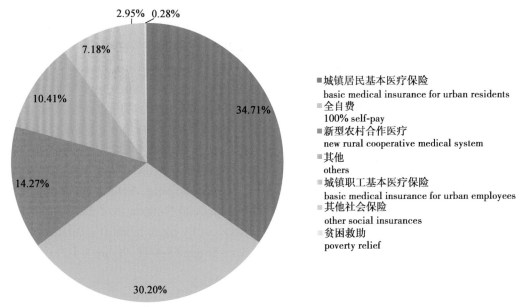

图 8-4-39　2017—2018 年西南地区骨肿瘤患儿住院费用医疗付费方式构成

Figure 8-4-39　Composition of medical payment methods for hospitalization expenses of children with bone cancer in Southwest China in 2017-2018

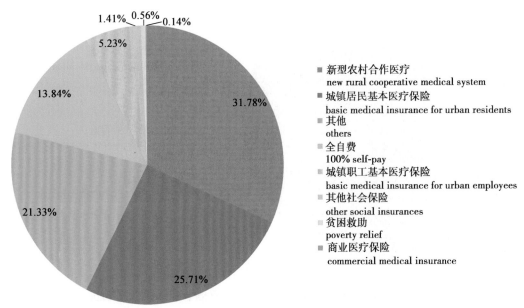

图 8-4-40　2017—2018 年西北地区骨肿瘤患儿住院费用医疗付费方式构成

Figure 8-4-40　Composition of medical payment methods for hospitalization expenses of children with bone cancer in Northwest China in 2017-2018

4.4.3 各省份骨肿瘤患儿住院费用医疗付费方式构成情况

内蒙古、江苏、江西、湖南、广西、海南、四川、贵州、云南和西藏10个省份均以全自费所占比例最高。辽宁、吉林、黑龙江、上海、河南、陕西、甘肃和新疆8个省份的新型农村合作医疗占比最高;北京、河北、山西、浙江、安徽、山东、重庆、青海和宁夏9个省份的城镇居民基本医疗保险占比最高(图8-4-41~图8-4-71)。

4.4.3 Composition of medical payment methods for hospitalization expenses of children with bone cancer in each provincial-level region

The proportion of 100% self-pay was the highest in the following 10 provincial-level regions: Inner Mongolia, Jiangsu, Jiangxi, Hunan, Guangxi, Hainan, Sichuan, Guizhou, Yunnan and Xizang. Liaoning, Jilin, Heilongjiang, Shanghai, Henan, Shaanxi, Gansu and Xinjiang had the highest proportion of new rural cooperative medical system. The following 9 provincial-level regions--Beijing, Hebei, Shanxi, Zhejiang, Anhui, Shandong, Chongqing, Qinghai and Ningxia--had the highest proportion of payment by basic medical insurance for urban residents (Figure 8-4-41~Figure 8-4-71).

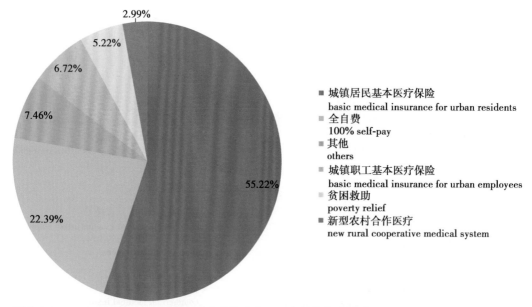

图 8-4-41　2017—2018 年北京骨肿瘤患儿住院费用医疗付费方式构成

Figure 8-4-41　Composition of medical payment methods for hospitalization expenses of children with bone cancer in Beijing in 2017-2018

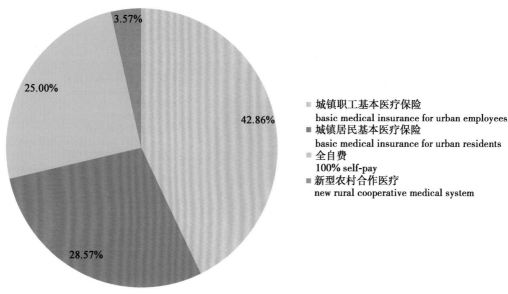

图 8-4-42　2017—2018 年天津骨肿瘤患儿住院费用医疗付费方式构成

Figure 8-4-42　Composition of medical payment methods for hospitalization expenses of children with bone cancer in Tianjin in 2017-2018

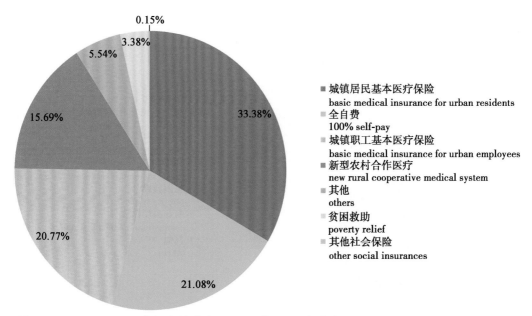

图 8-4-43　2017—2018 年河北骨肿瘤患儿住院费用医疗付费方式构成

Figure 8-4-43　Composition of medical payment methods for hospitalization expenses of children with bone cancer in Hebei in 2017-2018

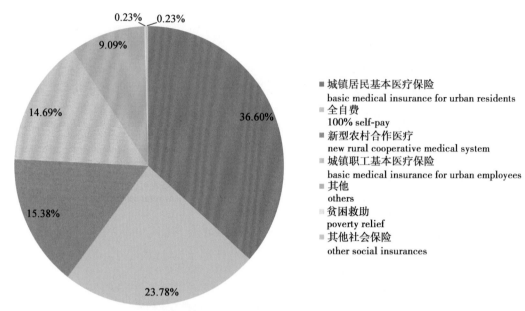

图 8-4-44　2017—2018 年山西骨肿瘤患儿住院费用医疗付费方式构成

Figure 8-4-44　Composition of medical payment methods for hospitalization expenses of children with bone cancer in Shanxi in 2017-2018

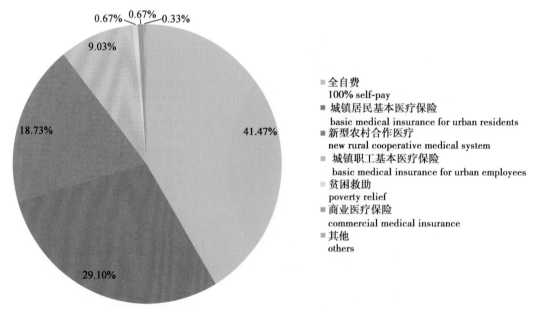

图 8-4-45　2017—2018 年内蒙古骨肿瘤患儿住院费用医疗付费方式构成

Figure 8-4-45　Composition of medical payment methods for hospitalization expenses of children with bone cancer in Inner Mongolia in 2017-2018

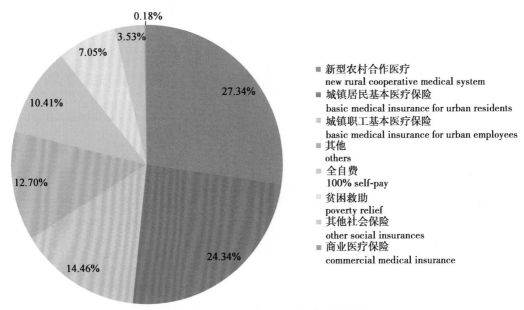

图 8-4-46　2017—2018 年辽宁骨肿瘤患儿住院费用医疗付费方式构成

Figure 8-4-46　Composition of medical payment methods for hospitalization expenses of children with bone cancer in Liaoning in 2017-2018

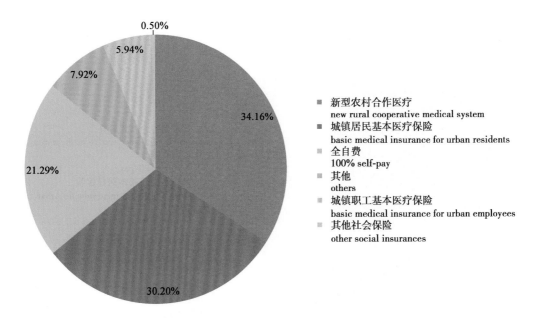

图 8-4-47　2017—2018 年吉林骨肿瘤患儿住院费用医疗付费方式构成

Figure 8-4-47　Composition of medical payment methods for hospitalization expenses of children with bone cancer in Jilin in 2017-2018

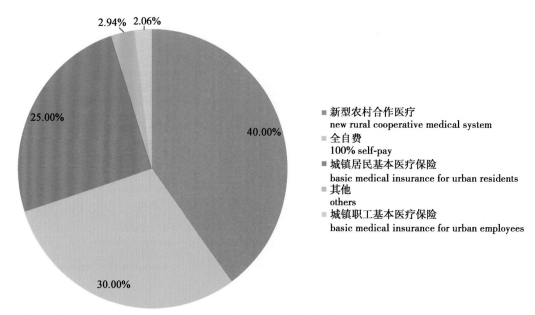

图 8-4-48　2017—2018 年黑龙江骨肿瘤患儿住院费用医疗付费方式构成

Figure 8-4-48　Composition of medical payment methods for hospitalization expenses of children with bone cancer in Heilongjiang in 2017-2018

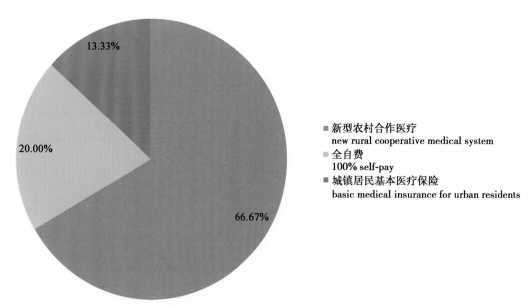

图 8-4-49　2017—2018 年上海骨肿瘤患儿住院费用医疗付费方式构成

Figure 8-4-49　Composition of medical payment methods for hospitalization expenses of children with bone cancer in Shanghai in 2017-2018

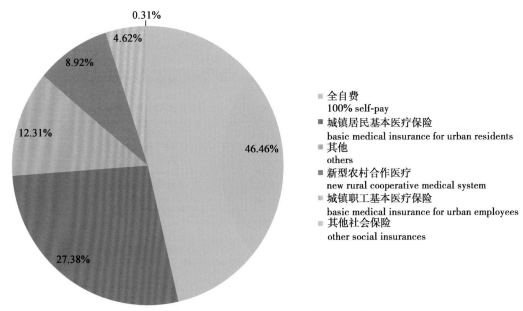

图 8-4-50　2017—2018 年江苏骨肿瘤患儿住院费用医疗付费方式构成

Figure 8-4-50　Composition of medical payment methods for hospitalization expenses of children with bone cancer in Jiangsu in 2017-2018

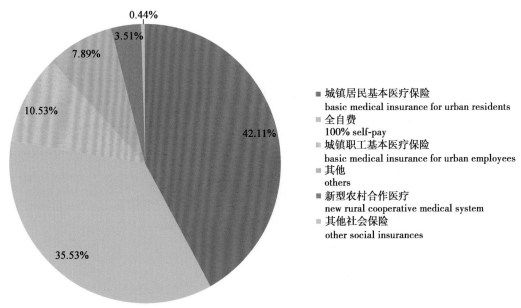

图 8-4-51　2017—2018 年浙江骨肿瘤患儿住院费用医疗付费方式构成

Figure 8-4-51　Composition of medical payment methods for hospitalization expenses of children with bone cancer in Zhejiang in 2017-2018

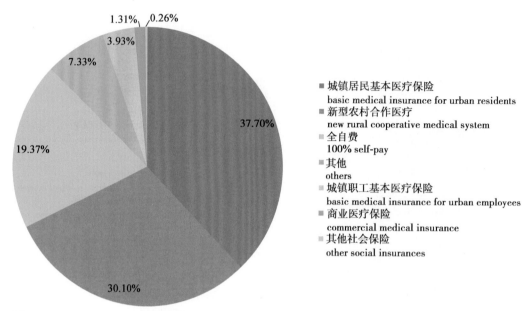

图 8-4-52　2017—2018 年安徽骨肿瘤患儿住院费用医疗付费方式构成

Figure 8-4-52　Composition of medical payment methods for hospitalization expenses of children with bone cancer in Anhui in 2017-2018

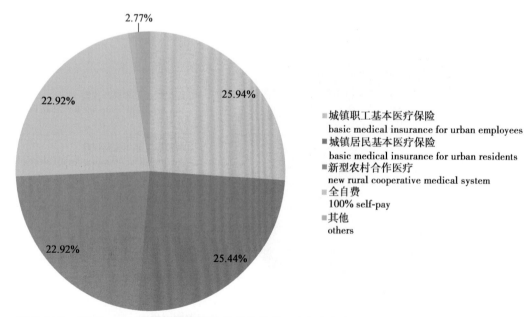

图 8-4-53　2017—2018 年福建骨肿瘤患儿住院费用医疗付费方式构成

Figure 8-4-53　Composition of medical payment methods for hospitalization expenses of children with bone cancer in Fujian in 2017-2018

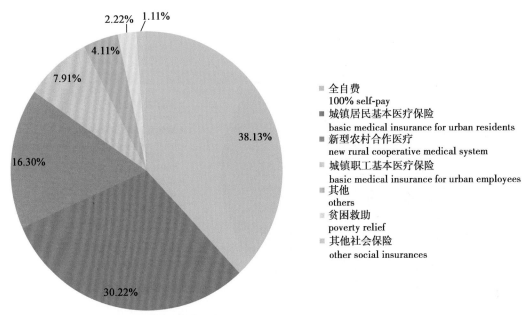

图 8-4-54　2017—2018 年江西骨肿瘤患儿住院费用医疗付费方式构成

Figure 8-4-54　Composition of medical payment methods for hospitalization expenses of children with bone cancer in Jiangxi in 2017-2018

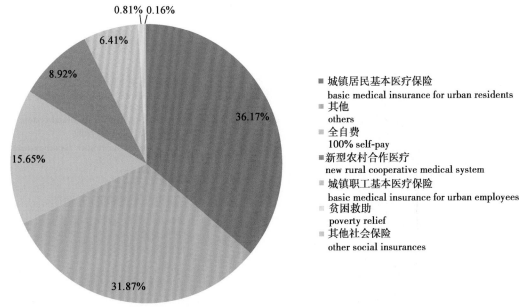

图 8-4-55　2017—2018 年山东骨肿瘤患儿住院费用医疗付费方式构成

Figure 8-4-55　Composition of medical payment methods for hospitalization expenses of children with bone cancer in Shandong in 2017-2018

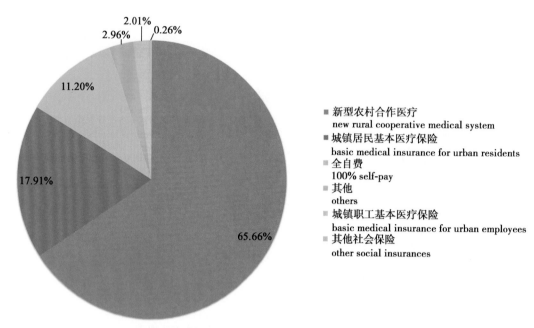

图 8-4-56　2017—2018 年河南骨肿瘤患儿住院费用医疗付费方式构成

Figure 8-4-56　Composition of medical payment methods for hospitalization expenses of children with bone cancer in Henan in 2017-2018

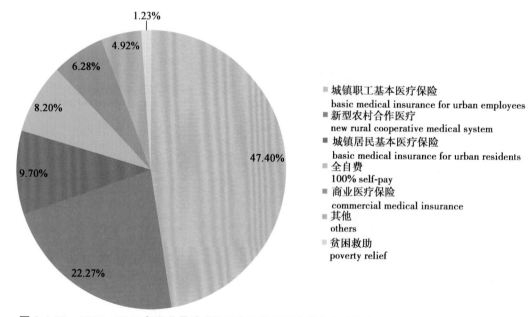

图 8-4-57　2017—2018 年湖北骨肿瘤患儿住院费用医疗付费方式构成

Figure 8-4-57　Composition of medical payment methods for hospitalization expenses of children with bone cancer in Hubei in 2017-2018

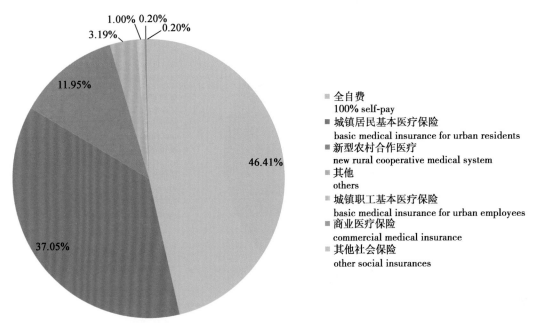

图 8-4-58　2017—2018 年湖南骨肿瘤患儿住院费用医疗付费方式构成

Figure 8-4-58　Composition of medical payment methods for hospitalization expenses of children with bone cancer in Hunan in 2017-2018

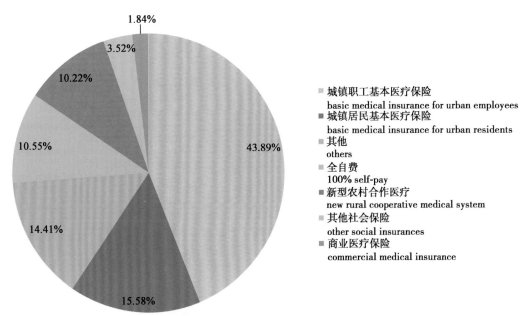

图 8-4-59　2017—2018 年广东骨肿瘤患儿住院费用医疗付费方式构成

Figure 8-4-59　Composition of medical payment methods for hospitalization expenses of children with bone cancer in Guangdong in 2017-2018

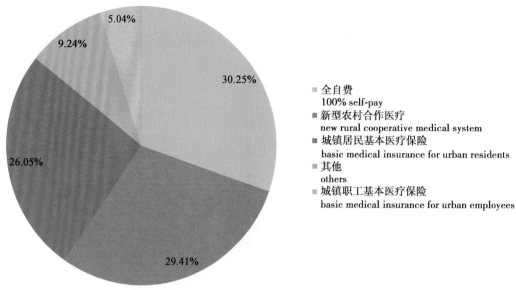

图 8-4-60 2017—2018 年广西骨肿瘤患儿住院费用医疗付费方式构成

Figure 8-4-60 Composition of medical payment methods for hospitalization expenses of children with bone cancer in Guangxi in 2017-2018

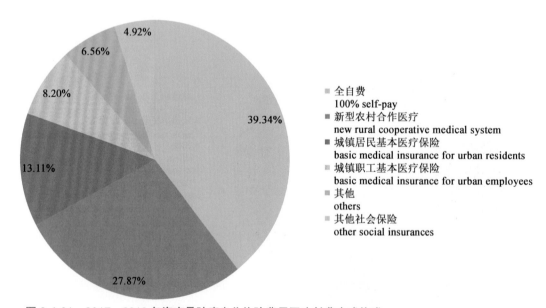

图 8-4-61 2017—2018 年海南骨肿瘤患儿住院费用医疗付费方式构成

Figure 8-4-61 Composition of medical payment methods for hospitalization expenses of children with bone cancer in Hainan in 2017-2018

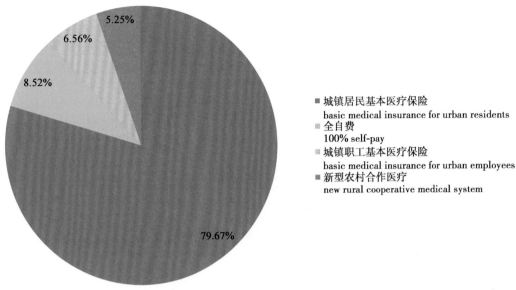

图 8-4-62   2017—2018 年重庆骨肿瘤患儿住院费用医疗付费方式构成

Figure 8-4-62   Composition of medical payment methods for hospitalization expenses of children with bone cancer in Chongqing in 2017-2018

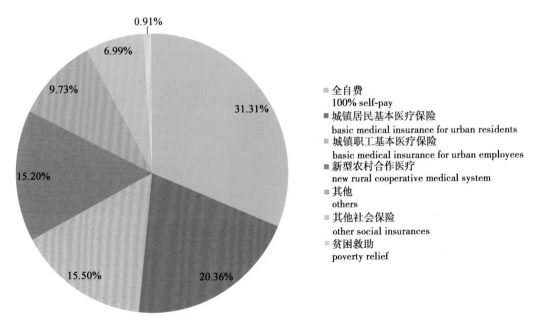

图 8-4-63   2017—2018 年四川骨肿瘤患儿住院费用医疗付费方式构成

Figure 8-4-63   Composition of medical payment methods for hospitalization expenses of children with bone cancer in Sichuan in 2017-2018

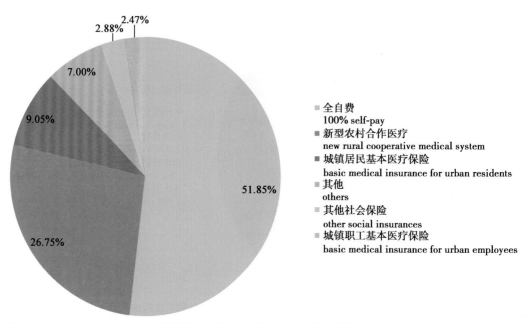

图 8-4-64　2017—2018 年贵州骨肿瘤患儿住院费用医疗付费方式构成

Figure 8-4-64　Composition of medical payment methods for hospitalization expenses of children with bone cancer in Guizhou in 2017-2018

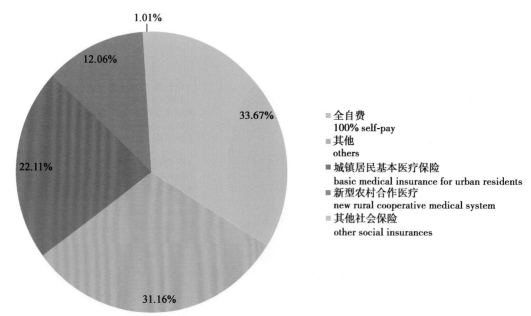

图 8-4-65　2017—2018 年云南骨肿瘤患儿住院费用医疗付费方式构成

Figure 8-4-65　Composition of medical payment methods for hospitalization expenses of children with bone cancer in Yunnan in 2017-2018

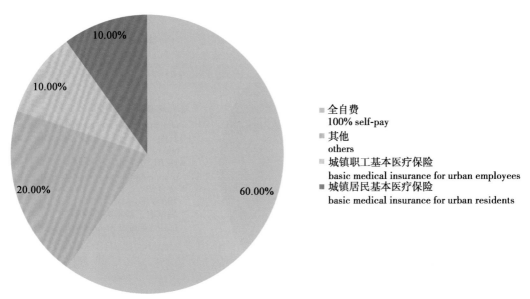

图 8-4-66　2017—2018 年西藏骨肿瘤患儿住院费用医疗付费方式构成

Figure 8-4-66　Composition of medical payment methods for hospitalization expenses of children with bone cancer in Xizang in 2017-2018

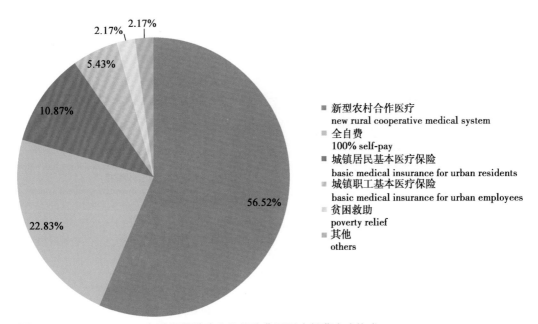

图 8-4-67　2017—2018 年陕西骨肿瘤患儿住院费用医疗付费方式构成

Figure 8-4-67　Composition of medical payment methods for hospitalization expenses of children with bone cancer in Shaanxi in 2017-2018

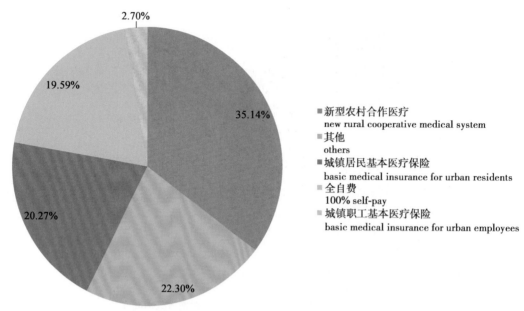

图 8-4-68　2017—2018 年甘肃骨肿瘤患儿住院费用医疗付费方式构成

Figure 8-4-68　Composition of medical payment methods for hospitalization expenses of children with bone cancer in Gansu in 2017-2018

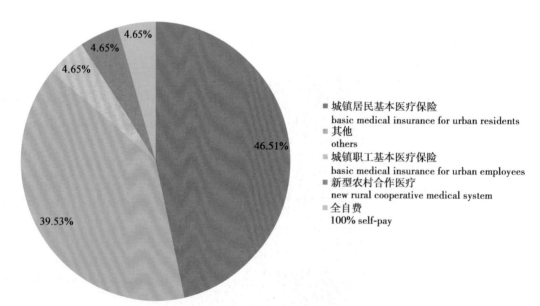

图 8-4-69　2017—2018 年青海骨肿瘤患儿住院费用医疗付费方式构成

Figure 8-4-69　Composition of medical payment methods for hospitalization expenses of children with bone cancer in Qinghai in 2017-2018

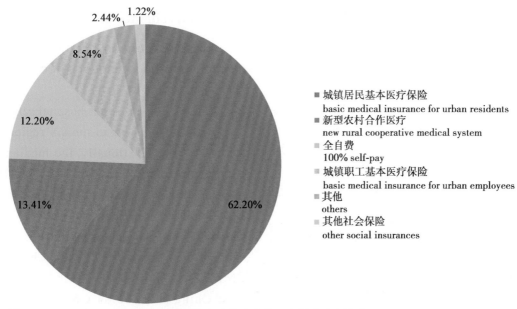

图 8-4-70 2017—2018 年宁夏骨肿瘤患儿住院费用医疗付费方式构成

Figure 8-4-70 Composition of medical payment methods for hospitalization expenses of children with bone cancer in Ningxia in 2017-2018

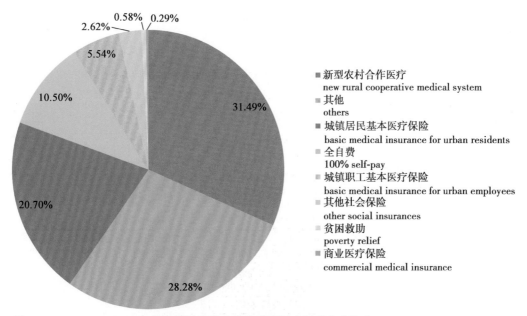

图 8-4-71 2017—2018 年新疆骨肿瘤患儿住院费用医疗付费方式构成

Figure 8-4-71 Composition of medical payment methods for hospitalization expenses of children with bone cancer in Xinjiang in 2017-2018

4.5 全国儿童肿瘤监测机构骨肿瘤患儿住院费用分析

4.5.1 全国儿童肿瘤监测机构骨肿瘤患儿次均住院费用情况

4.5.1.1 全国及六大区骨肿瘤患儿次均住院费用情况　全国骨肿瘤患儿次均住院费用(中位数)为 12 757.55 元。高于全国中位数水平的地区分别为中南地区(15 234.49 元)和华北地区(12 831.45 元),低于全国中位数水平的地区分别为西南地区(9 499.41 元)、华东地区(10 499.85 元)、西北地区(11 886.84 元)和东北地区(11 949.46 元)(图 8-4-72)。

4.5 Analysis of hospitalization expenses of children with bone cancer in pediatric cancer surveillance sites in China

4.5.1 Expenses per hospitalization of children with bone cancer in pediatric cancer surveillance sites in China

4.5.1.1 Expenses per hospitalization of children with bone cancer in the six regions and the whole country　Nationally, the median expense per hospitalization was 12, 757.55 CNY. The regions above the national median were Central and Southern China (15, 234.49 CNY) and North China (12, 831.45 CNY), while those below the national median were Southwest China (9 499.41 CNY), East China (10, 499.85 CNY), Northwest China (11, 886.84 CNY) and Northeast China (11, 949.46 CNY) (Figure 8-4-72).

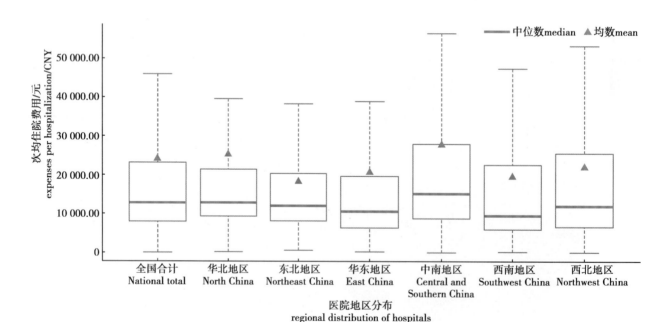

图 8-4-72　2017—2018 年全国及六大区骨肿瘤患儿次均住院费用

Figure 8-4-72　Expenses per hospitalization of children with bone cancer in the six regions and the whole country in 2017-2018

4.5.1.2　各省份骨肿瘤患儿次均住院费用情况　根据骨肿瘤患儿次均住院费用（中位数），前3位的省份分别为天津（25 085.93 元）、广东（24 370.31 元）和云南（21 839.95 元），后3位分别为陕西（6 107.01 元）、上海（6 885.46 元）和重庆（7 042.53 元）（图8-4-73）。

4.5.2　全国儿童肿瘤监测机构骨肿瘤患儿次均住院分项费用情况

4.5.2.1　全国及六大区骨肿瘤患儿次均住院分项费用情况　根据全国骨肿瘤患儿次均住院分项费用（中位数），前3位分别为西药类费用（5 507.14 元）、综合医疗服务类费用（1 471.50 元）和诊断类费用（1 254.75 元）。六大区分项费用中位数的顺位与全国相比略有不同。如西南地区，次均住院分项费用（中位数）前3位分别为西药类费用（3 259.85 元）、诊断类费用（2 531.80 元）和综合医疗服务类费用（1 512.90 元）（图8-4-74）。按均数统计的结果详见图8-4-75。

4.5.2.2　各省份骨肿瘤患儿次均住院分项费用情况　根据各省份骨肿瘤患儿次均住院分项费用（中位数），以西药类费用为例，前3位的省份依次为北京（7 899.54 元）、海南（7 031.99 元）和湖北（6 337.85 元），后3位依次为江苏（1 020.93 元）、陕西（1 269.54 元）和上海（1 322.82 元）（图8-4-76）。按均数统计的结果详见图8-4-77。

4.5.1.2　Expenses per hospitalization of children with bone cancer in each provincial-level region　In terms of the median expenses per hospitalization of children with bone cancer, the top three provincial-level regions were Tianjin (25, 085.93 CNY), Guangdong (24, 370.31 CNY) and Yunnan (21, 839.95 CNY), and the last three were Shaanxi (6, 107.01 CNY), Shanghai (6, 885.46 CNY) and Chongqing (7, 042.53 CNY) (Figure 8-4-73).

4.5.2　Expenses of each item per hospitalization of children with bone cancer in pediatric cancer surveillance sites in China

4.5.2.1　Expenses of each item per hospitalization of children with bone cancer in the six regions and the whole country　In terms of the median expenses of each item per hospitalization of children with bone cancer, the top three were western medication expenses (5, 507.14 CNY), comprehensive medical services expenses (1, 471.50 CNY), and diagnostic expenses (1, 254.75 CNY). The ranking of the median expenses of each item in the six regions was slightly different from that of the whole country. For example, in Southwest China, the three items with the highest median expenses were western medication expenses (3, 259.85 CNY), diagnostic expenses (2, 531.80 CNY) and comprehensive medical services expenses (1, 512.90 CNY) (Figure 8-4-74). Data by the mean expenses in Figure 8-4-75.

4.5.2.2　Expenses of each item per hospitalization of children with bone cancer in each provincial-level region　In terms of the median expenses of each item per hospitalization of children with bone cancer in each provincial-level region, taking western medication expenses as an example, the top three provincial-level regions were Beijing (7 899.54 CNY), Hainan (7 031.99 CNY) and Hubei (6 337.85 CNY), and the last three were Jiangsu (1 020.93 CNY), followed by Shaanxi (1 269.54 CNY) and Shanghai (1 322.82 CNY) (Figure 8-4-76). Data by the mean expenses in Figure 8-4-77.

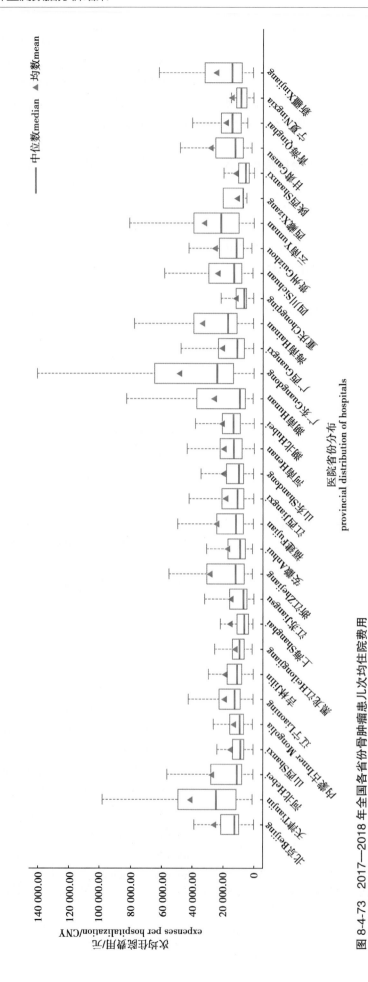

图 8-4-73　2017—2018 年全国各省份骨肿瘤患儿次均住院费用

Figure 8-4-73　Expenses per hospitalization of children with bone cancer in each provincial-level region in 2017-2019

医院地区分布 regional distribution of hospitals	分项费用/元 expenses of each item/CNY									
	综合医疗服务类费用 comprehensive medical service expenses	诊断类费用 diagnostic expenses	治疗类费用 treatment expenses	康复类费用 rehabilitation expenses	中医类费用 traditional chinese medicine service expenses	西药类费用 western medication expenses	中药类费用 traditional chinese medication expenses	血液和血液制品类费用 blood and blood product expenses	耗材类费用 medical consumable expenses	其他类费用 others
全国合计 National total	1 471.50	1 254.75	5.00	0	0	5 507.14	0	82.00	545.21	27.00
华北地区 North China	1 445.00	681.50	0	20.00	0	7 384.63	0	378.00	490.67	36.00
东北地区 Northeast China	1 467.89	1 969.44	9.95	0	0	4 800.85	558.02	0	1 019.70	42.60
华东地区 East China	1 552.00	1 845.50	107.00	0	0	3 498.66	0	0	552.32	0
中南地区 Central and Southern China	1 629.55	1 366.50	168.00	0	0	5 524.91	0	0	725.22	56.00
西南地区 Southwest China	1 512.90	2 531.80	25.05	0	0	3 259.85	15.89	0	466.26	6.00
西北地区 Northwest China	1 437.00	1 903.00	100.00	0	0	3 484.17	0	0	410.37	22.00

图 8-4-74　2017—2018 年全国及六大区骨肿瘤患儿次均住院分项费用（按中位数计）

Figure 8-4-74　Expenses of each item per hospitalization of children with bone cancer in the six regions and the whole country in 2017-2018（by the median）

医院地区分布 regional distribution of hospitals	分项费用/元 expenses of each item/CNY									
	综合医疗服务类费用 comprehensive medical service expenses	诊断类费用 diagnostic expenses	治疗类费用 treatment expenses	康复类费用 rehabilitation expenses	中医类费用 traditional chinese medicine service expenses	西药类费用 western medication expenses	中药类费用 traditional chinese medication expenses	血液和血液制品类费用 blood and blood product expenses	耗材类费用 medical consumable expenses	其他类费用 others
全国合计 National total	2 111.13	2 463.37	1 712.55	23.47	26.81	7 162.47	327.71	714.52	7 602.18	1 588.31
华北地区 North China	1 785.07	1 839.70	848.57	25.54	27.05	8 832.35	160.87	938.02	10 040.88	108.18
东北地区 Northeast China	1 832.30	2 751.41	2 251.01	19.66	14.74	6 148.27	1 575.15	645.45	3 552.14	749.81
华东地区 East China	2 440.96	2 802.67	1 737.68	21.42	17.23	5 209.68	270.07	615.06	5 876.96	1 035.27
中南地区 Central and Southern China	2 203.52	2 628.31	3 187.27	19.24	42.42	7 056.72	246.12	586.14	7 944.34	5 974.22
西南地区 Southwest China	3 012.39	3 710.03	1 979.94	32.42	11.70	4 708.65	381.12	262.72	3 601.30	736.79
西北地区 Northwest China	2 089.49	2 929.22	1 697.27	19.24	28.92	6 806.79	373.55	406.64	5 512.38	235.69

图 8-4-75　2017—2018 年全国及六大区骨肿瘤患儿次均住院分项费用（按均数计）

Figure 8-4-75　Expenses of each item per hospitalization of children with bone cancer in the six regions and the whole country in 2017-2018（by the mean）

provincial distribution of hospitals	分项费用/元 expenses of each item/CNY									
	综合医疗服务类费用 comprehensive medical service expenses	诊断类费用 diagnostic expenses	治疗类费用 treatment expenses	康复类费用 rehabilitation expenses	中医类服务费用 traditional chinese medicine service expenses	西药类费用 western medication expenses	中药类费用 traditional chinese medication expenses	血液和血液制品类费用 blood and blood product expenses	耗材类费用 medical consumable expenses	其他类费用 others
北京Beijing	1 447.50	591.00	0	20.00	0	7 899.54	0	416.00	459.96	40.00
天津Tianjin	4 480.00	7 802.00	215.00	0	0	5 818.66	0	0	3 505.76	0
河北Hebei	612.70	840.00	0	0	0	4 916.76	0	1 410.00	639.60	0
山西Shanxi	1 426.00	1 347.00	0	0	0	3 375.91	0	0	784.50	0
内蒙古Inner Mongolia	500.50	1 341.00	0	0	0	4 705.83	0	0	8.66	63.00
辽宁Liaoning	1 468.20	2 038.30	369.60	0	0	5 900.05	1 437.90	401.50	1 036.01	36.00
吉林Jilin	1 690.80	2 094.00	0	0	0	3 252.78	42.16	0	692.60	0
黑龙江Heilongjiang	1 317.50	1 603.45	0	0	0	3 807.63	0	0	1 415.10	60.00
上海Shanghai	1 362.50	1 348.50	0	0	0	1 322.82	0	0	661.82	0
江苏Jiangsu	961.20	2 386.00	630.08	0	0	1 020.93	0	0	543.20	46.82
浙江Zhejiang	1 361.25	3 165.81	399.00	33.00	0	2 524.18	78.80	0	1 099.60	45.83
安徽Anhui	1 071.70	2 238.55	141.00	0	0	2 364.90	0	0	505.72	172.80
福建Fujian	2 348.00	1 962.00	0	0	0	3 549.96	0	1 172.00	252.11	0
江西Jiangxi	1 852.00	2 356.00	492.00	0	0	4 386.02	122.24	0	484.61	49.00
山东Shandong	1 562.50	1 387.50	101.50	0	0	4 305.00	26.98	0	648.65	0
河南Henan	1 800.50	0	0	0	0	6 074.25	0	0	144.53	0
湖北Hubei	1 894.25	1 716.65	134.00	0	0	6 337.85	0	0	578.68	48.00
湖南Hunan	1 450.50	1 370.25	0	0	0	3 253.89	0	0	1 147.95	578.00
广东Guangdong	1 231.54	3 355.12	2 826.19	0	0	5 638.68	0	0	1 730.22	652.13
广西Guangxi	1 642.95	1 762.70	678.80	0	0	1 962.70	0	0	352.11	6.92
海南Hainan	1 887.00	2 929.26	1 028.20	0	54.00	7 031.99	153.08	0	1 500.05	0
重庆Chongqing	1 153.47	1 691.45	0	0	0	3 057.48	0	0	327.43	5.00
四川Sichuan	2 487.65	2 763.50	355.00	24.00	0	3 030.91	7.50	0	822.36	6.00
贵州Guizhou	1 758.70	2 642.00	535.00	0	0	3 544.93	0	0	886.40	60.66
云南Yunnan	3 843.60	5 033.00	1 360.00	125.00	0	4 495.23	359.79	0	1 200.78	552.00
西藏Xizang	3 222.00	1 457.00	—	0	—	2 865.11	—	—	—	318.21
陕西Shaanxi	1 379.40	840.50	192.00	20.00	0	1 269.54	0	106.00	99.00	325.38
甘肃Gansu	1 612.50	2 512.00	77.50	0	0	3 221.41	543.50	94.47	311.75	0
青海Qinghai	1 240.00	4 233.00	88.29	0	0	4 991.30	42.63	470.65	682.68	18.00
宁夏Ningxia	964.00	1 751.70	0	0	0	1 386.42	42.63	0	542.22	0
新疆Xinjiang	1 573.00	2 071.00	156.00	0	0	5 563.30	0	0	517.97	34.00

图 8-4-76　2017—2018 年全国各省份骨肿瘤患儿次均住院分项费用（按中位数计）

Figure 8-4-76　Expenses of each item per hospitalization of children with bone cancer in each provincial-level region in 2017-2018 (by the median)

provincial distribution of hospitals	综合医疗服务类费用 comprehensive medical service expenses	诊断类费用 diagnostic expenses	治疗类费用 treatment expenses	康复类费用 rehabilitation expenses	中医类费用 traditional chinese medicine service expenses	西药类费用 western medication expenses	中药类费用 traditional chinese medication expenses	血液和血液制品类费用 blood and blood product expenses	耗材类费用 medical consumable expenses	其他类费用 others
北京Beijing	1 703.77	1 541.79	778.81	25.50	26.86	9 308.41	138.23	913.11	10 882.05	68.34
天津Tianjin	5 945.00	8 454.27	2 175.34	0	0	9 342.95	28.89	795.11	12 257.62	0
河北Hebei	2 111.77	4 364.88	1 256.09	27.22	59.72	8 473.30	234.11	2 134.95	6 849.51	752.52
山西Shanxi	1 949.48	2 143.97	1 040.65	19.54	4.77	4 328.65	290.66	444.49	4 497.52	23.45
内蒙古Inner Mongolia	1 198.75	1 963.70	1 381.89	88.10	69.00	4 997.76	786.10	150.65	325.76	595.05
辽宁Liaoning	1 773.93	2 948.27	4 161.39	0	0	7 361.82	2 271.03	1 023.50	3 801.10	786.24
吉林Jilin	2 234.87	2 891.23	1 569.12	43.02	32.35	4 815.62	1 458.23	944.45	2 767.28	1 274.30
黑龙江Heilongjiang	1 545.48	2 032.94	966.74	0	0	4 275.36	59.64	46.11	3 728.42	122.12
上海Shanghai	3 402.05	3 714.67	2 128.47	59.21	38.05	3 640.07	4.56	72.43	2 704.87	138.55
江苏Jiangsu	1 499.92	3 251.67	2 701.94	26.47	6.66	2 808.89	69.20	854.00	4 358.10	399.11
浙江Zhejiang	2 167.72	4 369.80	3 056.33	70.02	115.25	4 747.29	146.04	316.45	12 774.47	138.90
安徽Anhui	1 240.89	2 571.42	1 352.20	70.87	52.27	3 001.96	151.99	310.64	2 866.04	362.49
福建Fujian	3 582.94	2 796.46	1 462.41	10.69	8.65	5 558.53	84.36	1 972.16	6 982.26	336.21
江西Jiangxi	2 808.14	2 959.61	1 800.34	2.19	0	6 707.81	463.37	391.08	4 588.59	295.96
山东Shandong	2 312.60	2 310.89	1 428.64	9.65	2.43	5 482.00	383.14	264.04	5 713.84	1 902.13
河南Henan	2 412.56	841.18	848.32	23.12	97.34	6 527.38	347.68	501.59	1 811.67	78.66
湖北Hubei	2 111.43	2 918.30	1 736.48	11.87	4.67	7 264.80	276.82	239.85	2 562.73	2 946.07
湖南Hunan	2 327.53	2 588.43	1 633.59	4.11	131.98	5 781.32	231.75	865.73	9 822.69	1 361.16
广东Guangdong	1 845.16	4 656.40	5 989.47	33.93	23.96	7 447.22	183.80	871.30	14 418.57	13 469.55
广西Guangxi	3 997.31	3 407.92	2 104.02	18.67	0	6 064.22	83.46	945.91	3 092.74	620.49
海南Hainan	3 465.88	4 060.55	3 637.86	0	132.50	10 142.75	450.49	1 676.89	8 095.23	0
重庆Chongqing	1 711.10	3 215.30	943.34	9.87	3.39	3 507.89	180.96	112.32	1 280.88	22.31
四川Sichuan	3 619.49	3 432.98	4 352.25	113.63	52.90	4 518.35	222.50	564.09	4 756.83	225.90
贵州Guizhou	2 249.57	3 395.43	2 454.57	15.10	7.56	4 147.44	436.56	430.78	6 381.15	4 859.27
云南Yunnan	5 794.57	5 257.28	2 353.06	24.24	3.26	7 755.81	984.11	308.58	6 687.57	874.35
西藏Xizang	3 542.33	1 408.17	—	141.67	—	5 933.52	—	—	—	329.71
陕西Shaanxi	2 132.63	1 996.71	1 114.12	4.67	17.11	2 801.23	6.42	245.52	2 273.50	737.49
甘肃Gansu	2 156.58	3 041.86	2 106.15	63.72	105.60	4 894.87	901.57	899.56	10 580.58	63.60
青海Qinghai	1 437.96	4 270.24	605.18	65.45	0	7 000.73	162.56	338.18	1 815.63	700.04
宁夏Ningxia	1 274.08	2 997.72	1 486.13	39.10	2.56	2 083.50	119.39	1 136.78	5 215.90	36.72
新疆Xinjiang	2 245.95	3 029.27	1 834.11	3.89	12.99	9 223.40	352.79	229.41	5 348.27	125.20

图 8-4-77　2017—2018 年全国各省份骨肿瘤患儿次均住院分项费用（按均数计）

Figure 8-4-77　Expenses of each item per hospitalization of children with bone cancer in each provincial-level region in 2017-2018 (by the mean)

4.6 全国儿童肿瘤监测机构骨肿瘤患儿平均住院日分析

4.6.1 全国及六大区骨肿瘤患儿平均住院日情况

全国骨肿瘤患儿平均住院日的中位数为7天。高于全国中位数水平的地区分别为中南地区（10天）、西北地区（10天）、华东地区（9天）、西南地区（9天）和东北地区（8天），低于全国中位数水平的地区为华北地区（6天）（图8-4-78）。

4.6.2 各省份骨肿瘤患儿平均住院日情况

根据各省份骨肿瘤患儿平均住院日的中位数，骨肿瘤患儿平均住院日最长的省份是天津（23天），其次是云南（19天）、西藏（18天）和青海（15天），最短的是北京和上海（6天）（图8-4-79）。

4.6 Analysis of the average length of hospitalization of children with bone cancer in pediatric cancer surveillance sites in China

4.6.1 Average length of hospitalization of children with bone cancer in the six regions and the whole country

Nationally, the median of average length of hospitalization was 7 days. Central and Southern China (10 days), Northwest China (10 days), East China (9 days), Southwest China (9 days) and Northeast China (8 days) were above the national median, and North China (6 days) was below the national median (Figure 8-4-78).

4.6.2 Average length of hospitalization of children with bone cancer in each provincial-level region

In terms of the median of average length of hospitalization of children with bone cancer in each provincial-level region, the provincial-level region with the longest average hospital stay was Tianjin (23 days), followed by Yunnan (19 days), Xizang (18 days) and Qinghai (15 days), and the shortest were Beijing and Shanghai (6 days)(Figure 8-4-79).

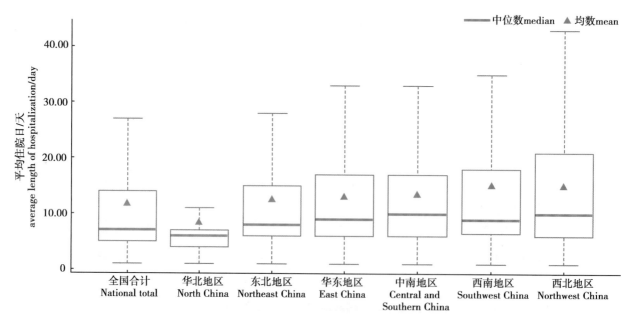

图 8-4-78 2017—2018 年全国及六大区骨肿瘤患儿平均住院日

Figure 8-4-78 Average length of hospitalization of children with bone cancer in the six regions and the whole country in 2017-2018

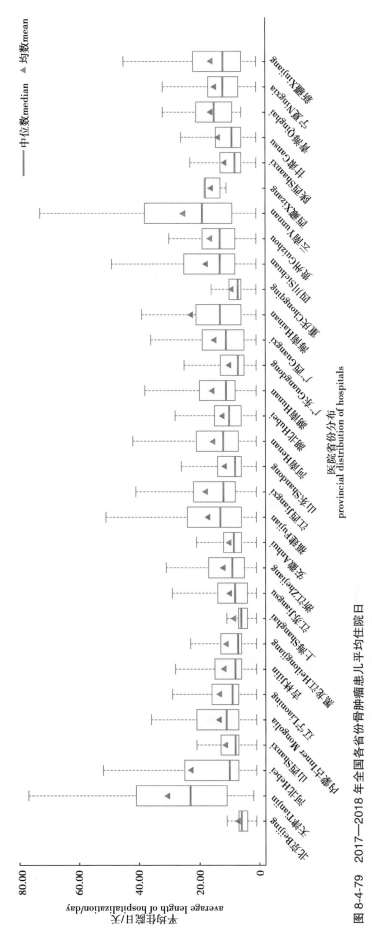

图 8-4-79 2017—2018 年全国各省份骨肿瘤患儿平均住院日

Figure 8-4-79 Average length of hospitalization of children with bone cancer in each provincial-level region in 2017-2018

5 肾癌

5.1 全国儿童肿瘤监测机构肾癌患儿出院人次分析

5.1.1 六大区肾癌患儿出院人次构成情况

在肾癌患儿出院人次中，各大区出院人次占全部出院人次的比例由高到低依次为华东地区（25.96%）、华北地区（25.06%）、中南地区（18.60%）、西北地区（12.31%）、西南地区（12.26%）和东北地区（5.81%）（图 8-5-1）。

5 Kidney cancer

5.1 Analysis of discharges among children with kidney cancer in pediatric cancer surveillance sites in China

5.1.1 Composition of discharges among children with kidney cancer in the six regions

In terms of the discharges among children with kidney cancer, the regions with the highest to the lowest proportions of discharges among children with kidney cancer in all discharges were East China (25.96%), North China (25.06%), Central and Southern China (18.60%), Northwest China (12.31%), Southwest China (12.26%) and Northeast China (5.81%) (Figure 8-5-1).

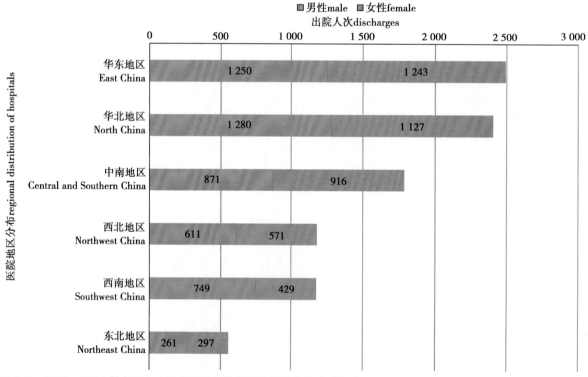

图 8-5-1 2017—2018 年全国六大区儿童肿瘤监测机构肾癌出院人次构成

Figure 8-5-1 Composition of discharges among children with kidney cancer in pediatric cancer surveillance sites in the six regions in 2017-2018

5.1.2　各省份肾癌患儿出院人次构成情况

在所有省份中,肾癌患儿出院人次占全部出院人次比例前 3 位的省份分别为北京(20.78%)、河南(8.21%)和江苏(7.12%),后 3 位分别为西藏(0.00%)、青海(0.06%)和内蒙古(0.12%)(图 8-5-2,图 8-5-3)。

5.1.2　Composition of discharges among children with kidney cancer in each provincial-level region

Among all provincial-level regions, Beijing (20.78%), Henan (8.21%) and Jiangsu (7.12%) were the three provincial-level regions with the highest proportions of discharges among children with kidney cancer in all discharges, and Xizang (0.00%), Qinghai (0.06%) and Inner Mongolia (0.12%) had the lowest proportions of discharges among children with kidney cancer (Figure 8-5-2~Figure 8-5-3).

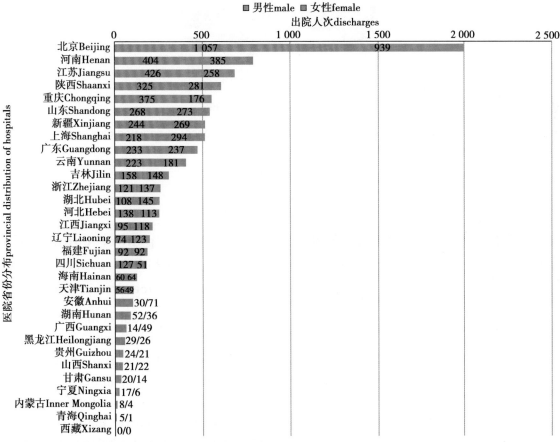

图 8-5-2　2017—2018 年全国各省份儿童肿瘤监测机构肾癌出院人次构成

Figure 8-5-2　Composition of discharges among children with kidney cancer in pediatric cancer surveillance sites in each provincial-level region in 2017-2018

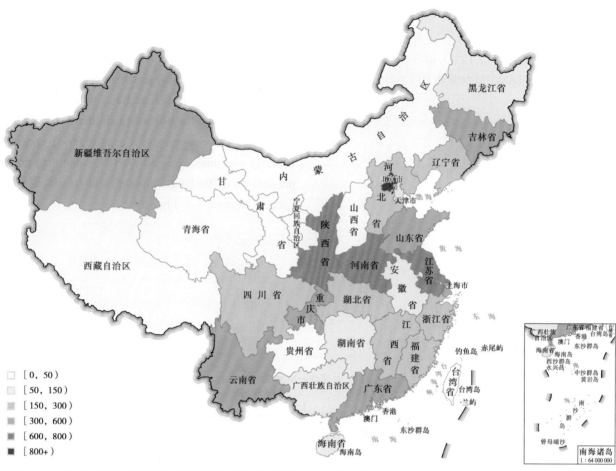

图 8-5-3　2017—2018 年全国各省份儿童肿瘤监测机构肾癌出院人次分布

Figure 8-5-3　Distribution of discharges among children with kidney cancer in pediatric cancer surveillance sites in each provincial-level region in 2017-2018

5.2　全国儿童肿瘤监测机构肾癌患儿年龄／性别构成

5.2.1　全国肾癌患儿年龄／性别构成情况

从性别分布来看，男性患儿占全部出院人次比例为 52.29%，女性患儿为 47.71%。从年龄分布来看，1 岁年龄组所占比例最高（19.83%），其次为 2 岁（18.43%）和 3 岁（15.10%）年龄组（图 8-5-4）。

5.2　Age/gender composition of children with kidney cancer in pediatric cancer surveillance sites in China

5.2.1　Age/gender composition of children with kidney cancer nationally

In terms of gender distribution, male children accounted for 52.29% of all discharges, and female for 47.71%. In terms of age distribution, the 1-year age group accounted for the highest proportion (19.83%), followed by the 2-year age group (18.43%) and 3-year age group (15.10%)(Figure 8-5-4).

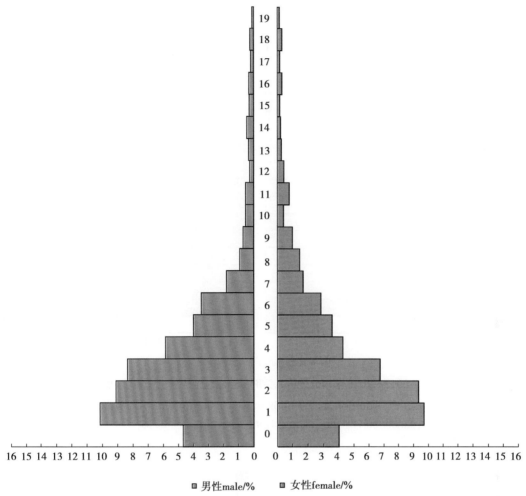

■男性male/%　　　■女性female/%

图 8-5-4　2017—2018 年全国儿童肿瘤监测机构肾癌患儿年龄 / 性别构成

Figure 8-5-4　Age/gender composition of children with kidney cancer in pediatric cancer surveillance sites in China in 2017-2018

5.2.2　六大区肾癌患儿年龄 / 性别构成情况

从性别分布来看,除东北地区和中南地区外的其他四大区均显示男性患儿占全部出院人次比例高于女性患儿。从年龄分布来看,六大区的比例各有不同,其中华北地区、东北地区和中南地区的 1 岁年龄组所占比例最高;华东地区、西南地区和西北地区的 2 岁年龄组所占比例最高(图 8-5-5~图 8-5-10)。

5.2.2　Age/gender composition of children with kidney cancer in the six regions

In terms of gender distribution, male children accounted for a higher proportion of all discharges than female in all the six regions, with the exceptions of Northeast China, and Central and Southern China. In terms of age distribution, the proportions of the six regions were different, among which the proportions of the 1-year age group in North China, Northeast China and Central and Southern China were the highest. The proportions of the 2-year age group in East China, Southwest China and Northwest China were the highest (Figure 8-5-5~Figure 8-5-10).

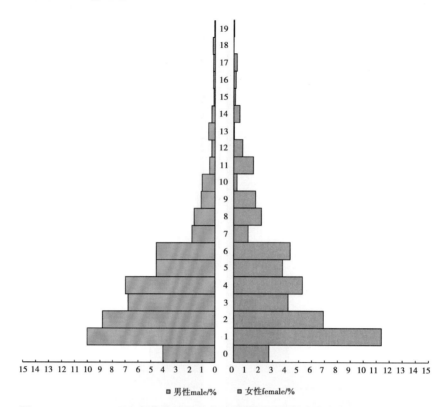

图 8-5-5　2017—2018 年华北地区儿童肿瘤监测机构肾癌患儿年龄／性别构成

Figure 8-5-5　Age/gender composition of children with kidney cancer in pediatric cancer surveillance sites in North China in 2017-2018

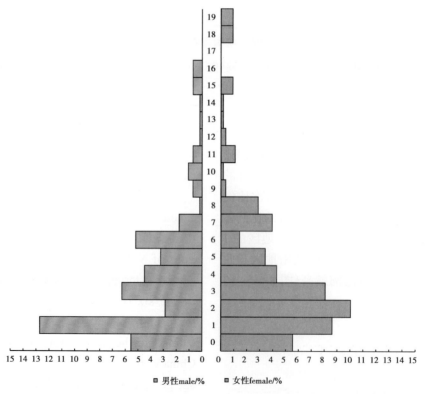

图 8-5-6　2017—2018 年东北地区儿童肿瘤监测机构肾癌患儿年龄／性别构成

Figure 8-5-6　Age/gender composition of children with kidney cancer in pediatric cancer surveillance sites in Northeast China in 2017-2018

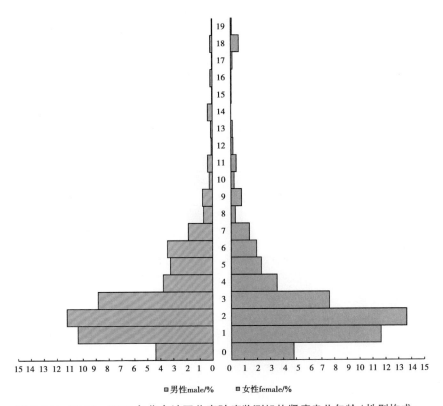

图 8-5-7　2017—2018 年华东地区儿童肿瘤监测机构肾癌患儿年龄/性别构成

Figure 8-5-7　Age/gender composition of children with kidney cancer in pediatric cancer surveillance sites in East China in 2017-2018

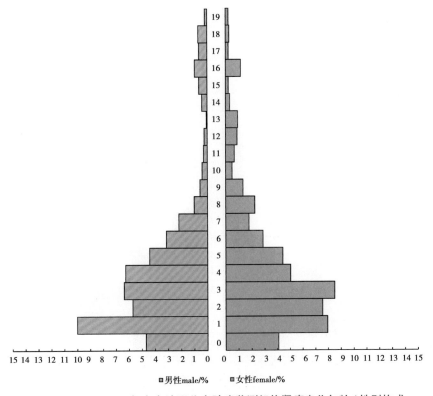

图 8-5-8　2017—2018 年中南地区儿童肿瘤监测机构肾癌患儿年龄/性别构成

Figure 8-5-8　Age/gender composition of children with kidney cancer in pediatric cancer surveillance sites in Central and Southern China in 2017-2018

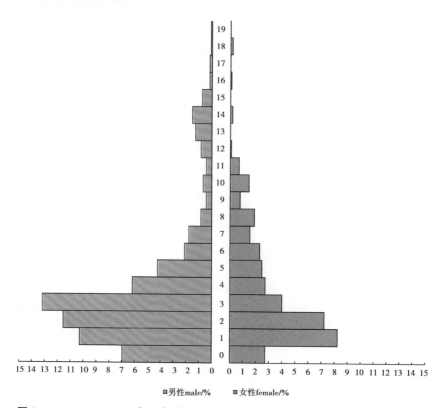

图 8-5-9　2017—2018 年西南地区儿童肿瘤监测机构肾癌患儿年龄／性别构成

Figure 8-5-9　Age/gender composition of children with kidney cancer in pediatric cancer surveillance sites in Southwest China in 2017-2018

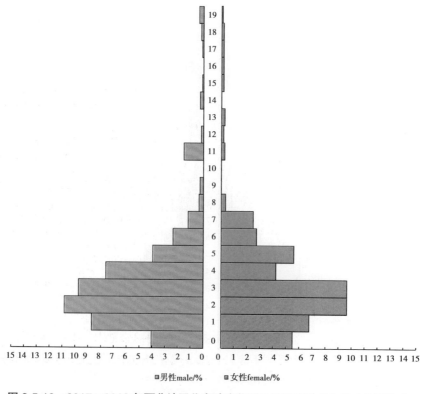

图 8-5-10　2017—2018 年西北地区儿童肿瘤监测机构肾癌患儿年龄／性别构成

Figure 8-5-10　Age/gender composition of children with kidney cancer in pediatric cancer surveillance sites in Northwest China in 2017-2018

5.2.3　各省份肾癌患儿年龄／性别构成情况

从性别和年龄分布来看,各省份出院患儿分布比例各有不同。如陕西,从性别分布来看,男性患儿占全部出院人次比例为53.63%,女性患儿为46.37%;从年龄分布来看,2岁年龄组所占比例最高(25.25%),其次为3岁(20.30%)和4岁(14.85%)年龄组。再如新疆,从性别分布来看,女性患儿占全部出院人次比例为52.44%,男性患儿为47.56%;从年龄分布来看,3岁年龄组所占比例最高(19.10%),其次为1岁(18.71%)和2岁(15.01%)年龄组(图8-5-11~图8-5-31)。

5.2.3　Age/gender composition of children with kidney cancer in each provincial-level region

The gender and age distributions of discharges in each provincial-level region were different. Taking Shaanxi as an example, in terms of gender distribution, male children accounted for 53.63%, and female for 46.37% of all discharges. In terms of age distribution, the 2-year age group accounted for the highest proportion (25.25%), followed by the 3-year age group (20.30%) and 4-year age group (14.85%). In Xinjiang, in terms of gender distribution, female children accounted for 52.44%, and male 47.56% of total discharges. In terms of age distribution, the 3-year age group accounted for the highest proportion (19.10%), followed by the 1-year age group (18.71%) and 2-year age group (15.01%) (Figure 8-5-11~Figure 8-5-31).

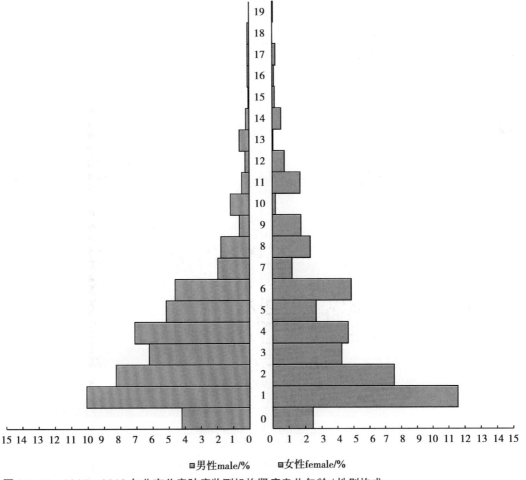

图 8-5-11　2017—2018 年北京儿童肿瘤监测机构肾癌患儿年龄／性别构成

Figure 8-5-11　Age/gender composition of children with kidney cancer in pediatric cancer surveillance sites in Beijing in 2017-2018

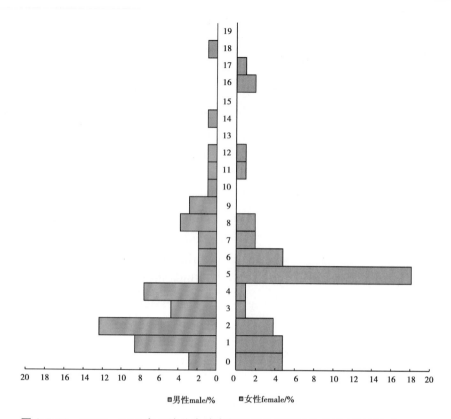

图 8-5-12　2017—2018 年天津儿童肿瘤监测机构肾癌患儿年龄／性别构成

Figure 8-5-12　Age/gender composition of children with kidney cancer in pediatric cancer surveillance sites in Tianjin in 2017-2018

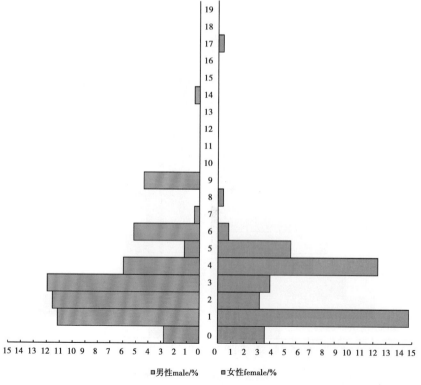

图 8-5-13　2017—2018 年河北儿童肿瘤监测机构肾癌患儿年龄／性别构成

Figure 8-5-13　Age/gender composition of children with kidney cancer in pediatric cancer surveillance sites in Hebei in 2017-2018

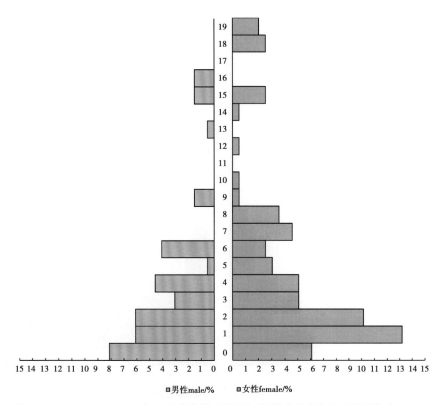

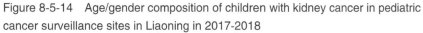

图 8-5-14　2017—2018 年辽宁儿童肿瘤监测机构肾癌患儿年龄 / 性别构成

Figure 8-5-14　Age/gender composition of children with kidney cancer in pediatric cancer surveillance sites in Liaoning in 2017-2018

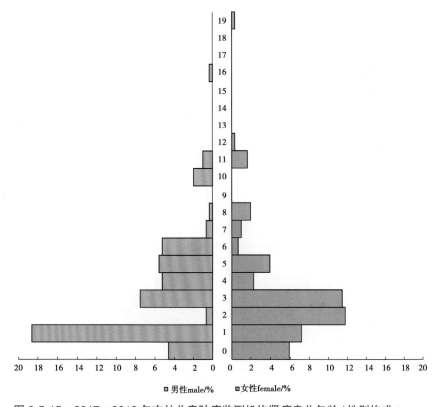

图 8-5-15　2017—2018 年吉林儿童肿瘤监测机构肾癌患儿年龄 / 性别构成

Figure 8-5-15　Age/gender composition of children with kidney cancer in pediatric cancer surveillance sites in Jilin in 2017-2018

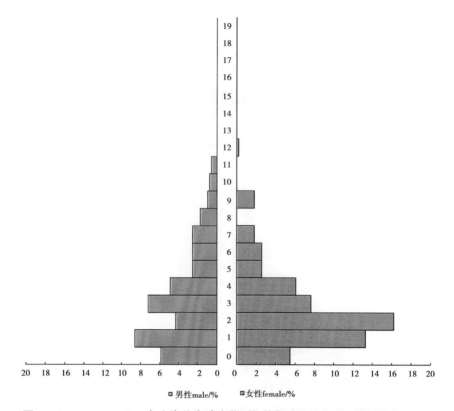

图 8-5-16 2017—2018 年上海儿童肿瘤监测机构肾癌患儿年龄 / 性别构成

Figure 8-5-16 Age/gender composition of children with kidney cancer in pediatric cancer surveillance sites in Shanghai in 2017-2018

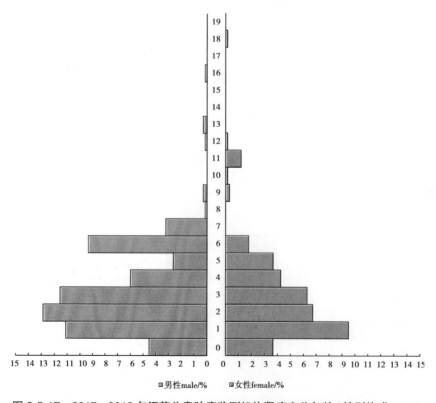

图 8-5-17 2017—2018 年江苏儿童肿瘤监测机构肾癌患儿年龄 / 性别构成

Figure 8-5-17 Age/gender composition of children with kidney cancer in pediatric cancer surveillance sites in Jiangsu in 2017-2018

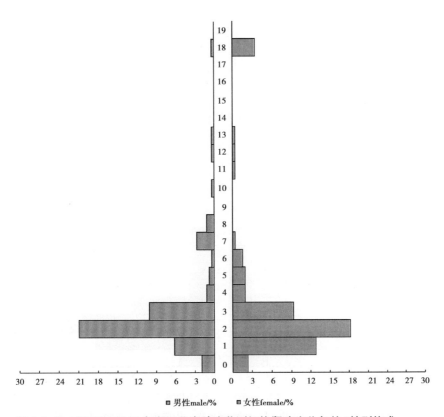

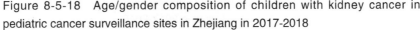

图 8-5-18　2017—2018 年浙江儿童肿瘤监测机构肾癌患儿年龄／性别构成

Figure 8-5-18　Age/gender composition of children with kidney cancer in pediatric cancer surveillance sites in Zhejiang in 2017-2018

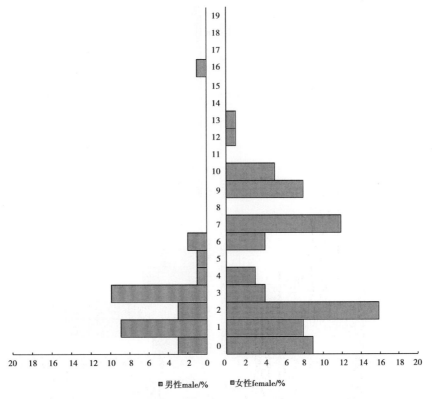

图 8-5-19　2017—2018 年安徽儿童肿瘤监测机构肾癌患儿年龄／性别构成

Figure 8-5-19　Age/gender composition of children with kidney cancer in pediatric cancer surveillance sites in Anhui in 2017-2018

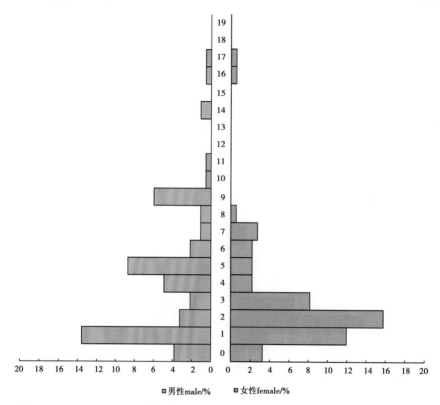

图 8-5-20　2017—2018 年福建儿童肿瘤监测机构肾癌患儿年龄／性别构成

Figure 8-5-20　Age/gender composition of children with kidney cancer in pediatric cancer surveillance sites in Fujian in 2017-2018

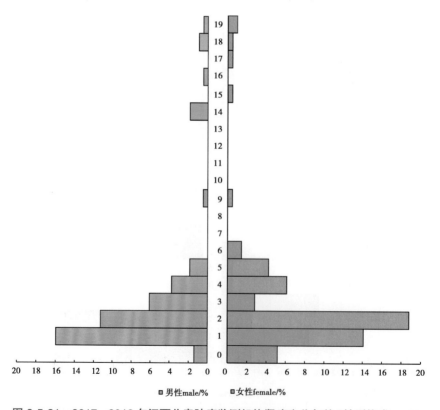

图 8-5-21　2017—2018 年江西儿童肿瘤监测机构肾癌患儿年龄／性别构成

Figure 8-5-21　Age/gender composition of children with kidney cancer in pediatric cancer surveillance sites in Jiangxi in 2017-2018

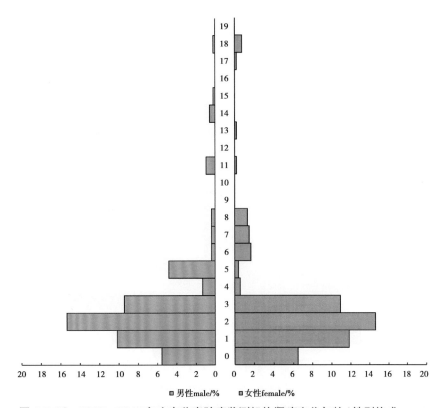

图 8-5-22　2017—2018 年山东儿童肿瘤监测机构肾癌患儿年龄 / 性别构成

Figure 8-5-22　Age/gender composition of children with kidney cancer in pediatric cancer surveillance sites in Shandong in 2017-2018

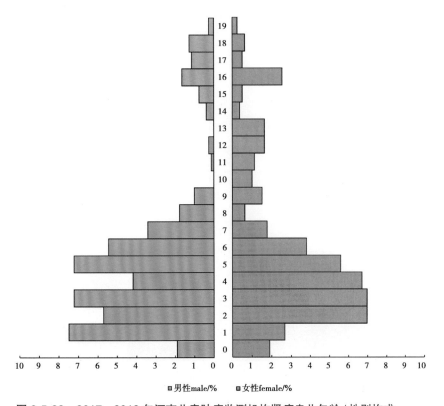

图 8-5-23　2017—2018 年河南儿童肿瘤监测机构肾癌患儿年龄 / 性别构成

Figure 8-5-23　Age/gender composition of children with kidney cancer in pediatric cancer surveillance sites in Henan in 2017-2018

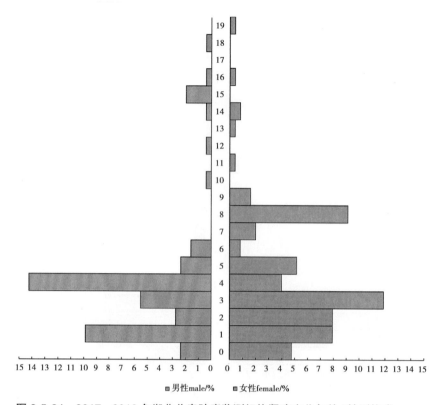

图 8-5-24　2017—2018 年湖北儿童肿瘤监测机构肾癌患儿年龄 / 性别构成

Figure 8-5-24　Age/gender composition of children with kidney cancer in pediatric cancer surveillance sites in Hubei in 2017-2018

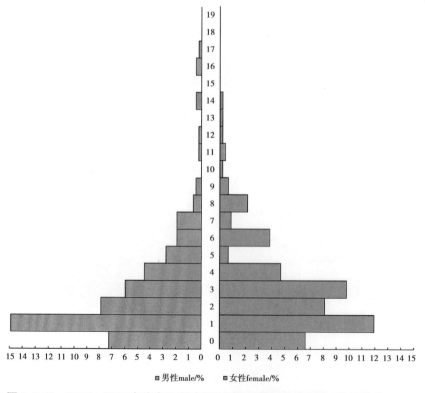

图 8-5-25　2017—2018 年广东儿童肿瘤监测机构肾癌患儿年龄 / 性别构成

Figure 8-5-25　Age/gender composition of children with kidney cancer in pediatric cancer surveillance sites in Guangdong in 2017-2018

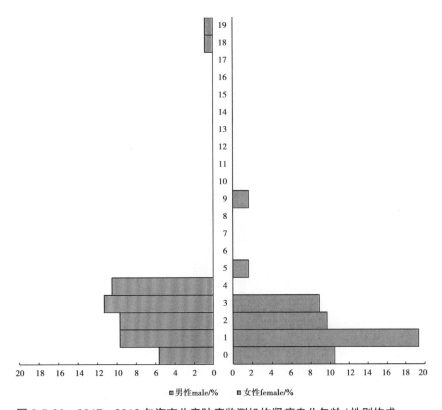

图 8-5-26　2017—2018 年海南儿童肿瘤监测机构肾癌患儿年龄 / 性别构成

Figure 8-5-26　Age/gender composition of children with kidney cancer in pediatric cancer surveillance sites in Hainan in 2017-2018

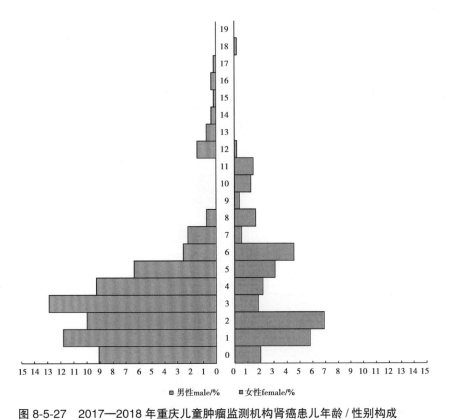

图 8-5-27　2017—2018 年重庆儿童肿瘤监测机构肾癌患儿年龄 / 性别构成

Figure 8-5-27　Age/gender composition of children with kidney cancer in pediatric cancer surveillance sites in Chongqing in 2017-2018

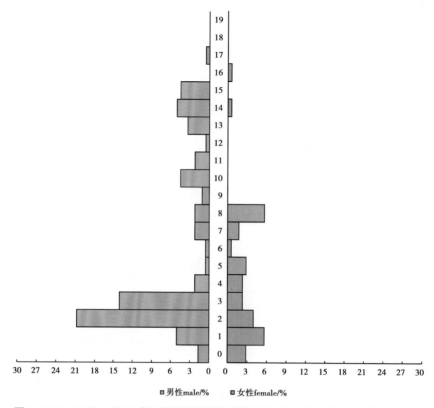

图 8-5-28 2017—2018 年四川儿童肿瘤监测机构肾癌患儿年龄／性别构成

Figure 8-5-28 Age/gender composition of children with kidney cancer in pediatric cancer surveillance sites in Sichuan in 2017-2018

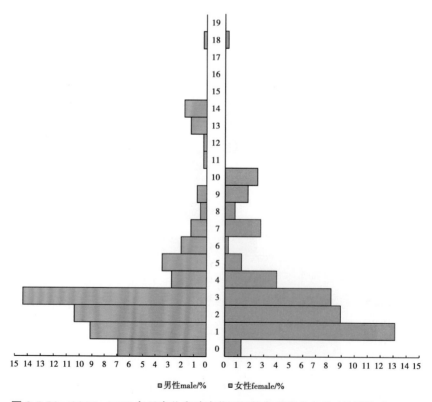

图 8-5-29 2017—2018 年云南儿童肿瘤监测机构肾癌患儿年龄／性别构成

Figure 8-5-29 Age/gender composition of children with kidney cancer in pediatric cancer surveillance sites in Yunnan in 2017-2018

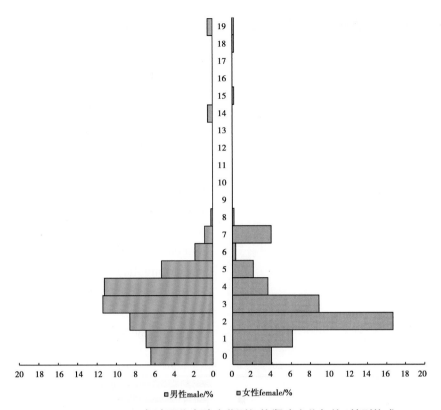

图 8-5-30　2017—2018 年陕西儿童肿瘤监测机构肾癌患儿年龄 / 性别构成

Figure 8-5-30　Age/gender composition of children with kidney cancer in pediatric cancer surveillance sites in Shaanxi in 2017-2018

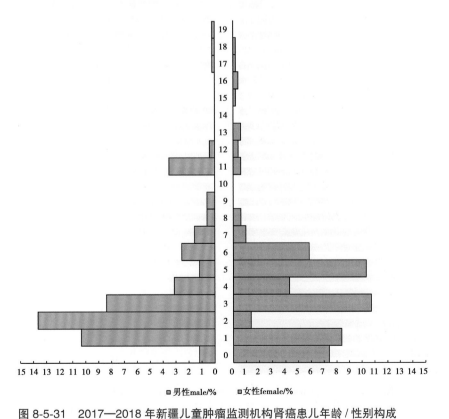

图 8-5-31　2017—2018 年新疆儿童肿瘤监测机构肾癌患儿年龄 / 性别构成

Figure 8-5-31　Age/gender composition of children with kidney cancer in pediatric cancer surveillance sites in Xinjiang in 2017-2018

5.3　全国儿童肿瘤监测机构肾癌患儿就医省份分布

5.3.1　全国各省份肾癌患儿本省就医与省外就医的分布情况

总体而言,肾癌患儿本省就医的比例为63.06%。在所有省份中,本省就医比例前3位的省份分别为北京(99.68%)、上海(96.43%)和吉林(91.27%)。省外就医比例前3位分别为西藏(100.00%)、内蒙古(91.72%)和甘肃(86.73%)(图8-5-32)。

5.3　Distribution of provincial-level regions visited by children with kidney cancer in pediatric cancer surveillance sites in China

5.3.1　Distribution of children with kidney cancer receiving medical treatment in and out of their own provincial-level regions

In general, 63.06% of all children with kidney cancer sought medical treatment in their own provincial-level regions. Beijing (99.68%), Shanghai (96.43%) and Jilin (91.27%) were the top three recipients of patients from other provincial-level regions. Xizang (100.00%), Inner Mongolia (91.72%) and Gansu (86.73%) were the top three provincial-level regions in terms of the proportion of patients going to other provincial-level regions for medical treatment (Figure 8-5-32).

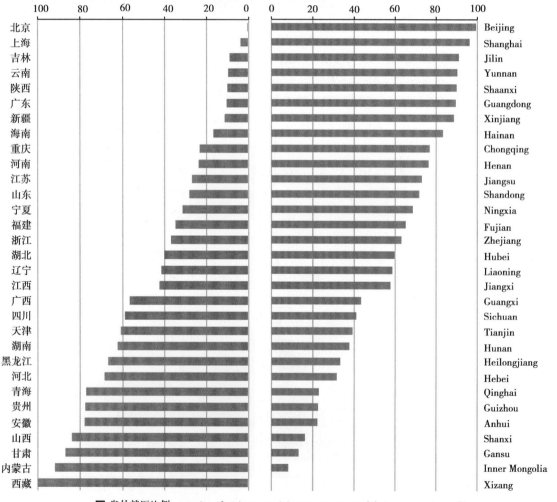

■ 省外就医比例proportion of patients receiving treatment out of their own provinces /%

■ 本省就医比例proportion of patients receiving treatment in their own provinces /%

图 8-5-32　2017—2018 年全国各省份肾癌患儿本省就医与省外就医比例 /%

Figure 8-5-32　Proportion of children with kidney cancer receiving medical treatment in and out of their own provincial-level regions in 2017-2018/%

5.3.2　全国各省份肾癌患儿省外就医的去向省份分布情况

各省份肾癌患儿选择省外就医的去向分布呈现明显的规律，主要的去向省份为北京、上海、重庆、江苏和广东。如户籍地为福建的肾癌患儿，选择省外就医的主要去向为上海、北京和广东，分别占户籍地为福建的肾癌患儿选择省外就医总数的46.4%、25.8%和21.6%。再如户籍地为四川的肾癌患儿，选择省外就医的主要去向为重庆和北京，分别占户籍地为四川的肾癌患儿选择省外就医总数的81.7%和14.6%（图8-5-33，按行方向查看）。

5.3.3　全国各省份收治肾癌患儿来源的省份分布情况

各省份儿童肿瘤监测机构收治的省外就医肾癌患儿来源分布略有差异，多数省份收治的肾癌患儿来源以其相邻省份为主。如天津，其收治的省外就医肾癌患儿主要来源于河北和山东，分别占天津收治的省外就医肾癌患儿总数的43.6%和22.3%。再如湖北，其收治的省外就医肾癌患儿主要来源于河南，占湖北收治的省外就医肾癌患儿总数的87.9%（图8-5-34，按列方向查看）。

5.3.2　Distribution of provincial-level regions receiving children with kidney cancer from other provincial-level regions

The distribution of provincial-level regions receiving children with kidney cancer from other provincial-level regions showed obvious regularity. The main destinations were Beijing, Shanghai, Chongqing, Jiangsu and Guangdong. For Fujian children with kidney cancer, their main destinations were Shanghai, Beijing and Guangdong, accounting for 46.4%, 25.8% and 21.6%, respectively, of the total number of children with kidney cancer going outside Fujian. For Sichuan children with kidney cancer, their main destinations were Chongqing (81.7%) and Beijing (14.6%) (Figure 8-5-33, view in rows).

5.3.3　Distribution of the provincial-level regions of origin of children receiving treatment for kidney cancer out of their own provincial-level regions

There was a slight difference in the distribution of the provincial-level regions of origin of children with kidney cancer admitted to surveillance sites in different provincial-level regions, and most of the children were mainly from their neighboring provincial-level regions. For example, in Tianjin, the children hospitalized from other provincial-level regions were mainly from Hebei and Shandong, accounting for 43.6% and 22.3% of the total children hospitalized from other provincial-level regions in Tianjin, respectively. In Hubei, children from other provincial-level regions hospitalized for kidney cancer were mainly from Henan, accounting for 87.9% of the total (Figure 8-5-34, view in lines).

收治省外就医肿瘤患儿的医院省份分布
provincial distribution of hospitals receiving children with cancer from outside the province

患儿户籍所在省份分布 distribution of the provinces of origin of children with cancer receiving treatment out of their own provinces	北京 Beijing	天津 Tianjin	河北 Hebei	山西 Shanxi	内蒙古 Inner Mongolia	辽宁 Liaoning	吉林 Jilin	黑龙江 Heilongjiang	上海 Shanghai	江苏 Jiangsu	浙江 Zhejiang	安徽 Anhui	福建 Fujian	江西 Jiangxi	山东 Shandong	河南 Henan	湖北 Hubei	湖南 Hunan	广东 Guangdong	广西 Guangxi	海南 Hainan	重庆 Chongqing	四川 Sichuan	贵州 Guizhou	云南 Yunnan	西藏 Xizang	陕西 Shaanxi	甘肃 Gansu	青海 Qinghai	宁夏 Ningxia	新疆 Xinjiang	合计 total
北京 Beijing	100.0	0	0	0	0	0	0	0	0	0	0	0	0	0	0	0	0	0	0	0	0	0	0	0	0	0	0	0	0	0	0	100
天津 Tianjin	84.0	10.2	5.9	0	0	0	0	0	0	0	0	0	0	0	0	0	0	0	0	0	0	0	0	0	0	0	0	0	0	0	0	100
河北 Hebei	64.5	6.3	0	0	0	0	0	0	0	0	0	0	0	0	0	0	0	0	0	0	0	0	0	0	0	0	0	0	0	0	0	100
山西 Shanxi	46.5	1.5	7.5	0	0	0	0	0	1.0	0	0	0	0	0	4.8	0	0	0	0	0	0	0.5	0	0	0	0	20.9	0	0	0.8	8.2	100
内蒙古 Inner Mongolia	99.2	0	0	0	0	0	0	0	0	0	0	0	0	0	0	0	0	0	0	0	0	0	0	0	0	0	0	0	0	0	0	100
辽宁 Liaoning	54.1	4.2	0	0	0	33.3	0	0	0.8	0	0	0	0	0	4.2	0	0	0	0	0	0	0	0	0	0	0	0	0	0	0	0	100
吉林 Jilin	80.0	0	0	0	0	0	0	0	0	0	0	0	0	0	0	0	0	0	0	0	0	0	0	0	0	0	0	0	0	0	0	100
黑龙江 Heilongjiang	0	0	0.9	0	0	0	39.1	0	5.5	0	0	0	0	0	0	0	0	0	0	0	0	0	0	0	0	0	0	0	0	0	0	100
上海 Shanghai	28.5	0	0	0	0	0	0	0	70.4	0	0	0	0	0	0	0	0	0	0	0	0	0	0	0	0	0	0	0	0	0	0	100
江苏 Jiangsu	15.3	1.1	0	0	0	0	0	0	70.2	0	0	0	0	0	11.8	0	0	0	0	0	0	0	0	0	0	0	0	0	0	0	0	100
浙江 Zhejiang	16.8	1.0	0	0	0	0	0	0	22.0	49.7	0	0	0	0	0	0	0	0	0	0	0	0	0	0	0	0	0	0	0	0	0	100
安徽 Anhui	25.7	1.4	2.0	0	0	0	0	0	46.4	0	7.2	0	0	0	0	0	0	0	0	0	0	0	0	0	0	0	0	0	0	0	0.3	100
福建 Fujian	15.6	0	0	0	0	0	0	0	52.6	0	1.0	0	0	1.0	0	0	0	0	21.6	0	0	0	0	0	0	0	3.1	0	0	0	0	100
江西 Jiangxi	69.2	0	0	0	0	0	0	0	4.5	0	3.9	0	0	0	0	0.3	0.3	11.7	16.2	0	0	0	0	0	0	0	3.8	0	0	0	0	100
山东 Shandong	67.1	10.6	5.6	0	0	0	0	0	0	0	0.5	0	0	0	0	0	0	0	0	0	0	0	0	0	0	0	0	0	0	0	0.5	100
河南 Henan	37.8	2.5	5.5	0	0	0	0	0	16.4	0	2.1	0.4	0	0	7.1	0	12.2	0	0	0	0	0	0	0	0	0	0.4	0	0	0	0	100
湖北 Hubei	34.5	2.7	5.5	0	0	0	0	0	15.0	0	20.5	0	0	0	0	0	0	3.1	3.8	0	0	0	0	0	0	0	3.4	0	0	0	0	100
湖南 Hunan	40.7	1.9	0	0	0	0	0	0	0	0	5.6	0	0	0	0	0	1.4	0	8.9	0	0	0	0	0	0	0	0	1.9	0	0	0	100
广东 Guangdong	13.4	0	0	0	0	0	0	0	8.5	0	3.1	0	0	0	0	0	0	0	40.2	0	0	0	0	0	0	0	0	0	0	0	0	100
广西 Guangxi	0	6.1	0	0	0	0	0	0	4.2	0	0	0	0	0	0	0	0	0	68.3	0	0	3.7	0	0	0	0	0	0	0	0	0	100
海南 Hainan	0	0	0	0	0	0	0	0	4.2	0	0	0	0	0	0	0	0	0	37.5	0	0	0	0	0	0	0	0	0	0	0	0	100
重庆 Chongqing	14.7	0	0	0	0	0	0	0	0	0	0	0	0.4	0	0	0	0	0	0.4	0	0.8	81.7	1.6	0	0	0	0	0	0	0	0	100
四川 Sichuan	4.6	0	0	0	0	0	0	0	0	0	0	0	0	0	0	0	0	0	0	0	0	90.7	0	0	0.7	0	0.8	0	0	0	0	100
贵州 Guizhou	57.2	0	0	0	0	0	0	0	0	0	0	0	0	0	0	0	0	2.0	14.2	0	0	11.9	0	0	0	0	0	0	0	0	0	100
云南 Yunnan	0	0	0	0	0	0	0	0	0	0	9.5	0	0	0	0	0	0	0	0	0	0	42.9	42.9	0	0	0	0	0	0	0	0	100
西藏 Xizang	87.4	0	0	0	0	0	0	0	0	0	0	0	0	0	0	0	0	0	0	0	0	0	0	0	0	0	0	0	0	0	0	100
陕西 Shaanxi	42.8	0	0	0	0	0	0	0	2.4	0	0	0	0	0	0	0	0	0	0	0	0	0	0	0	0	0	51.8	0	0	0	0	100
甘肃 Gansu	25.0	0	0	0	0	0	0	0	0	0	0	0	0	0	5.0	0	0	0	0	0	0	0	0	0	0	0	30.0	30.0	5.0	0	0.6	100
青海 Qinghai	20.0	0	0	0	0	0	0	0	0	0	0	0	0	0	0	0	0	0	0	0	0	0	0	0	0	0	80.0	0	0	0	0	100
宁夏 Ningxia	0	0	0	0	0	0	0	0	0	0	0	0	0	0	0	0	0	0	0	0	0	0	0	0	0	0	0	0	0	0	0	100
新疆 Xinjiang	93.2	0	0	0	0	0	0	0	1.7	0	0	0	0	0	0	0	0	0	3.4	0	0	0	1.7	0	0	0	0	0	0	0	0	100

图 8-5-33　2017—2018 年全国各省份户籍地肾癌患儿选择省外就医的省份分布/%

Figure 8-5-33　Distribution of provincial-level regions receiving children with kidney cancer from other provincial-level regions in 2017-2018/%

收治省外就医肿瘤患儿的医院省份分布 / provincial distribution of hospitals receiving children with cancer from outside the province

患儿就医所在省份来源分布 / distribution of the provinces of origin of children with cancer receiving treatment out of their own provinces（%）

来源省份＼就医医院省份	北京 Beijing	天津 Tianjin	河北 Hebei	山西 Shanxi	内蒙古 Inner Mongolia	辽宁 Liaoning	吉林 Jilin	黑龙江 Heilongjiang	上海 Shanghai	江苏 Jiangsu	浙江 Zhejiang	安徽 Anhui	福建 Fujian	江西 Jiangxi	山东 Shandong	河南 Henan	湖北 Hubei	湖南 Hunan	广东 Guangdong	广西 Guangxi	海南 Hainan	重庆 Chongqing	四川 Sichuan	贵州 Guizhou	云南 Yunnan	西藏 Xizang	陕西 Shaanxi	甘肃 Gansu	青海 Qinghai	宁夏 Ningxia	新疆 Xinjiang
北京 Beijing	1.0	0	1.5	0	0	0	0	0	0	0	0	0	0	0	0	0	0	0	0	0	0	0	0	0	0	0	0	0	0	0	0
天津 Tianjin	19.8	0	0	0	0	0	0	0	0	0	0	0	0	0	0	0	0	0	0	0	0	0	0	0	0	0	0	0	0	0	0
河北 Hebei	8.4	43.6	0	0	0	0	0	0	0.9	0	0	0	0	0	55.9	16.7	0	0	0	0	0	0	0	0	0	0	0	0	0	0	0
山西 Shanxi	3.7	2.1	19.7	0	0	0	0	0	0	0	0	0	0	0	0	0	3.0	0	0	0	0	0	10.0	0	0	0	27.8	0	0	0	47.4
内蒙古 Inner Mongolia	7.6	0	15.2	0	0	25.0	94.5	0	0	0	0	0	0	0	0	0	0	0	0	0	0	0	0	0	0	0	1.8	0	0	100.0	0
辽宁 Liaoning	0.8	1.1	1.5	0	0	0	5.5	0	0	0	0	0	0	0	0	0	0	0	0	0	0	0	0	0	0	0	0	0	0	0	2.7
吉林 Jilin	5.2	0	0	0	0	66.7	0	0	0	0	0	0	0	0	2.9	0	0	0	0	0	0	0	0	0	0	0	0	0	0	0	0
黑龙江 Heilongjiang	0	2.1	0	0	0	8.3	0	0	0	0	0	0	0	0	0	0	0	0	0	0	0	0	0	0	0	0	0	0	0	0	0
上海 Shanghai	3.0	1.1	0	0	0	0	0	0	26.0	0	0	0	0	0	0	0	0	0	0	0	0	0	0	0	0	0	0	0	0	0	2.6
江苏 Jiangsu	0.9	5.3	0	0	0	0	0	0	15.1	0	0	0	0	0	38.3	0	0	0	0	0	0	0	0	0	0	0	0	0	0	0	0
浙江 Zhejiang	3.4	0	10.6	0	0	0	0	0	15.7	4.6	0	0	0	50.0	0	0	3.1	0	0	0	0	0	0	100.0	0	0	2.4	0	0	0	0
安徽 Anhui	1.5	0	0	0	0	0	0	0	9.3	88.2	31.5	0	0	0	0	0	0	0	0	0	0	0	0	0	0	0	0	0	0	0	2.6
福建 Fujian	1.4	0	0	0	0	0	0	0	16.7	0	1.3	0	0	0	0	0	0	0	11.2	0	0	0	0	0	0	0	0	0	0	0	0
江西 Jiangxi	8.1	0	0	0	0	0	0	0	1.9	0	7.6	0	0	0	0	0	0	78.3	13.4	0	0	0	0	0	0	0	1.8	0	0	0	0
山东 Shandong	9.4	22.3	16.7	0	0	0	0	0	1.6	0	1.3	0	0	0	0	0	0	0	0	0	0	0	0	0	0	0	0	0	0	0	0
河南 Henan	3.3	6.4	19.7	0	0	0	0	0	4.9	2.1	6.3	100.0	0	0	0	0	87.9	0	4.8	0	0	0	0	0	0	0	0.6	0	0	0	0
湖北 Hubei	2.2	4.3	12.1	0	0	0	0	0	3.3	1.5	38.0	0	0	50.0	0	5.5	0	8.7	7.0	0	0	0	0	0	0	0	3.0	0	0	0	0
湖南 Hunan	0.8	2.1	0	0	0	0	0	0	1.4	2.1	7.6	0	0	0	0	0	0	0	23.0	0	0	0.9	0	0	0	0	0	0	0	0	0
广东 Guangdong	0.7	0	0	0	0	0	0	0	1.4	0.5	1.3	0	0	0	0	0	0	13.0	0	0	0	0.3	0	0	0	0	0	0	0	0	42.1
广西 Guangxi	0.8	5.3	0	0	0	0	0	0	0.2	0	0	0	0	0	0	0	0	0	29.9	0	0	0	0	0	0	0	0	0	0	0	0
海南 Hainan	3.6	0	0	0	0	0	0	0	0	0	0	0	0	0	0	0	0	0	4.8	0	0	0	0	0	0	0	0	0	0	0	0
重庆 Chongqing	2.1	0	0	0	0	0	0	0	0	0	0	0	0	0	0	0	0	0	0	0	0	0	10.0	0	0	0	0	0	0	0	0
四川 Sichuan	0.4	0	0	0	0	0	0	0	0.6	1.0	0	0	100.0	0	0	0	3.0	0	0.5	0	100.0	56.5	0	0	100.0	0	1.2	0	0	0	0
贵州 Guizhou	1.4	0	0	0	0	0	0	0	0	0	0	0	0	0	0	0	0	0	0	0	0	39.2	0	0	0	0	0	0	0	0	0
云南 Yunnan	0	0	0	0	0	0	0	0	0	0	5.1	0	0	0	0	0	0	0	2.7	0	0	1.4	40.0	0	0	0	0	0	0	0	0
西藏 Xizang	2.5	3.2	0	0	0	0	0	0	0	0	0	0	0	0	0	0	0	0	0	0	0	0	30.0	0	0	0	0	0	0	0	0
陕西 Shaanxi	4.3	1.1	0	0	0	0	0	0	0	0	0	0	0	0	0	0	0	0	0	0	0	0.6	0	0	0	0	0	0	0	0	0
甘肃 Gansu	0.3	0	0	0	0	0	0	0	0.8	0	0	0	0	0	0	0	3.0	0	0	0	0	0.9	0	0	0	0	53.0	0	0	0	2.6
青海 Qinghai	0.1	0	3.0	0	0	0	0	0	0	0	0	0	0	0	2.9	0	0	0	0	0	0	0	0	0	0	0	3.6	75.0	0	0	0
宁夏 Ningxia	3.3	0	0	0	0	0	0	0	0	0	0	0	0	0	0	0	0	0	0	0	0	0	0	0	0	0	4.8	25.0	0	0	0
新疆 Xinjiang	0	0	0	0	0	0	0	0	0	0	0	0	0	0	0	0	0	0	0	0	0	0	10.0	0	0	0	0	0	0	0	0
合计 Total	100	100	100			100	100		100	100	100	100	100	100	100	100	100	100	100	100	100	100	100	100	100		100	100		100	100

图 8-5-34　2017—2018 年全国各省省份儿童肿瘤监测机构省外就医肾癌患儿来源分布 /%

Figure 8-5-34　Distribution of provincial-level regions of origin of children with kidney cancer going outside their provincial-level regions for medical treatment in 2017-2018/%

5.4 全国儿童肿瘤监测机构肾癌患儿住院费用医疗付费方式构成

5.4.1 全国肾癌患儿住院费用医疗付费方式构成情况

全国肾癌患儿住院费用的医疗付费方式中，占比最高的前3种类型分别为全自费（32.03%）、新型农村合作医疗（22.34%）和城镇居民基本医疗保险（19.06%）（图8-5-35）。

5.4 Composition of medical payment methods for hospitalization expenses of children with kidney cancer in pediatric cancer surveillance sites in China

5.4.1 Composition of medical payment methods for hospitalization expenses of children with kidney cancer nationally

Among the medical payment methods of children with kidney cancer nationally, the top three methods were 100% self-pay (32.03%), new rural cooperative medical system (22.34%) and basic medical insurance for urban residents (19.06%) (Figure 8-5-35).

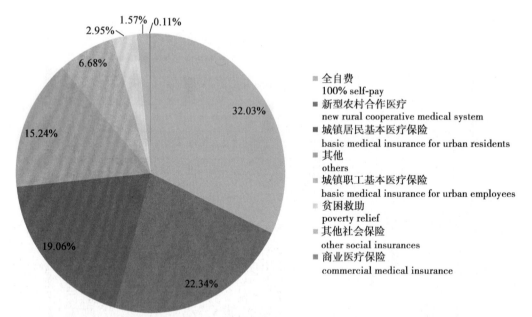

图 8-5-35　2017—2018 年全国肾癌患儿住院费用医疗付费方式构成

Figure 8-5-35　Composition of medical payment methods for hospitalization expenses of children with kidney cancer nationally in 2017-2018

5.4.2 六大区肾癌患儿住院费用医疗付费方式构成情况

六大区的医疗付费方式所占比例各不相同，西南地区和华东地区均以全自费占比最高，分别为 60.05% 和 38.81%；中南地区和东北地区均以新型农村合作医疗占比最高，分别为 40.31% 和 30.33%；华北地区以城镇居民基本医疗保险占比最高，为 29.44%；西北地区以其他占比最高，为 32.29%（图 8-5-36~ 图 8-5-41）。

5.4.2 Composition of medical payment methods for hospitalization expenses of children with kidney cancer in the six regions

The proportions of medical payment methods in the six regions were different, and the proportion of 100% self-pay was the highest in Southwest China and East China, which were 60.05% and 38.81%. In Central and Southern China and Northeast China, the proportions of new rural cooperative medical system was the highest, accounting for 40.31% and 30.33%. In North China, the proportion of basic medical insurance for urban residents was the highest, accounting for 29.44%. In Northwest China, other payment methods had the highest proportion, accounting for 32.29% (Figure 8-5-36~Figure 8-5-41).

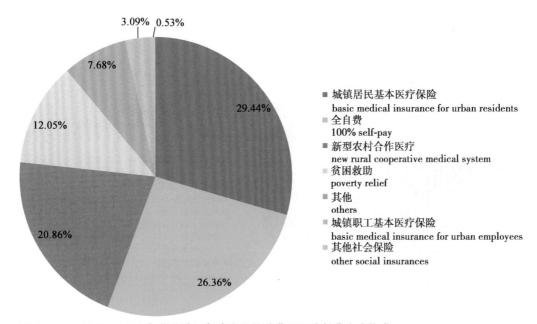

图 8-5-36　2017—2018 年华北地区肾癌患儿住院费用医疗付费方式构成

Figure 8-5-36　Composition of medical payment methods for hospitalization expenses of children with kidney cancer in North China in 2017-2018

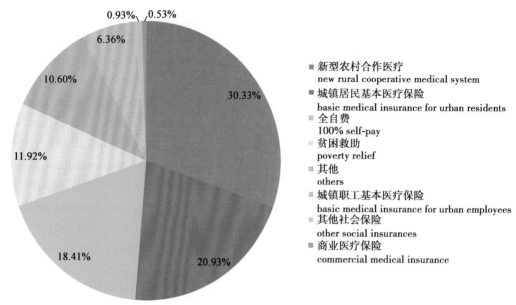

图 8-5-37　2017—2018 年东北地区肾癌患儿住院费用医疗付费方式构成

Figure 8-5-37　Composition of medical payment methods for hospitalization expenses of children with kidney cancer in Northeast China in 2017-2018

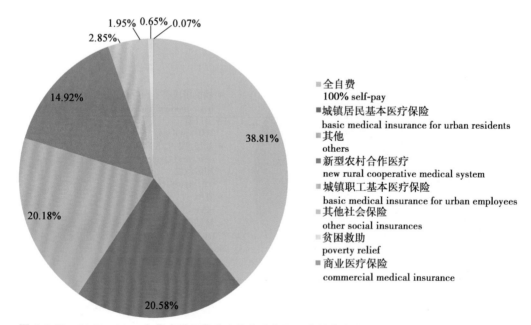

图 8-5-38　2017—2018 年华东地区肾癌患儿住院费用医疗付费方式构成

Figure 8-5-38　Composition of medical payment methods for hospitalization expenses of children with kidney cancer in East China in 2017-2018

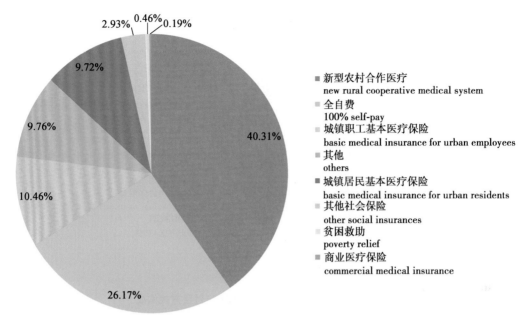

图 8-5-39   2017—2018 年中南地区肾癌患儿住院费用医疗付费方式构成

Figure 8-5-39   Composition of medical payment methods for hospitalization expenses of children with kidney cancer in Central and Southern China in 2017-2018

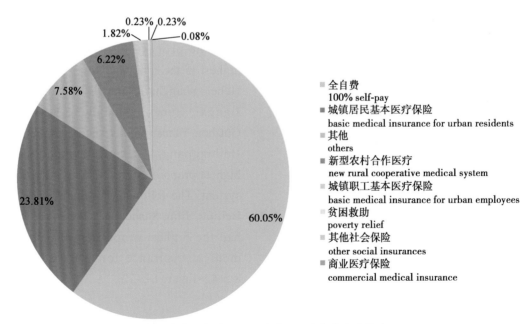

图 8-5-40   2017—2018 年西南地区肾癌患儿住院费用医疗付费方式构成

Figure 8-5-40   Composition of medical payment methods for hospitalization expenses of children with kidney cancer in Southwest China in 2017-2018

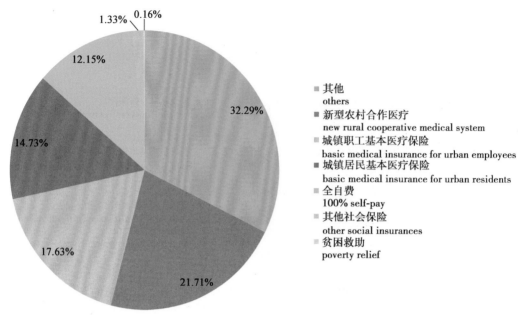

图 8-5-41 2017—2018 年西北地区肾癌患儿住院费用医疗付费方式构成

Figure 8-5-41 Composition of medical payment methods for hospitalization expenses of children with kidney cancer in Northwest China in 2017-2018

5.4.3 各省份肾癌患儿住院费用医疗付费方式构成情况

河北、上海、江苏、浙江、安徽、福建、江西、湖南、广东、广西、四川、贵州、云南和西藏 14 个省份均以全自费所占比例最高。山西、内蒙古、黑龙江、河南、海南和甘肃 6 个省份的新型农村合作医疗保险占比最高。北京、吉林、山东、重庆和宁夏 5 个省份的城镇居民基本医疗保险占比最高(图 8-5-42~图 8-5-72)。

5.4.3 Composition of medical payment methods for hospitalization expenses of children with kidney cancer in each provincial-level region

The proportion of 100% self-pay was the highest in the following 14 provincial-level regions: Hebei, Shanghai, Jiangsu, Zhejiang, Anhui, Fujian, Jiangxi, Hunan, Guangdong, Guangxi, Sichuan, Guizhou, Yunnan and Xizang. Shanxi, Inner Mongolia, Heilongjiang, Henan, Hainan and Gansu had the highest proportion of new rural cooperative medical system. The following 5 provincial-level regions—Beijing, Jilin, Shandong, Chongqing and Ningxia—had the highest proportion of payment by basic medical insurance for urban residents (Figure 8-5-42~Figure 8-5-72).

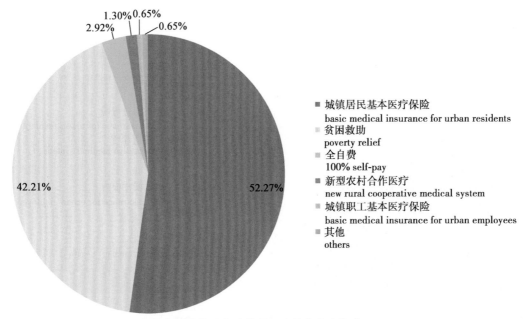

图 8-5-42　2017—2018 年北京肾癌患儿住院费用医疗付费方式构成

Figure 8-5-42　Composition of medical payment methods for hospitalization expenses of children with kidney cancer in Beijing in 2017-2018

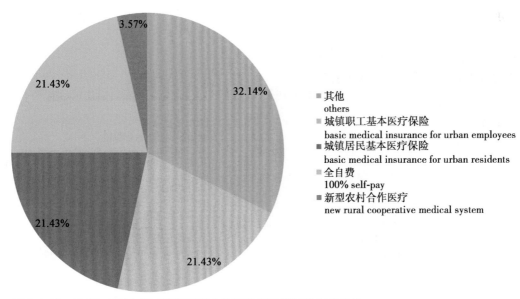

图 8-5-43　2017—2018 年天津肾癌患儿住院费用医疗付费方式构成

Figure 8-5-43　Composition of medical payment methods for hospitalization expenses of children with kidney cancer in Tianjin in 2017-2018

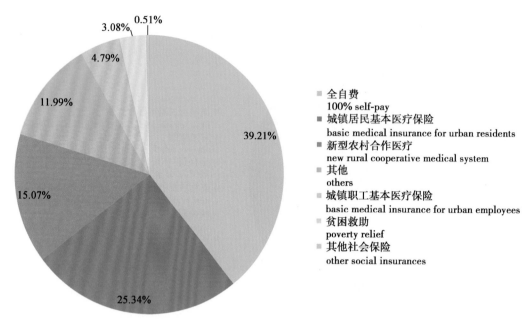

图 8-5-44　2017—2018 年河北肾癌患儿住院费用医疗付费方式构成

Figure 8-5-44　Composition of medical payment methods for hospitalization expenses of children with kidney cancer in Hebei in 2017-2018

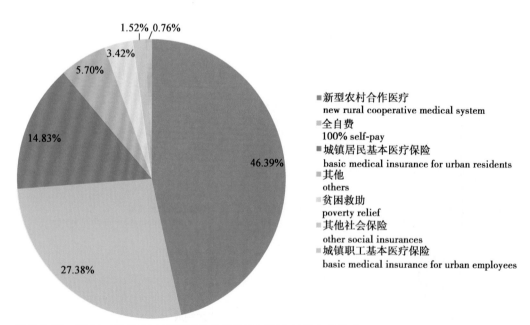

图 8-5-45　2017—2018 年山西肾癌患儿住院费用医疗付费方式构成

Figure 8-5-45　Composition of medical payment methods for hospitalization expenses of children with kidney cancer in Shanxi in 2017-2018

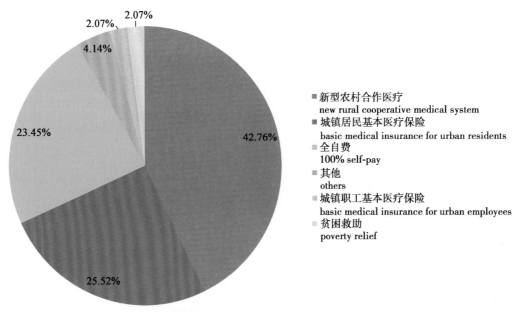

图 8-5-46　2017—2018 年内蒙古肾癌患儿住院费用医疗付费方式构成

Figure 8-5-46　Composition of medical payment methods for hospitalization expenses of children with kidney cancer in Inner Mongolia in 2017-2018

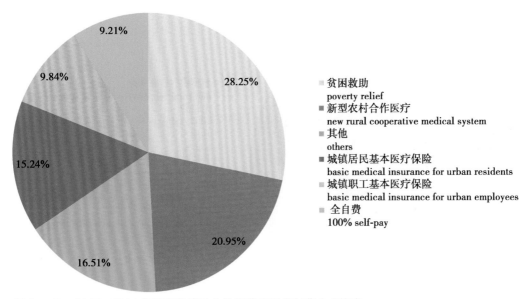

图 8-5-47　2017—2018 年辽宁肾癌患儿住院费用医疗付费方式构成

Figure 8-5-47　Composition of medical payment methods for hospitalization expenses of children with kidney cancer in Liaoning in 2017-2018

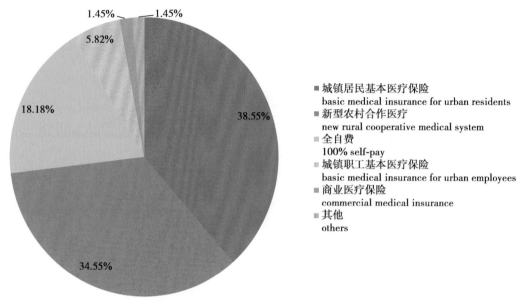

图 8-5-48 　2017—2018 年吉林肾癌患儿住院费用医疗付费方式构成

Figure 8-5-48 　Composition of medical payment methods for hospitalization expenses of children with kidney cancer in Jilin in 2017-2018

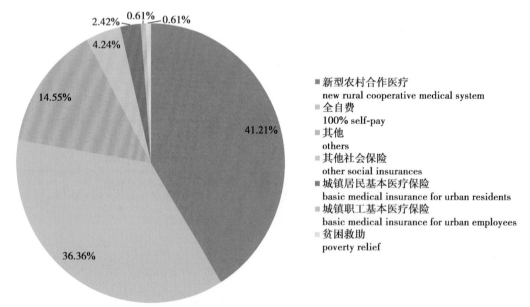

图 8-5-49 　2017—2018 年黑龙江肾癌患儿住院费用医疗付费方式构成

Figure 8-5-49 　Composition of medical payment methods for hospitalization expenses of children with kidney cancer in Heilongjiang in 2017-2018

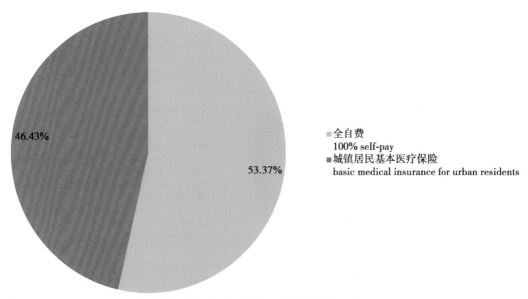

图 8-5-50　2017—2018 年上海肾癌患儿住院费用医疗付费方式构成

Figure 8-5-50　Composition of medical payment methods for hospitalization expenses of children with kidney cancer in Shanghai in 2017-2018

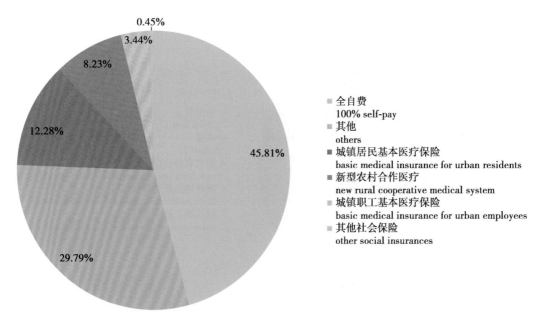

图 8-5-51　2017—2018 年江苏肾癌患儿住院费用医疗付费方式构成

Figure 8-5-51　Composition of medical payment methods for hospitalization expenses of children with kidney cancer in Jiangsu in 2017-2018

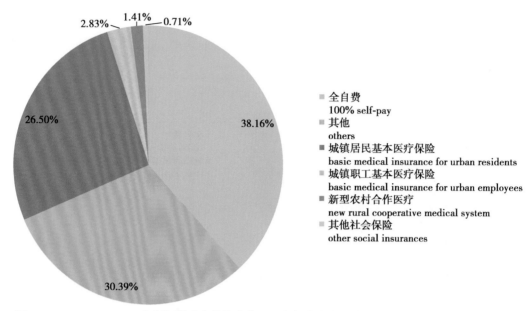

图 8-5-52　2017—2018 年浙江肾癌患儿住院费用医疗付费方式构成

Figure 8-5-52　Composition of medical payment methods for hospitalization expenses of children with kidney cancer in Zhejiang in 2017-2018

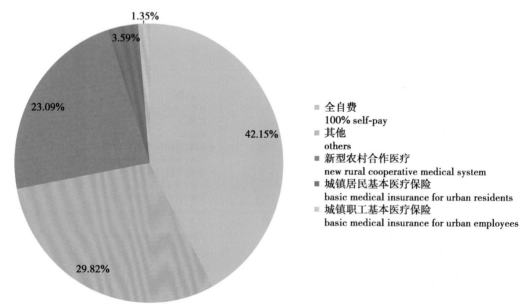

图 8-5-53　2017—2018 年安徽肾癌患儿住院费用医疗付费方式构成

Figure 8-5-53　Composition of medical payment methods for hospitalization expenses of children with kidney cancer in Anhui in 2017-2018

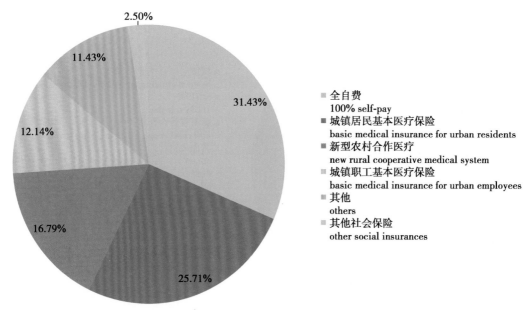

图 8-5-54　2017—2018 年福建肾癌患儿住院费用医疗付费方式构成

Figure 8-5-54　Composition of medical payment methods for hospitalization expenses of children with kidney cancer in Fujian in 2017-2018

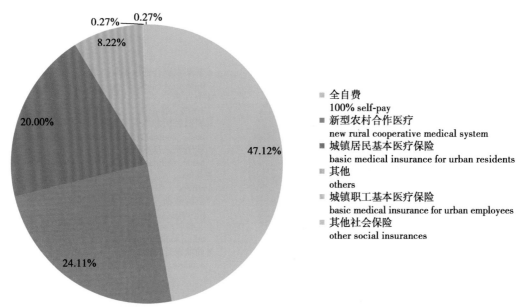

图 8-5-55　2017—2018 年江西肾癌患儿住院费用医疗付费方式构成

Figure 8-5-55　Composition of medical payment methods for hospitalization expenses of children with kidney cancer in Jiangxi in 2017-2018

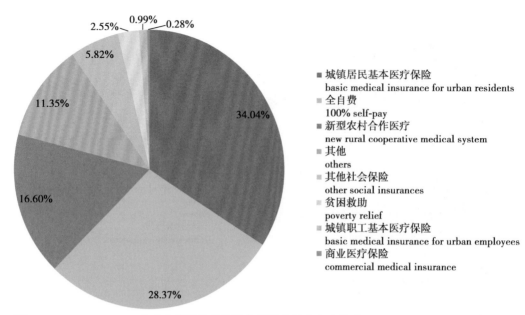

图 8-5-56　2017—2018 年山东肾癌患儿住院费用医疗付费方式构成

Figure 8-5-56　Composition of medical payment methods for hospitalization expenses of children with kidney cancer in Shandong in 2017-2018

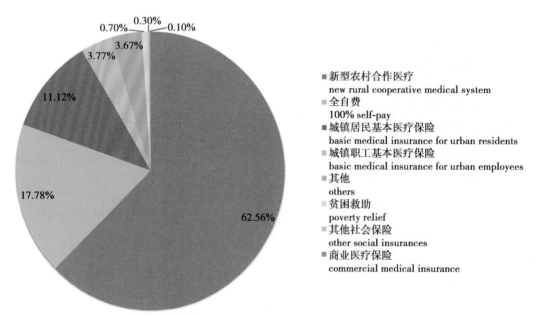

图 8-5-57　2017—2018 年河南肾癌患儿住院费用医疗付费方式构成

Figure 8-5-57　Composition of medical payment methods for hospitalization expenses of children with kidney cancer in Henan in 2017-2018

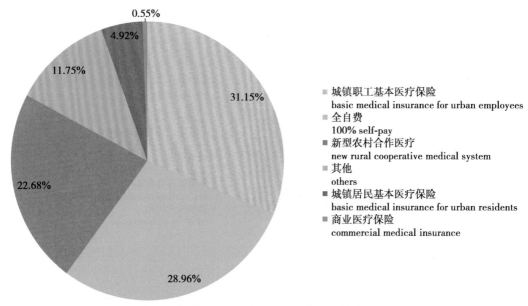

图 8-5-58   2017—2018 年湖北肾癌患儿住院费用医疗付费方式构成

Figure 8-5-58   Composition of medical payment methods for hospitalization expenses of children with kidney cancer in Hubei in 2017-2018

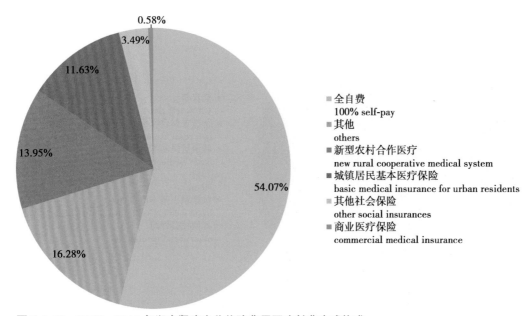

图 8-5-59   2017—2018 年湖南肾癌患儿住院费用医疗付费方式构成

Figure 8-5-59   Composition of medical payment methods for hospitalization expenses of children with kidney cancer in Hunan in 2017-2018

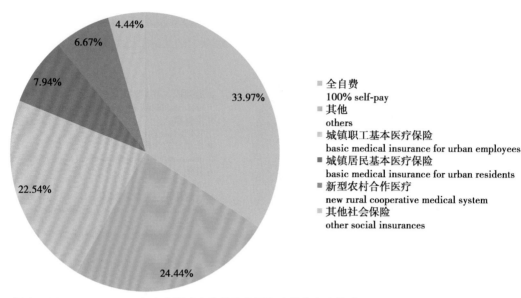

图 8-5-60　2017—2018 年广东肾癌患儿住院费用医疗付费方式构成

Figure 8-5-60　Composition of medical payment methods for hospitalization expenses of children with kidney cancer in Guangdong in 2017-2018

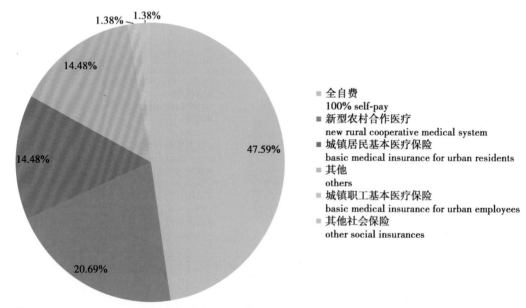

图 8-5-61　2017—2018 年广西肾癌患儿住院费用医疗付费方式构成

Figure 8-5-61　Composition of medical payment methods for hospitalization expenses of children with kidney cancer in Guangxi in 2017-2018

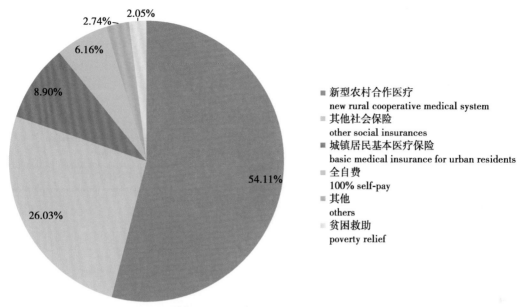

图 8-5-62　2017—2018 年海南肾癌患儿住院费用医疗付费方式构成

Figure 8-5-62　Composition of medical payment methods for hospitalization expenses of children with kidney cancer in Hainan in 2017-2018

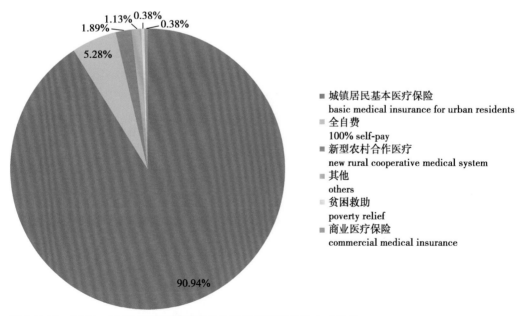

图 8-5-63　2017—2018 年重庆肾癌患儿住院费用医疗付费方式构成

Figure 8-5-63　Composition of medical payment methods for hospitalization expenses of children with kidney cancer in Chongqing in 2017-2018

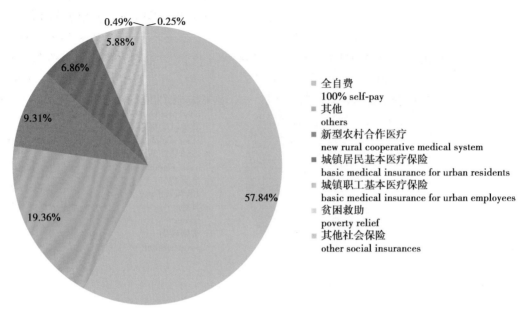

图 8-5-64　2017—2018 年四川肾癌患儿住院费用医疗付费方式构成

Figure 8-5-64　Composition of medical payment methods for hospitalization expenses of children with kidney cancer in Sichuan in 2017-2018

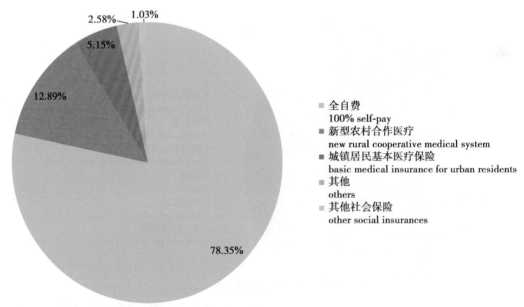

图 8-5-65　2017—2018 年贵州肾癌患儿住院费用医疗付费方式构成

Figure 8-5-65　Composition of medical payment methods for hospitalization expenses of children with kidney cancer in Guizhou in 2017-2018

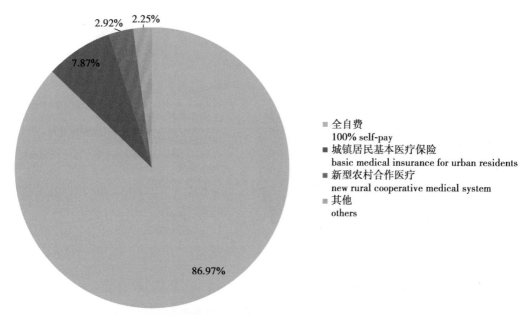

图 8-5-66   2017—2018 年云南肾癌患儿住院费用医疗付费方式构成

Figure 8-5-66   Composition of medical payment methods for hospitalization expenses of children with kidney cancer in Yunnan in 2017-2018

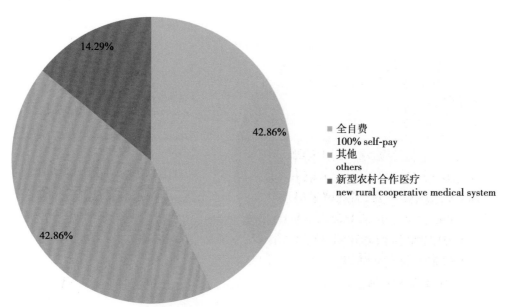

图 8-5-67   2017—2018 年西藏肾癌患儿住院费用医疗付费方式构成

Figure 8-5-67   Composition of medical payment methods for hospitalization expenses of children with kidney cancer in Xizang in 2017-2018

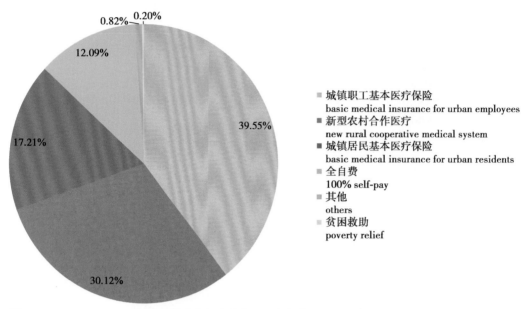

图 8-5-68 2017—2018 年陕西肾癌患儿住院费用医疗付费方式构成

Figure 8-5-68 Composition of medical payment methods for hospitalization expenses of children with kidney cancer in Shaanxi in 2017-2018

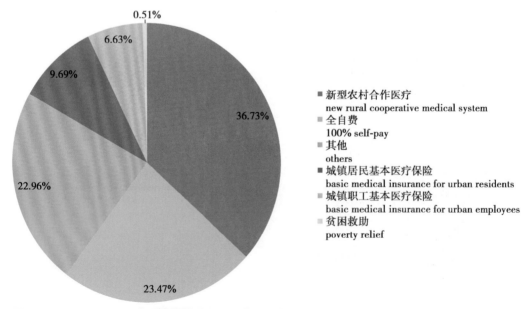

图 8-5-69 2017—2018 年甘肃肾癌患儿住院费用医疗付费方式构成

Figure 8-5-69 Composition of medical payment methods for hospitalization expenses of children with kidney cancer in Gansu in 2017-2018

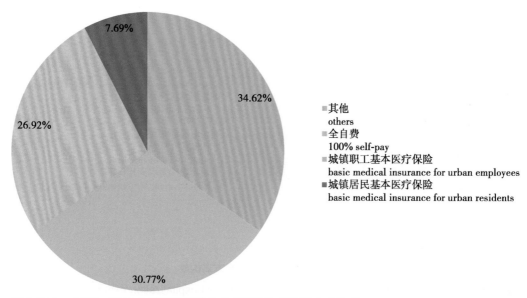

图 8-5-70　2017—2018 年青海肾癌患儿住院费用医疗付费方式构成

Figure 8-5-70　Composition of medical payment methods for hospitalization expenses of children with kidney cancer in Qinghai in 2017-2018

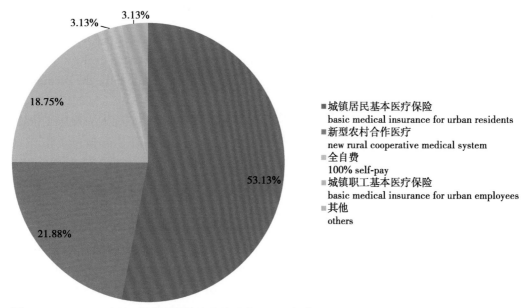

图 8-5-71　2017—2018 年宁夏肾癌患儿住院费用医疗付费方式构成

Figure 8-5-71　Composition of medical payment methods for hospitalization expenses of children with kidney cancer in Ningxia in 2017-2018

377

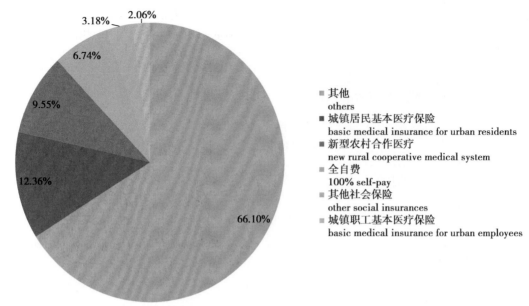

3.18% 2.06%

6.74%

9.55%

12.36%

66.10%

■ 其他
others
■ 城镇居民基本医疗保险
basic medical insurance for urban residents
■ 新型农村合作医疗
new rural cooperative medical system
■ 全自费
100% self-pay
■ 其他社会保险
other social insurances
■ 城镇职工基本医疗保险
basic medical insurance for urban employees

图 8-5-72　2017—2018 年新疆肾癌患儿住院费用医疗付费方式构成

Figure 8-5-72　Composition of medical payment methods for hospitalization expenses of children with kidney cancer in Xinjiang in 2017-2018

5.5 全国儿童肿瘤监测机构肾癌患儿住院费用分析

5.5.1 全国儿童肿瘤监测机构肾癌患儿次均住院费用情况

5.5.1.1　全国及六大区肾癌患儿次均住院费用情况　全国肾癌患儿次均住院费用（中位数）为4 398.35 元。高于全国中位数水平的地区分别为东北地区（8 384.70 元）、中南地区（6 932.19 元）、华北地区（4 917.77 元）和西南地区（4 853.96 元），低于全国中位数水平的地区分别为西北地区（2 804.03 元）和华东地区（3 003.77 元）（图 8-5-73）。

5.5.1.2　各省份肾癌患儿次均住院费用情况　根据肾癌患儿次均住院费用（中位数），前 3 位的省份分别为内蒙古（24 318.17 元）、天津（15 729.20 元）和贵州（14 647.84 元），后 3 位分别为海南（1 193.73 元）、宁夏（1 259.85 元）和山东（2 281.00 元）（图 8-5-74）。

5.5 Analysis of hospitalization expenses of children with kidney cancer in pediatric cancer surveillance sites in China

5.5.1 Expenses per hospitalization of children with kidney cancer in pediatric cancer surveillance sites in China

5.5.1.1　Expenses per hospitalization of children with kidney cancer in the six regions and the whole country　Nationally, the median expense per hospitalization was 4, 398.35 CNY. The regions above the national median were Northeast China (8, 384.70 CNY), Central and Southern China (6, 932.19 CNY), North China (4, 917.77 CNY) and Southwest China (4, 853.96 CNY). Regions lower than the national median were Northwest China (2, 804.03 CNY) and East China (3, 003.77 CNY) (Figure 8-5-73).

5.5.1.2　Expenses per hospitalization of children with kidney cancer in each provincial-level region　In terms of the median expenses per hospitalization of children with kidney cancer, the top three provincial-level regions were Inner Mongolia (24, 318.17 CNY), Tianjin (15, 729.20 CNY) and Guizhou (14, 647.84 CNY), while the last three were Hainan (1, 193.73 CNY), Ningxia (1, 259.85 CNY) and Shandong (2, 281.00 CNY) (Figure 8-5-74).

5.5.2　全国儿童肿瘤监测机构肾癌患儿次均住院分项费用情况

5.5.2.1　全国及六大区肾癌患儿次均住院分项费用情况　根据全国肾癌患儿次均住院分项费用(中位数)，前 3 位分别为诊断类费用(980.00 元)、西药类费用(780.75 元)和综合医疗服务类费用(739.90 元)。六大区分项费用中位数的顺位与全国相比略有不同。如东北地区，次均住院分项费用(中位数)前 3 位分别为诊断类费用(1 850.00 元)、综合医疗服务类费用(1 538.00 元)和西药类费用(1 007.47 元)(图 8-5-75)。按均数统计的结果详见图 8-5-76。

5.5.2　Expenses of each item per hospitalization of children with kidney cancer in pediatric cancer surveillance sites in China

5.5.2.1　Expenses of each item per hospitalization of children with kidney cancer in the six regions and the whole country　In terms of the median expenses of each item per hospitalization of children with kidney cancer, the top three items were diagnostic expenses (980.00 CNY), western medication expenses (780.75 CNY) and comprehensive medical services expenses (739.90 CNY). The ranking of the median expenses of each item per hospitalization in the six regions was slightly different from the national median. For example, in Northeast China, the top three median expenses of each item per hospitalization were diagnostic expenses (1 850.00 CNY), comprehensive medical services expenses (1 538.00 CNY) and western medication expenses (1 007.47 CNY) (Figure 8-5-75). Data by the mean expenses in Figure 8-5-76.

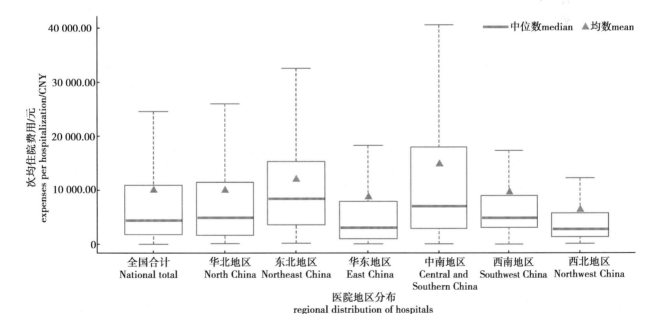

图 8-5-73　2017—2018 年全国及六大区肾癌患儿次均住院费用

Figure 8-5-73　Expenses per hospitalization of children with kidney cancer in the six regions and the whole country in 2017-2018

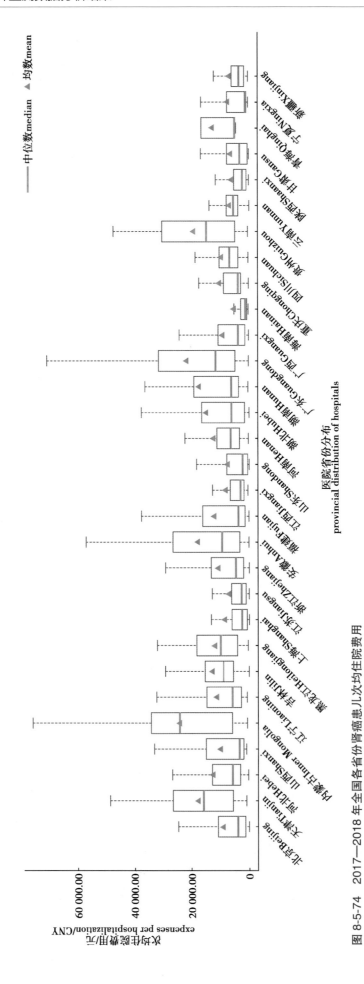

图 8-5-74　2017—2018 年全国各省份肾癌患儿次均住院费用

Figure 8-5-74　Expenses per hospitalization of children with kidney cancer in each provincial-level region in 2017-2018

分项费用/元
expenses of each item/CNY

regional distribution of hospitals 图按区分布	综合医疗服务类费用 comprehensive medical service expenses	诊断类费用 diagnostic expenses	治疗类费用 treatment expenses	康复类费用 rehabilitation expenses	中医类费用 traditional chinese medicine service expenses	西药类费用 western medication expenses	中药类费用 traditional chinese medication expenses	血液和血液制品类费用 blood and blood product expenses	耗材类费用 medical consumable expenses	其他类费用 others
全国合计 National total	739.90	980.00	0	0	0	780.75	0	0	301.85	0
华北地区 North China	680.55	590.25	0	0	0	816.94	0	0	553.45	0
东北地区 Northeast China	1 538.00	1 850.00	0	0	0	1 007.47	0	369.65	708.80	0
华东地区 East China	492.80	851.01	22.00	0	0	601.65	0	0	204.02	15.00
中南地区 Central and Southern China	896.50	1 638.60	38.80	0	0	865.42	0	0	381.89	0
西南地区 Southwest China	1 038.00	1 555.00	70.00	0	0	1 145.68	0	0	364.21	0
西北地区 Northwest China	331.00	931.00	0	0	0	645.27	0	0	110.44	4.00

图 8-5-75　2017—2018 年全国及六大区肾癌患儿次均住院分项费用（按中位数计）

Figure 8-5-75　Expenses of each item per hospitalization of children with kidney cancer in the six regions and the whole country in 2017-2018 (by the median)

分项费用/元
expenses of each item/CNY

regional distribution of hospitals 图按区分布	综合医疗服务类费用 comprehensive medical service expenses	诊断类费用 diagnostic expenses	治疗类费用 treatment expenses	康复类费用 rehabilitation expenses	中医类费用 traditional chinese medicine service expenses	西药类费用 western medication expenses	中药类费用 traditional chinese medication expenses	血液和血液制品类费用 blood and blood product expenses	耗材类费用 medical consumable expenses	其他类费用 others
全国合计 National total	1 472.73	2 261.71	1 261.54	6.43	3.41	2 093.33	72.70	353.54	1 538.40	446.64
华北地区 North China	1 486.36	1 613.97	575.68	0.38	0.19	2 548.18	141.93	398.12	1 968.46	414.85
东北地区 Northeast China	1 959.59	2 858.15	1 650.13	1.06	0	2 028.91	107.18	778.06	1 717.10	1 002.61
华东地区 East China	1 337.75	2 164.58	1 645.56	12.95	4.60	1 468.98	41.85	245.11	1 389.88	364.14
中南地区 Central and Southern China	1 677.04	3 087.74	2 750.49	9.18	9.71	3 050.09	53.16	247.34	2 105.33	924.17
西南地区 Southwest China	1 750.78	2 915.57	817.61	15.79	6.57	1 875.36	28.53	595.42	1 207.15	90.14
西北地区 Northwest China	971.15	1 773.33	635.62	0.75	0.90	1 598.73	9.95	155.52	585.16	105.19

图 8-5-76　2017—2018 年全国及六大区肾癌患儿次均住院分项费用（按均数计）

Figure 8-5-76　Expenses of each item per hospitalization of children with kidney cancer in the six regions and the whole country in 2017-2018 (by the mean)

5.5.2.2 各省份肾癌患儿次均住院分项费用情况 根据各省份肾癌患儿次均住院分项费用(中位数),以综合医疗服务类费用为例,前3位的省份依次为天津(2 301.50 元)、吉林(2 145.50 元)和贵州(2 040.18 元),后3位依次为海南(173.70 元)、宁夏(173.83 元)和青海(221.00 元)(图 8-5-77)。按均数统计的结果详见图 8-5-78。

5.6 全国儿童肿瘤监测机构肾癌患儿平均住院日分析

5.6.1 全国及六大区肾癌患儿平均住院日情况

全国肾癌患儿平均住院日的中位数为 5 天。高于全国中位数水平的地区分别为东北地区(8 天)、中南地区(6 天)和西南地区(6 天),低于全国中位数水平的地区分别为华北地区(4 天)、西北地区(4 天)和华东地区(3 天)(图 8-5-79)。

5.5.2.2 Expenses of each item per hospitalization of children with kidney cancer in each provincial-level region In terms of the median expenses of each item for each hospitalization of children with kidney cancer in each provincial-level region, taking comprehensive medical services expenses as an example, the top three provincial-level regions were Tianjin (2, 301.50 CNY), Jilin (2, 145.50 CNY) and Guizhou (2, 040.18 CNY). The last three were Hainan (173.70 CNY), Ningxia (173.83 CNY) and Qinghai (221.00 CNY)(Figure 8-5-77). Data by the mean expenses in Figure 8-5-78.

5.6 Analysis of the average length of hospitalization of children with kidney cancer in pediatric cancer surveillance sites in China

5.6.1 Average length of hospitalization of children with kidney cancer in the six regions and the whole country

Nationally, the median of average length of hospitalization was 5 days. Northeast China (8 days), Central and Southern China (6 days) and Southwest China (6 days) were above the national median. North China (4 days), Northwest China (4 days) and East China (3 days) were below the national median (Figure 8-5-79).

医院省份分布 provincial distribution of hospitals	综合医疗服务类费用 comprehensive medical service expenses	诊断类费用 diagnostic expenses	治疗类费用 treatment expenses	康复类费用 rehabilitation expenses	中医类费用 traditional chinese medicine service expenses	西药类费用 western medication expenses	中药类费用 traditional chinese medication expenses	血液和血液制品类费用 blood and blood product expenses	耗材类费用 medical consumable expenses	其他类费用 others
北京Beijing	626.23	543.00	0	0	0	734.62	0	0	568.91	0
天津Tianjin	2 301.50	3 931.00	200.00	0	0	1 323.39	0	240.00	2 396.38	0
河北Hebei	359.32	925.50	0	0	0	1 782.87	0	0	181.18	217.16
山西Shanxi	823.00	1 227.30	20.00	0	0	613.96	0	0	356.10	7.25
内蒙古Inner Mongolia	1 305.75	4 585.00	2 743.25	0	-	2 107.55	34.34	40.00	939.58	849.00
辽宁Liaoning	1 100.12	1 066.18	24.59	0	0	736.87	0	135.00	260.56	1 386.90
吉林Jilin	2 145.50	2 659.50	0	0	0	1 277.26	0	525.00	1 022.95	92.00
黑龙江Heilongjiang	1 032.00	1 150.00	0	0	0	3 630.30	0	0	690.70	0
上海Shanghai	631.25	519.00	0	0	0	528.34	0	0	213.64	120.00
江苏Jiangsu	324.80	706.00	144.60	6.00	0	699.60	23.42	0	163.10	14.88
浙江Zhejiang	780.23	1 076.51	124.00	0	0	1 020.15	0	52.57	281.98	48.35
安徽Anhui	1 641.00	2 844.10	2 614.40	60.00	0	945.23	30.36	0	477.40	0
福建Fujian	771.00	1 589.00	0	0	0	572.18	0	0	48.99	14.98
江西Jiangxi	562.80	1 218.00	0	30.00	0	585.10	63.20	115.23	149.79	24.51
山东Shandong	400.00	694.00	18.00	0	0	350.36	0	0	160.55	0
河南Henan	860.25	952.00	0	0	0	2 526.67	0	0	282.36	0
湖北Hubei	970.00	1 853.97	0	0	0	755.52	0	0	369.73	8.00
湖南Hunan	1 054.00	1 603.75	0	0	0	1 054.61	0	0	791.92	486.68
广东Guangdong	1 265.85	2 786.40	4 955.55	0	0	858.73	0	0	1 108.84	0
广西Guangxi	661.10	999.90	91.70	0	0	585.42	0	0	212.18	0
海南Hainan	173.70	460.48	45.00	0	0	389.61	0	0	75.71	0
重庆Chongqing	969.81	1 108.40	0	0	0	922.84	0	0	473.87	0
四川Sichuan	1 413.35	2 053.00	130.00	24.00	0	904.55	0	0	470.55	0
贵州Guizhou	2 040.18	3 386.20	450.20	0	0	1 695.98	0	274.80	914.26	91.00
云南Yunnan	1 031.00	2 327.50	180.00	0	0	1 754.18	55.69	230.00	93.24	0.05
陕西Shaanxi	266.50	431.00	0	0	0	628.57	0	0	109.07	0
甘肃Gansu	781.50	765.50	0	6.00	0	272.26	0	0	0	0
青海Qinghai	221.00	3 945.50	0	0	0	800.00	0	0	23.00	-
宁夏Ningxia	173.83	233.59	377.89	-	-	552.86	-	291.25	152.71	-
新疆Xinjiang	373.50	1 220.00	32.00	0	0	661.71	0	0	120.89	16.00

分项费用/元 expenses of each item/CNY

图 8-5-77　2017—2018 年全国各省省份肾癌患儿次均住院分项费用（按中位数计）

Figure 8-5-77　Expenses per item for each hospitalization of children with kidney cancer in each provincial-level region in 2017-2018（by the median）

383

医院省份分布 provincial distribution of hospitals	综合医疗服务类费用 comprehensive medical service expenses	诊断类费用 diagnostic expenses	治疗类费用 treatment expenses	康复类费用 rehabilitation expenses	中医类服务费用 traditional chinese medicine service expenses	西药类费用 western medication expenses	中药类费用 traditional chinese medication expenses	血液和血液制品类费用 blood and blood product expenses	耗材类费用 medical consumable expenses	其他类费用 others
北京Beijing	1 410.32	1 389.74	407.46	0.41	0	2 391.98	158.34	379.81	1 963.89	219.91
天津Tianjin	3 353.34	4 430.50	2 937.13	0	0	2 325.12	3.43	660.47	3 270.91	74.48
河北Hebei	1 213.98	1 939.27	617.27	0	2.87	3 999.57	61.14	465.99	1 523.82	2 268.88
山西Shanxi	1 716.60	2 327.24	1 681.70	0	0	1 461.24	39.11	234.18	1 318.57	406.08
内蒙古Inner Mongolia	2 669.38	5 041.67	3 334.63	12.00	–	4 018.22	459.27	958.33	2 960.11	1 104.11
辽宁Liaoning	1 572.89	1 591.38	3 379.76	1.88	0	1 764.70	54.15	360.03	1 285.77	2 614.00
吉林Jilin	2 316.52	3 884.05	1 047.10	0.99	0	1 783.19	131.88	1 017.65	1 951.49	0.66
黑龙江Heilongjiang	1 358.82	1 618.62	1 420.17	0	0	4 299.16	51.17	229.35	1 950.13	951.83
上海Shanghai	1 530.54	2 070.97	1 501.03	0	0	1 230.95	2.90	71.64	1 582.10	245.29
江苏Jiangsu	858.47	1 804.74	1 281.48	11.82	0	1 385.44	51.88	466.75	1 073.96	344.92
浙江Zhejiang	1 424.43	1 803.44	2 199.44	7.79	23.74	2 247.05	66.24	310.15	1 564.56	243.07
安徽Anhui	2 861.93	4 032.41	3 110.92	171.95	0	2 350.58	78.99	612.17	3 938.28	348.44
福建Fujian	2 865.49	2 692.10	3 146.88	0.45	0	1 736.84	19.37	457.89	684.59	539.46
江西Jiangxi	1 147.05	2 511.01	1 268.31	29.08	6.13	1 360.64	204.07	305.42	1 118.64	206.22
山东Shandong	1 089.70	2 247.00	1 495.06	1.18	1.44	1 233.67	27.87	173.91	1 312.74	593.87
河南Henan	1 350.97	1 458.60	583.12	2.77	6.93	3 348.03	107.43	96.61	547.44	150.97
湖北Hubei	2 055.47	3 361.85	1 754.51	18.14	5.02	3 500.44	63.55	111.18	2 902.69	389.02
湖南Hunan	1 835.43	3 913.93	2 928.82	42.58	31.12	3 278.34	110.29	305.03	3 810.29	711.92
广东Guangdong	2 003.58	4 703.54	5 219.99	2.52	2.55	3 324.71	16.75	449.42	2 739.82	2 039.30
广西Guangxi	1 642.55	2 932.26	1 643.64	9.32	4.62	1 369.56	6.18	231.47	1 142.01	114.52
海南Hainan	643.04	1 257.42	769.64	0	33.17	1 167.98	9.10	169.52	719.56	1.02
重庆Chongqing	2 089.86	3 064.26	728.11	13.74	0.80	1 623.43	4.04	574.98	1 510.48	7.09
四川Sichuan	2 062.78	2 640.88	1 115.64	22.51	26.62	1 824.96	53.40	621.91	1 021.87	283.94
贵州Guizhou	2 495.48	4 111.51	2 417.93	6.84	24.67	2 738.96	23.82	655.90	4 378.62	874.11
云南Yunnan	1 072.94	2 702.86	631.38	55.04	0	2 143.31	111.29	681.53	524.45	34.17
陕西Shaanxi	793.58	1 153.50	535.50	0	0.72	1 678.55	13.00	278.61	636.18	44.55
甘肃Gansu	1 155.46	2 008.17	1 444.38	13.81	4.61	1 020.94	35.47	44.91	654.45	108.80
青海Qinghai	991.00	6 320.33	1 312.57	23.33	0	1 506.54	0	210.08	1 761.96	282.48
宁夏Ningxia	910.58	1 953.66	2 024.11	–	–	1 031.86	–	444.08	2 014.21	–
新疆Xinjiang	1 178.03	2 186.23	657.28	0.16	0.82	1 602.20	5.50	61.48	437.27	151.45

分项费用/元
expenses of each item/CNY

图 8-5-78 2017—2018 年全国各省份肾癌患儿次均住院分项费用（按均数计）

Figure 8-5-78 Expenses per item for each hospitalization of children with kidney cancer in each provincial-level region in 2017-2018 (by the mean)

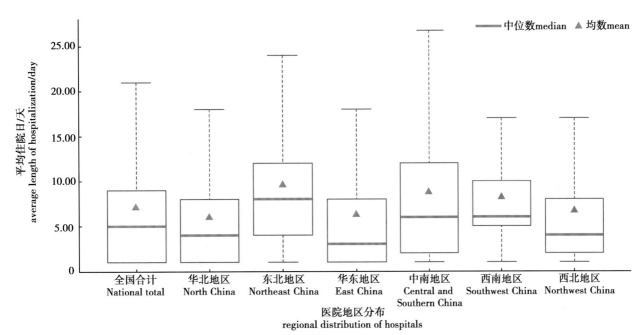

图 8-5-79　2017—2018 年全国及六大区肾癌患儿平均住院日

Figure 8-5-79   Average length of hospitalization of children with kidney cancer in the six regions and the whole country in 2017-2018

5.6.2　各省份肾癌患儿平均住院日情况

根据各省份肾癌患儿平均住院日的中位数,肾癌患儿平均住院日最长的省份为内蒙古(17 天),其次是贵州(14 天)、天津(12 天)、黑龙江(9 天)和安徽(9 天),最短的是海南(1 天)(图 8-5-80)。

5.6.2　Average length of hospitalization of children with kidney cancer in each provincial-level region

In terms of the median of average length of hospitalization of children with kidney cancer in each provincial-level region, the provincial-level region with the longest average hospital stay was Inner Mongolia (17 days), followed by Guizhou (14 days), Tianjin (12 days), Heilongjiang (9 days) and Anhui (9 days), and the shortest was Hainan (1 day)(Figure 8-5-80).

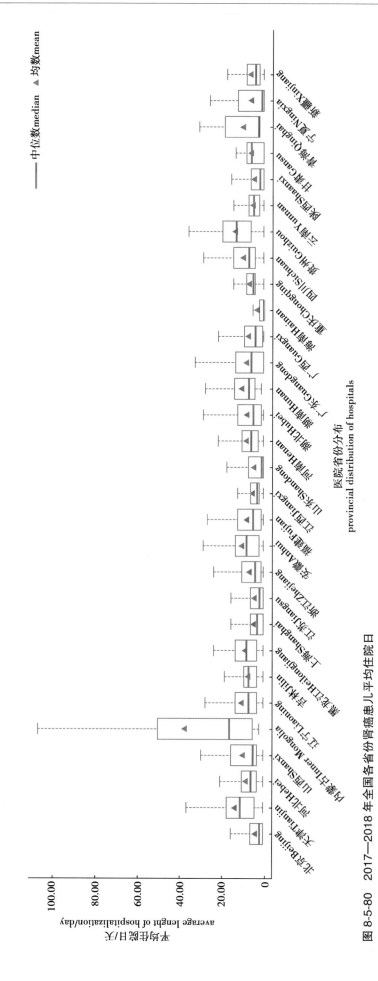

图 8-5-80　2017—2018 年全国各省份肾癌患儿平均住院日

Figure 8-5-80　Average length of hospitalization of children with kidney cancer in each provincial-level region in 2017-2018

6　肝癌

6.1　全国儿童肿瘤监测机构肝癌患儿出院人次分析

6.1.1　六大区肝癌患儿出院人次构成情况

在肝癌患儿出院人次中,各大区出院人次占全部出院人次的比例由高到低依次为华北地区(43.57%)、中南地区(18.48%)、华东地区(17.41%)、西南地区(11.74%)、东北地区(5.95%)和西北地区(2.85%)(图 8-6-1)。

6　Liver cancer

6.1　Analysis of discharges among children with liver cancer in pediatric cancer surveillance sites in China

6.1.1　Composition of discharges among children with liver cancer in the six regions

In terms of the discharges among children with liver cancer, the regions with the highest to the lowest proportion of the discharges among children with liver cancer in all discharges were North China (43.57%), Central and Southern China (18.48%), East China (17.41%), Southwest China (11.74%), Northeast China (5.95%) and Northwest China (2.85%) (Figure 8-6-1).

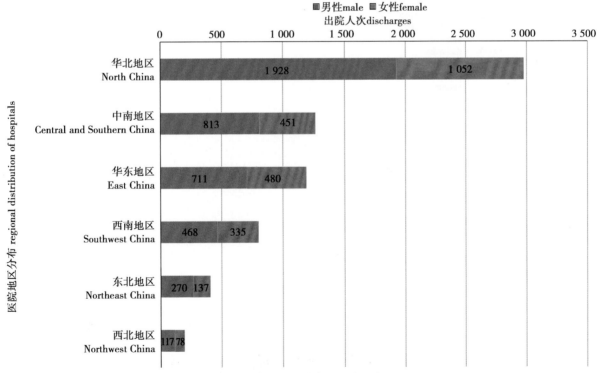

图 8-6-1　2017—2018 年全国六大区儿童肿瘤监测机构肝癌出院人次构成

Figure 8-6-1　Composition of discharges among children with liver cancer in pediatric cancer surveillance sites in the six regions in 2017-2018

6.1.2　各省份肝癌患儿出院人次构成情况

在所有省份中,肝癌患儿出院人次占全部出院人次比例前3位的省份分别为北京(39.23%)、重庆(7.88%)和广东(7.31%),后3位分别为西藏(0.00%)、青海(0.01%)和宁夏(0.07%)(图8-6-2,图8-6-3)。

6.1.2　Composition of discharges among children with liver cancer in each provincial-level region

Among all provincial-level regions, Beijing (39.23%), Chongqing (7.88%) and Guangdong (7.31%) were the three provincial-level regions with the highest proportions of discharges among children with liver cancer, and Xizang (0.00%), Qinghai (0.01%), and Ningxia (0.07%) had the lowest proportions of discharges among children with liver cancer (Figure 8-6-2~Figure 8-6-3).

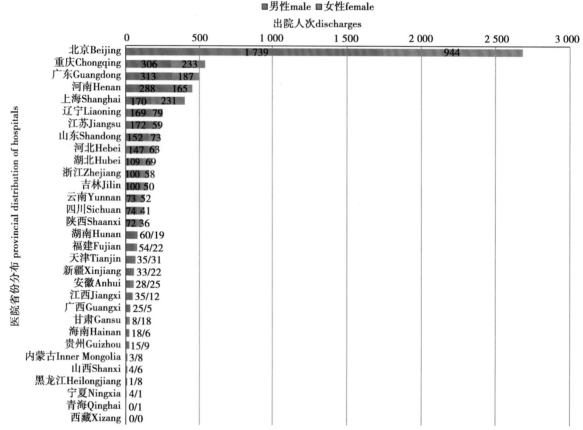

图 8-6-2　2017—2018 年全国各省份儿童肿瘤监测机构肝癌出院人次构成

Figure 8-6-2　Composition of discharges among children with liver cancer in pediatric cancer surveillance sites in each provincial-level region in 2017-2018

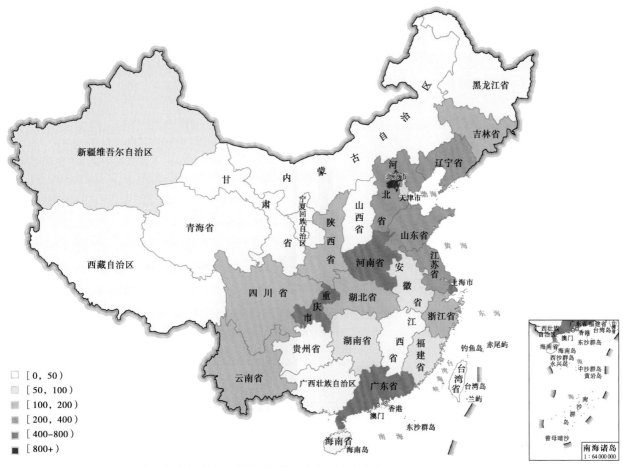

图 8-6-3   2017—2018 年全国各省份儿童肿瘤监测机构肝癌出院人次分布

Figure 8-6-3   Distribution of discharges among children with liver cancer in pediatric cancer surveillance sites in each provincial-level region in 2017-2018

6.2   全国儿童肿瘤监测机构肝癌患儿年龄／性别构成

6.2.1   全国肝癌患儿年龄／性别构成情况

从性别分布来看，男性患儿占全部出院人次比例为 62.97%，女性患儿为 37.03%。从年龄分布来看，1 岁年龄组所占比例最高（24.71%），其次为 2 岁（17.25%）和 1 岁以下（17.24%）年龄组（图 8-6-4）。

6.2   Age/gender composition of children with liver cancer in pediatric cancer surveillance sites in China

6.2.1   Age/gender composition of children with liver cancer nationally

In terms of gender distribution, male patients accounted for 62.97% of all discharges, and female for 37.03%. In terms of age distribution, the 1-year age group had the highest proportion (24.71%), followed by the 2-year age group (17.25%) and under-1-year age group (17.24%)(Figure 8-6-4).

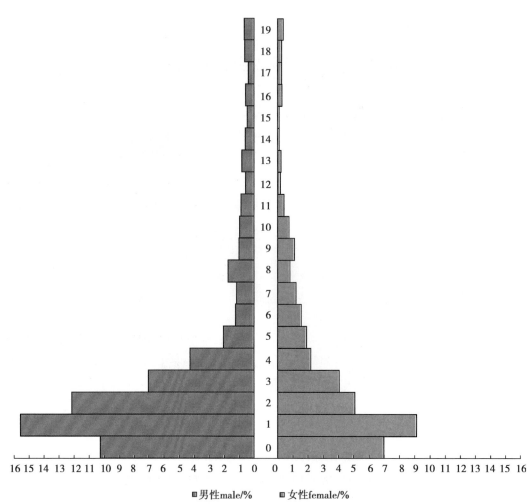

■男性male/%　■女性female/%

图 8-6-4　2017—2018 年全国儿童肿瘤监测机构肝癌患儿年龄 / 性别构成

Figure 8-6-4　Age/gender composition of children with liver cancer in pediatric cancer surveillance sites in China in 2017-2018

6.2.2　六大区肝癌患儿年龄 / 性别构成情况

从性别分布来看,六大区均显示男性患儿占全部出院人次比例高于女性患儿。从年龄分布来看,六大区的比例各有不同,其中华北地区、华东地区、中南地区、西南地区和西北地区的 1 岁年龄组所占比例最高;东北地区的 1 岁以下年龄组所占比例最高(图 8-6-5~ 图 8-6-10)。

6.2.2　Age/gender composition of children with liver cancer in the six regions

In terms of gender distribution, male children accounted for a higher proportion of all discharges than female in all the six regions. In terms of age distribution, the proportions of the six regions were different, among which the proportions of the 1-year age group in North China, East China, Central and Southern China, Southwest China and Northwest China were the highest. The proportion of the under-1-year age group in Northeast China was the highest (Figure 8-6-5~Figure 8-6-10).

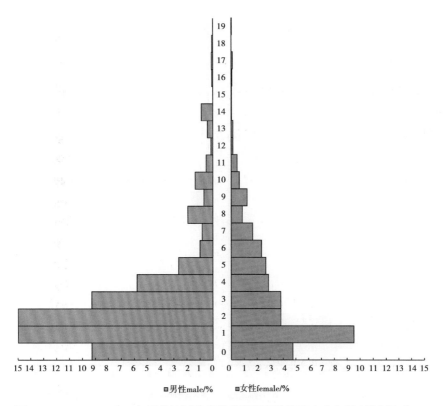

图 8-6-5　2017—2018 年华北地区儿童肿瘤监测机构肝癌患儿年龄／性别构成

Figure 8-6-5　Age/gender composition of children with liver cancer in pediatric cancer surveillance sites in North China in 2017-2018

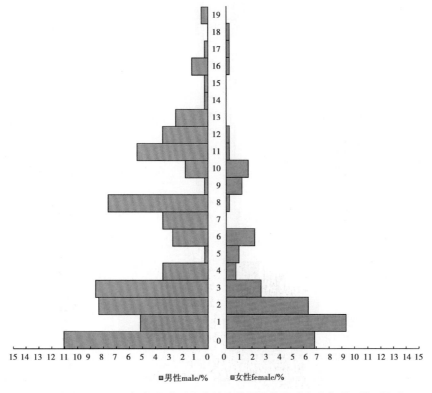

图 8-6-6　2017—2018 年东北地区儿童肿瘤监测机构肝癌患儿年龄／性别构成

Figure 8-6-6　Age/gender composition of children with liver cancer in pediatric cancer surveillance sites in Northeast China in 2017-2018

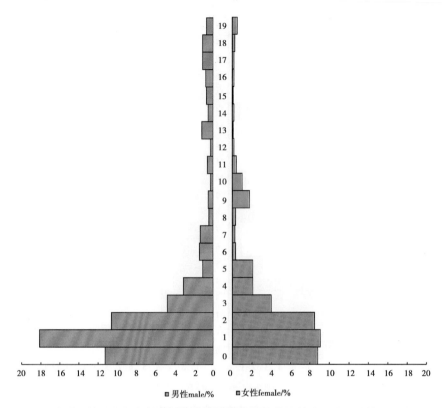

图 8-6-7　2017—2018 年华东地区儿童肿瘤监测机构肝癌患儿年龄 / 性别构成

Figure 8-6-7　Age/gender composition of children with liver cancer in pediatric cancer surveillance sites in East China in 2017-2018

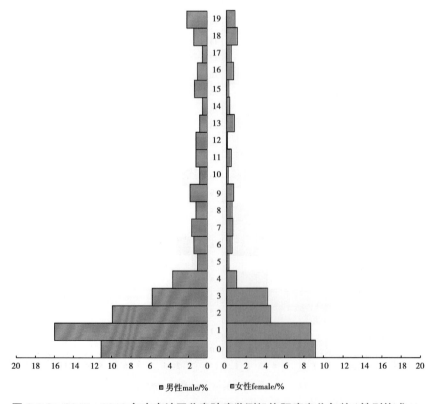

图 8-6-8　2017—2018 年中南地区儿童肿瘤监测机构肝癌患儿年龄 / 性别构成

Figure 8-6-8　Age/gender composition of children with liver cancer in pediatric cancer surveillance sites in Central and Southern China in 2017-2018

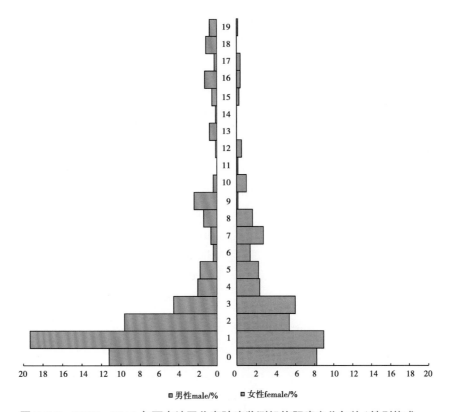

图 8-6-9   2017—2018 年西南地区儿童肿瘤监测机构肝癌患儿年龄 / 性别构成

Figure 8-6-9   Age/gender composition of children with liver cancer in pediatric cancer surveillance sites in Southwest China in 2017-2018

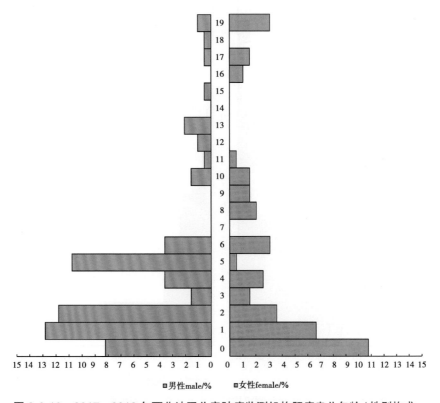

图 8-6-10   2017—2018 年西北地区儿童肿瘤监测机构肝癌患儿年龄 / 性别构成

Figure 8-6-10   Age/gender composition of children with liver cancer in pediatric cancer surveillance sites in Northwest China in 2017-2018

393

6.2.3 各省份肝癌患儿年龄/性别构成情况

从性别分布来看,除甘肃、黑龙江、内蒙古、青海、山西、上海和西藏外的其他24个省份出院患儿的性别分布均呈现男性比例高于女性;从年龄分布来看,各省份出院患儿的年龄分布各有不同。以重庆为例,从性别分布来看,男性患儿占全部出院人次比例为56.77%,女性患儿为43.23%;从年龄分布来看,1岁年龄组所占比例最高(26.16%),其次为1岁以下年龄组(19.48%)和2岁年龄组(13.36%)(图8-6-11~图8-6-25)。

6.2.3 Age/gender composition of children with liver cancer in each provincial-level region

In terms of gender distribution, the proportions of discharged male children in the other 24 provincial-level regions except Gansu, Heilongjiang, Inner Mongolia, Qinghai, Shanxi, Shanghai and Xizang were higher than those of female; in terms of age distribution, the proportions of all the provincial-level regions were different. Taking Chongqing as an example, in terms of gender distribution, male children accounted for 56.77%, and female 43.23% of the total discharges. In terms of age distribution, the 1-year age group accounted for the highest proportion (26.16%), followed by the under-1-year age group (19.48%) and the 2-year age group (13.36%) (Figure 8-6-11~Figure 8-6-25).

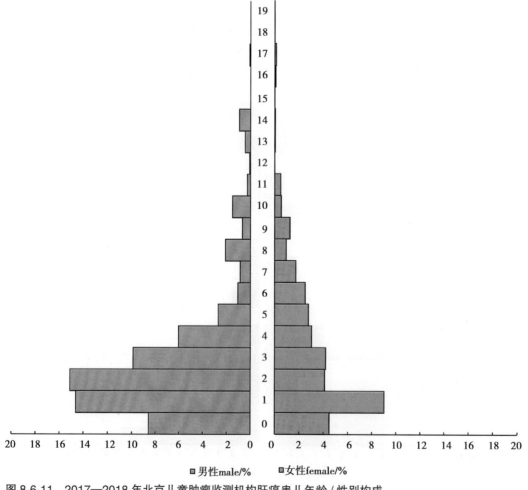

图 8-6-11　2017—2018 年北京儿童肿瘤监测机构肝癌患儿年龄/性别构成

Figure 8-6-11　Age/gender composition of children with liver cancer in pediatric cancer surveillance sites in Beijing in 2017-2018

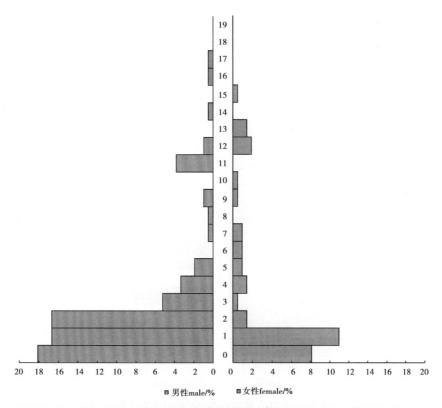

图 8-6-12　2017—2018 年河北儿童肿瘤监测机构肝癌患儿年龄／性别构成

Figure 8-6-12　Age/gender composition of children with liver cancer in pediatric cancer surveillance sites in Hebei in 2017-2018

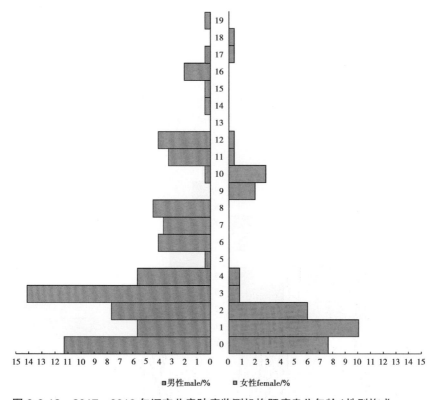

图 8-6-13　2017—2018 年辽宁儿童肿瘤监测机构肝癌患儿年龄／性别构成

Figure 8-6-13　Age/gender composition of children with liver cancer in pediatric cancer surveillance sites in Liaoning in 2017-2018

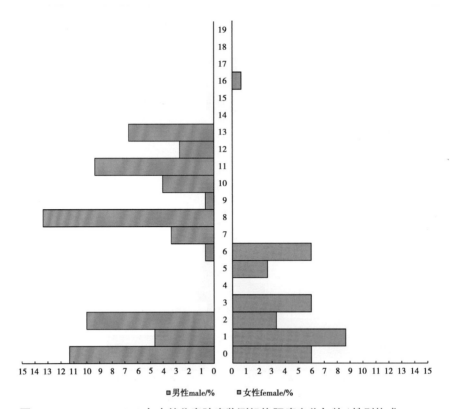

图 8-6-14　2017—2018 年吉林儿童肿瘤监测机构肝癌患儿年龄／性别构成

Figure 8-6-14　Age/gender composition of children with liver cancer in pediatric cancer surveillance sites in Jilin in 2017-2018

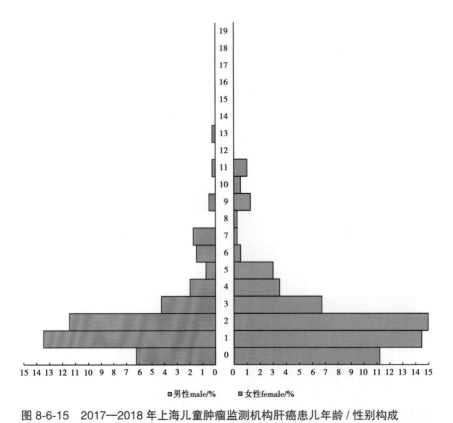

图 8-6-15　2017—2018 年上海儿童肿瘤监测机构肝癌患儿年龄／性别构成

Figure 8-6-15　Age/gender composition of children with liver cancer in pediatric cancer surveillance sites in Shanghai in 2017-2018

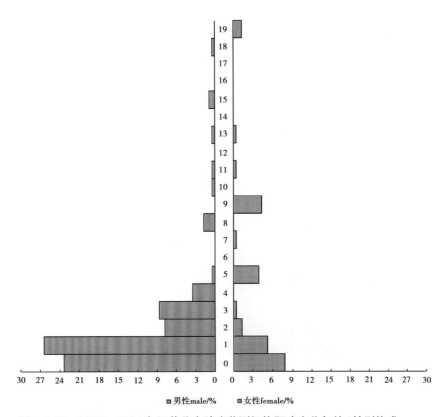

图 8-6-16　2017—2018 年江苏儿童肿瘤监测机构肝癌患儿年龄／性别构成

Figure 8-6-16　Age/gender composition of children with liver cancer in pediatric cancer surveillance sites in Jiangsu in 2017-2018

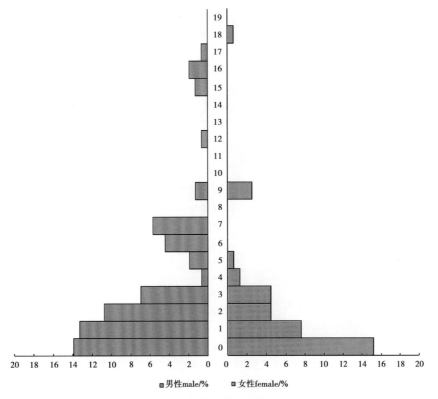

图 8-6-17　2017—2018 年浙江儿童肿瘤监测机构肝癌患儿年龄／性别构成

Figure 8-6-17　Age/gender composition of children with liver cancer in pediatric cancer surveillance sites in Zhejiang in 2017-2018

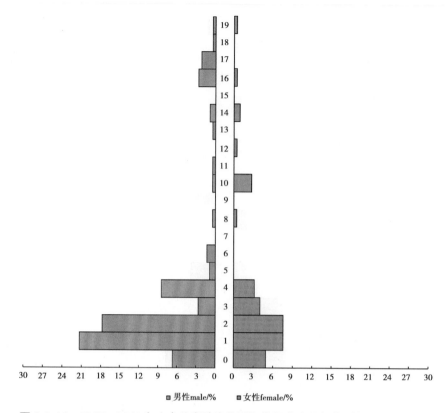

图 8-6-18　2017—2018 年山东儿童肿瘤监测机构肝癌患儿年龄 / 性别构成

Figure 8-6-18　Age/gender composition of children with liver cancer in pediatric cancer surveillance sites in Shandong in 2017-2018

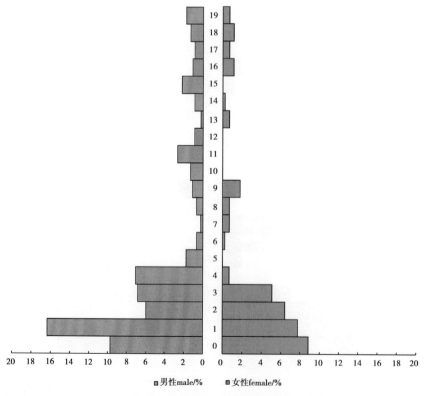

图 8-6-19　2017—2018 年河南儿童肿瘤监测机构肝癌患儿年龄 / 性别构成

Figure 8-6-19　Age/gender composition of children with liver cancer in pediatric cancer surveillance sites in Henan in 2017-2018

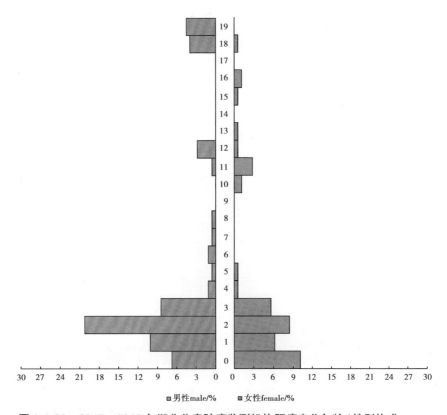

图 8-6-20　2017—2018 年湖北儿童肿瘤监测机构肝癌患儿年龄 / 性别构成

Figure 8-6-20　Age/gender composition of children with liver cancer in pediatric cancer surveillance sites in Hubei in 2017-2018

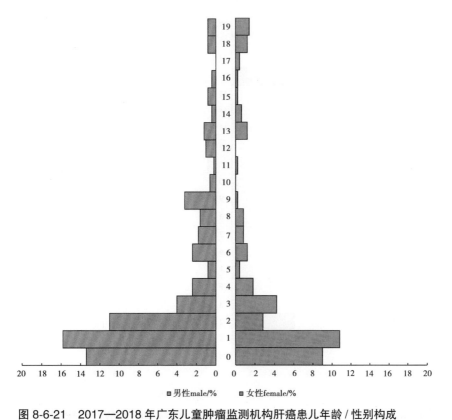

图 8-6-21　2017—2018 年广东儿童肿瘤监测机构肝癌患儿年龄 / 性别构成

Figure 8-6-21　Age/gender composition of children with liver cancer in pediatric cancer surveillance sites in Guangdong in 2017-2018

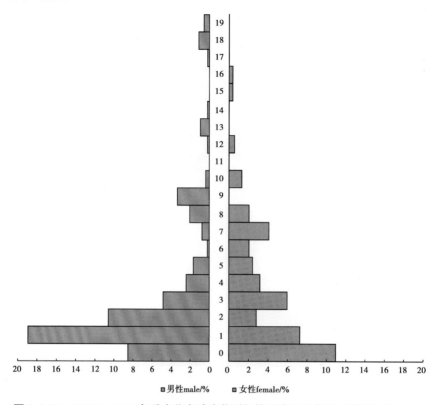

图 8-6-22 2017—2018 年重庆儿童肿瘤监测机构肝癌患儿年龄／性别构成

Figure 8-6-22 Age/gender composition of children with liver cancer in pediatric cancer surveillance sites in Chongqing in 2017-2018

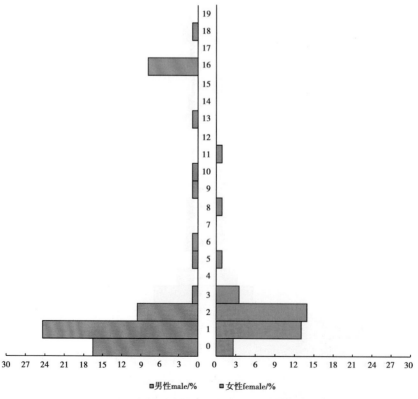

图 8-6-23 2017—2018 年四川儿童肿瘤监测机构肝癌患儿年龄／性别构成

Figure 8-6-23 Age/gender composition of children with liver cancer in pediatric cancer surveillance sites in Sichuan in 2017-2018

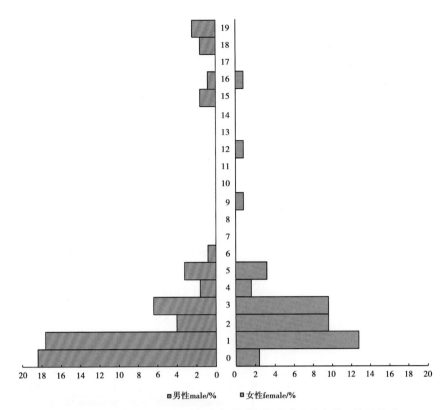

图 8-6-24　2017—2018 年云南儿童肿瘤监测机构肝癌患儿年龄 / 性别构成

Figure 8-6-24　Age/gender composition of children with liver cancer in pediatric cancer surveillance sites in Yunnan in 2017-2018

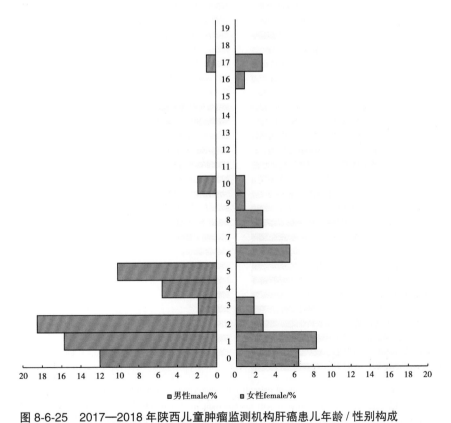

图 8-6-25　2017—2018 年陕西儿童肿瘤监测机构肝癌患儿年龄 / 性别构成

Figure 8-6-25　Age/gender composition of children with liver cancer in pediatric cancer surveillance sites in Shaanxi in 2017-2018

6.3 全国儿童肿瘤监测机构肝癌患儿就医省份分布

6.3.1 全国各省份肝癌患儿本省就医与省外就医的分布情况

总体而言,肝癌患儿本省就医的比例为45.20%。在所有省份中,本省就医比例前3位的省份分别为北京(98.73%)、广东(93.47%)和重庆(86.96%)。省外就医比例前3位分别为西藏(100.00%)、黑龙江(93.66%)和山西(92.74%)(图8-6-26)。

6.3 Distribution of provincial-level regions visited by children with liver cancer in pediatric cancer surveillance sites in China

6.3.1 Distribution of children with liver cancer receiving medical treatment in and out of their own provincial-level regions

In general, 45.20% of all children with liver cancer sought medical treatment in their own provincial-level regions. Beijing (98.73%), Guangdong (93.47%) and Chongqing (86.96%) were the top three recipients of patients from other provincial-level regions. Xizang (100.00%), Heilongjiang (93.66%) and Shanxi (92.74%) were the top three provincial-level regions in terms of the proportion of patients going to other provincial-level regions for medical treatment (Figure 8-6-26).

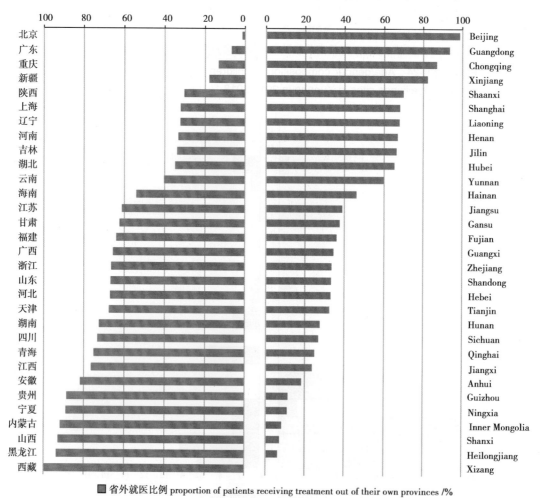

■ 省外就医比例 proportion of patients receiving treatment out of their own provinces /%
■ 本省就医比例 proportion of patients receiving treatment in their own provinces /%

图 8-6-26　2017—2018 年全国各省份肝癌患儿本省就医与省外就医比例 /%

Figure 8-6-26　Proportion of children with liver cancer receiving medical treatment in and out of their own provincial-level regions in 2017-2018/%

6.3.2　全国各省份肝癌患儿省外就医的去向省份分布情况

各省份肝癌患儿选择省外就医的去向分布呈现明显的规律,主要的去向省份为北京、上海、广东、天津和河北。如户籍地为浙江的肝癌患儿,选择省外就医的主要去向为北京和上海,分别占户籍地为浙江的肝癌患儿选择省外就医总数的 66.4% 和 25.5%。再如户籍地为海南的肝癌患儿,选择省外就医的主要去向为北京、广东和河北,分别占户籍地为海南的肝癌患儿选择省外就医总数的51.9%、25.9% 和 14.8%(图 8-6-27,按行方向查看)。

6.3.3　全国各省份收治肝癌患儿来源的省份分布情况

各省份儿童肿瘤监测机构收治的省外就医肝癌患儿来源分布略有差异,多数省份收治的肝癌患儿来源以其相邻省份为主。如上海,其收治的省外就医肝癌患儿主要来源于江苏、浙江和安徽,分别占上海收治的省外就医肝癌患儿总数的 21.6%、16.4% 和 15.6%。再如广东,其收治的省外就医肝癌患儿主要来源于湖南、江西和广西,分别占广东收治的省外就医肝癌患儿总数的 35.7%、17.8% 和14.1%(图 8-6-28,按列方向查看)。

6.3.2　Distribution of provincial-level regions receiving children with liver cancer from outside their provincial-level regions

The distribution of provincial-level regions receiving children with liver cancer from outside the provincial-level regions showed obvious regularity. The main destinations were Beijing, Shanghai, Guangdong, Tianjin and Hebei. For Zhejiang children with liver cancer, the main destinations were Beijing and Shanghai, accounting for 66.4% and 25.5%, respectively, of the total number of Zhejiang children with liver cancer going outside Zhejiang. For Hainan children with liver cancer, Beijing, Guangdong, and Hebei were the main destinations, accounting for 51.9%, 25.9% and 14.8%, respectively, of the total number of Hainan children with liver cancer going outside (Figure 8-6-27, view in rows).

6.3.3　Distribution of the provincial-level regions of origin of children receiving treatment out of their own provincial-level regions

There was a slight difference in the distribution of the provincial-level regions of origin of children with liver cancer admitted to surveillance sites in different provincial-level regions, and most of the children were mainly from their neighboring provincial-level regions. For example, in Shanghai, the children hospitalized from other provincial-level regions were mainly from Jiangsu, Zhejiang and Anhui, accounting for 21.6%, 16.4% and 15.6%, respectively, of the total number of children hospitalized from other provincial-level regions in Shanghai. In Guangdong, children hospitalized from other provincial-level regions were mainly from Hunan, Jiangxi and Guangxi, accounting for 35.7%, 17.8% and 14.1% of the total number of children hospitalized from other provincial-level regions in Guangdong, respectively (Figure 8-6-28, view in lines).

患者户籍所在地的省份分布 / distribution of the province of origin of children receiving treatment out of their own provinces

收治省外级医院肿瘤患儿的医院省份分布 / provincial distribution of hospitals receiving children with cancer from outside the province

户籍 Origin	北京 Beijing	天津 Tianjin	河北 Hebei	山西 Shanxi	内蒙古 Inner Mongolia	辽宁 Liaoning	吉林 Jilin	黑龙江 Heilongjiang	上海 Shanghai	江苏 Jiangsu	浙江 Zhejiang	安徽 Anhui	福建 Fujian	江西 Jiangxi	山东 Shandong	河南 Henan	湖北 Hubei	湖南 Hunan	广东 Guangdong	广西 Guangxi	海南 Hainan	重庆 Chongqing	四川 Sichuan	贵州 Guizhou	云南 Yunnan	西藏 Xizang	陕西 Shaanxi	甘肃 Gansu	青海 Qinghai	宁夏 Ningxia	新疆 Xinjiang	合计 total
北京 Beijing	98.3	0	0	0	0	0	0	0	0	0	0	0	0	0	0	0	0	0	0	0	0	0	0	1.7	0	0	0	0	0	0	0	100
天津 Tianjin	92.3	4.1	0	0	0	0	0	0	3.3	0	0	0	0	0	0	0	0	0	0	0	0	0	0	0	0	0	0	0	0	0	0	100
河北 Hebei	86.0	0.9	0	0	0	0	0	0	3.3	0	0	0	0	0	0.2	0	0	0	0	0	0	0	0	0	0	0	0	0	0	0	0	100
山西 Shanxi	74.6	0	0	0	0	0	0	0	0.9	0	0	0	0	0	0	11.3	0	0	0	0	0	0	0	0	0	0	0	0	0	0	0	100
内蒙古 Inner Mongolia	96.1	0	0	0	0	9.8	15.6	0	0	0	0	0	0	0	0	0	0	0	0	0	0	0	0	0	0	0	0	0	0	0	0	100
辽宁 Liaoning	100.0	2.9	0	0	0	0	1.0	0	0	0	0	0	0	0	0	0	0	0	0	0	0	0	0	0	0	0	0	0	0	0	0	100
吉林 Jilin	82.0	4.4	0	0	0	0	0	0	0	0	0	0	0	0	0	0	0	0	0	0	0	0	0	0	0	0	0	0	0	0	0	100
黑龙江 Heilongjiang	100.0	0	2.3	0	0	8.3	3.0	0	0	0	0	0	0	0	0	0	0	0	0	0	0	0	0	0	0	0	0	0	0	0	0	100
上海 Shanghai	65.8	0	0	0	0	0	0	0	0	0	0	0	0	0	0	0	0	0	0	0	0	0	0	0	0	0	0	0	0	0	0	100
江苏 Jiangsu	66.5	0	0	0	0	0	0	0	0	0	0	0	0	0	0	0	0	0	0	0	0	0	0	0	0	0	0	0	0	0	0	100
浙江 Zhejiang	38.5	0	3.2	0	0	0	0	0	32.2	0	0	0	0	0	1.6	0	4.0	0	0.8	0	0	0	0	0	0	0	0	0	0	0	0	100
安徽 Anhui	52.6	0.4	0	0	0	2.5	0	0	25.5	24.1	6.3	0	0	0	0.8	0	0.4	0	1.7	0	0	0	0	0	0	0	0	0	0	0	0	100
福建 Fujian	57.0	0	0	0	0	0	0	0	34.6	0	0	0	0	0.7	0	0	0.7	0	12.8	0	0	0	0	0	0	0	0	0	0	0	0	100
江西 Jiangxi	88.7	0	0.2	0	0	0.2	2.8	0	18.4	0.2	1.3	0	0	0	0	0	0	0	21.9	0	0	0	0	0	0	0	0.4	0	0	0	0	100
山东 Shandong	82.5	0.9	0.2	0.5	0	0.2	0	0	6.5	0.2	0	0	0	0	0	0	0	0	0.5	0	0	0	0	0	0	0	0	0	0	0	0.5	100
河南 Henan	85.7	1.3	0	0	0	0	0	0	7.8	0.9	0	0	0	0	0.5	0	2.3	0	3.7	0	0	0	0	0	0	0	0	0	0	0	0	100
湖北 Hubei	53.7	2.4	0	0	0	0	0	0	7.0	0	5.0	0	0	0	1.0	0.5	0	4.5	8.3	0	0	2.4	1.2	0	0	0	0	0	0	0	0	100
湖南 Hunan	95.5	0	0	0	0	0	0	0	0	0	0	0	0	0	0	0	0	0	32.8	0	0	0	0	0	0	0	0	0	0	0	0	100
广东 Guangdong	38.2	0	0	0	0	0	0	0	0	0	0	0	0	0	0	0	0	0	0	0	0	0	0	0	0	0	0	0	0	0	0	100
广西 Guangxi	51.9	0	14.8	0	0	1.8	0	0	0	0	0	0	0	0	0	0	0	1.8	47.3	0	0	0	0	0	0	0	0	0	0	0	0	100
海南 Hainan	80.0	3.3	0	0	0	0	0	0	0	7.4	0	0	0	0	0	0	0	0	25.9	0	0	0	0.3	0	0	0	0	0	0	0	0	100
重庆 Chongqing	25.4	0	0	0	0	0	0	0	2.4	0	0	0	0	0	0	0	0	0	16.7	0	0	69.6	0	0	0	0	0	0	0	0	0	100
四川 Sichuan	17.5	0	0	0	0	0	0	0	2.4	1.7	2.8	0	0	0	0	0	0	0	0.3	0	0	0	0	1.1	3.8	0	0	0	0	0	0	100
贵州 Guizhou	68.7	0	0	0	0	0	0	0	4.0	0	2.8	0	0	0	0	0	0	0	2.3	0.6	0	68.9	0	0	2.8	0	0	0	0	0	0	100
云南 Yunnan	0	0	1.2	0	0	0	0	0	10.0	0	0	0	0	0	0	0	2.5	0	1.3	0	0	12.5	3.8	0	0	0	0	0	0	0	0	100
西藏 Xizang	78.5	0	14.3	0	0	0	0	0	0	0	0	0	0	0	0	0	0	0	0	0	0	0	50.0	0	0	0	0	0	0	0	0	100
陕西 Shaanxi	58.2	2.4	0	0	0	0	0	0	2.4	0	0	0	0	0	0	0	0	0	0	0	0	2.4	0	0	0	0	20.9	0	0	0	0	100
甘肃 Gansu	33.3	0	0	0	0	0	0	0	18.6	0	2.3	0	0	0	0	0	0	0	66.7	0	0	0	0	0	0	0	0	0	0	0	0	100
青海 Qinghai	97.5	0	2.5	0	0	0	0	0	0	0	0	0	0	0	0	0	0	0	0	0	0	0	0	0	0	0	0	0	0	0	0	100
宁夏 Ningxia	90.9	0	0	0	0	0	0	0	9.1	0	0	0	0	0	0	0	0	0	0	0	0	0	0	0	0	0	0	0	0	0	50.0	100
新疆 Xinjiang	90.9	0	0	0	0	0	0	0	9.1	0	0	0	0	0	0	0	0	0	0	0	0	0	0	0	0	0	0	0	0	0	0	100

图 8-6-27　2017—2018 年全国各省份户籍肝癌患儿选择省外就医的省份分布 /%

Figure 8-6-27　Distribution of provincial-level regions receiving children with liver cancer from other provincial-level regions in 2017-2018/%

Column group label: 收治省外就医肿瘤患儿的医院省份分布 / provincial distribution of hospitals receiving children with cancer from outside the province

Row group label: 省外就医肿瘤患儿的来源省份分布 / distribution of the provinces of origin of children with cancer receiving treatment out of their own provinces

来源省份 \ 收治医院省份	北京 Beijing	天津 Tianjin	河北 Hebei	山西 Shanxi	内蒙古 Inner Mongolia	辽宁 Liaoning	吉林 Jilin	黑龙江 Heilongjiang	上海 Shanghai	江苏 Jiangsu	浙江 Zhejiang	安徽 Anhui	福建 Fujian	江西 Jiangxi	山东 Shandong	河南 Henan	湖北 Hubei	湖南 Hunan	广东 Guangdong	广西 Guangxi	海南 Hainan	重庆 Chongqing	四川 Sichuan	贵州 Guizhou	云南 Yunnan	西藏 Xizang	陕西 Shaanxi	甘肃 Gansu	青海 Qinghai	宁夏 Ningxia	新疆 Xinjiang
北京 Beijing		0	0	0	0	0	0	0	0	0	0	0	0	0	0	0	0	0	0	0	0	0	0	0	0	0	0	0	0	0	50.0
天津 Tianjin	2.4		0	0	0	0	0	0	0	0	0	0	0	0	0	0	0	0	0	0	0	0	0	0	0	0	0	0	0	0	0
河北 Hebei	13.3	40.6		0	0	0	0	0	3.1	0	0	0	0	0	10.0	0	0	0	0	0	0	0	0	0	0	0	0	0	0	0	0
山西 Shanxi	3.9	2.7	0		0	0	0	0	0.3	0	0	0	0	0	0	100.0	0	0	0	0	0	0	0	0	0	0	9.1	0	0	0	0
内蒙古 Inner Mongolia	3.6	0	0	0		38.7	52.8	0	0	0	0	0	0	0	0	0	0	0	0	0	0	0	0	0	0	0	0	0	0	0	0
辽宁 Liaoning	3.9	8.1	0	0	0		2.8	0	0	0	0	0	0	0	0	0	0	0	0	0	0	0	0	0	0	0	0	0	0	0	0
吉林 Jilin	2.3	0	0	0	0	0		0	0	0	0	0	0	0	0	0	0	0	0	0	0	0	0	0	0	0	0	0	0	0	25.0
黑龙江 Heilongjiang	4.3	16.2	10.0	0	0	35.5	11.1		0	0	0	0	0	0	0	0	0	0	0	0	0	0	0	0	0	0	0	0	0	0	0
上海 Shanghai	0.3	0	0	0	0	0	0	0		0	0	0	0	0	0	0	0	0	0	0	0	0	0	0	0	0	0	0	0	0	0
江苏 Jiangsu	6.7	0	0	0	0	0	0	0	0		0	0	0	0	0	0	0	0	1.0	0	0	0	0	0	0	0	0	0	0	0	0
浙江 Zhejiang	6.5	0	26.8	0	0	0	0	0	21.6	0		0	0	0	40.0	0	50.0	0	2.2	0	0	0	0	0	0	0	0	0	0	0	0
安徽 Anhui	3.6	2.7	0	0	0	0	0	0	16.4	85.1	45.4		0	0	20.0	0	5.0	0	9.2	0	0	0	0	0	0	0	0	0	0	0	0
福建 Fujian	2.8	0	0	0	0	0	0	0	15.6	0	6.1	0		0	0	0	0	0	17.8	0	0	0	0	0	0	0	0	0	0	0	0
江西 Jiangxi	3.4	0	0	0	0	0	0	0	12.0	0	0	0	100.0		0	0	5.0	0	1.1	0	0	0	0	0	0	0	0	0	0	0	0
山东 Shandong	15.1	10.8	0	0	0	3.2	33.3	0	7.3	1.4	0	0	0	0		0	0	0	4.3	0	0	0	0	0	0	0	0	0	0	0	0
河南 Henan	7.1	8.1	0	100.0	0	0	0	0	7.3	3.0	0	0	0	0	10.0		25.0	0	3.8	0	0	0	0	0	0	0	9.1	0	0	0	0
湖北 Hubei	2.8	5.4	0	0	0	0	0	0	4.4	0	0	0	0	0	0	0		50.0	0	0	0	0.6	14.2	0	0	0	0	0	0	0	0
湖南 Hunan	4.3	0	0	0	0	0	0	0	3.6	3.0	30.3	0	0	0	20.0	0	5.0		35.7	0	0	0	0	0	0	0	0	0	0	0	0
广东 Guangdong	0.8	0	0	0	0	0	0	0	0	0	0	0	0	0	0	0	0	50.0		0	100.0	0	0	0	0	0	0	0	0	0	0
广西 Guangxi	0.8	0	20.0	0	0	3.2	0	0	0	0	0	0	0	0	0	0	0	0	14.1		0	0	0	0	0	0	0	0	0	0	0
海南 Hainan	0.6	0	13.3	0	0	0	0	0	0	0	0	0	0	0	0	0	0	0	3.8	0		0	0	0	0	0	0	0	0	0	0
重庆 Chongqing	0.9	0	0	0	0	0	0	0	0	0	0	0	0	0	0	0	0	0	2.7	0	0		0	100.0	0	0	0	0	0	0	0
四川 Sichuan	2.9	2.7	0	0	0	0	0	0	0	0	0	0	0	0	0	0	0	0	0.5	0	0	60.2		0	16.7	0	0	0	0	0	0
贵州 Guizhou	1.2	0	0	0	0	0	0	0	1.8	7.5	15.2	0	0	0	0	0	0	0	2.2	100.0	0	36.0	28.6		83.3	0	0	0	0	0	0
云南 Yunnan	2.2	0	3.3	0	0	0	0	0	2.1	0	0	0	0	0	0	0	10.0	0	0.5	0	0	2.9	42.9	0		0	0	0	0	0	0
西藏 Xizang	0	0	0	0	0	0	0	0	0	0	0	0	0	0	0	0	0	0	0	0	0	0	14.3	0	0		0	0	0	0	0
陕西 Shaanxi	1.3	2.7	20.0	0	0	0	0	0	0.3	0	0	0	0	0	0	0	0	0	0	0	0	0.3	0	0	0	0		0	0	0	0
甘肃 Gansu	1.0	0	0	0	0	0	0	0	2.1	0	0	0	0	0	0	0	0	0	0	0	0	0	0	0	0	0	81.8		0	0	25.0
青海 Qinghai	0.1	0	0	0	0	0	0	0	0	0	0	0	0	0	0	0	0	0	0	0	0	0	0	0	0	0	0	0		0	0
宁夏 Ningxia	1.5	0	3.3	0	0	0	0	0	0.3	0	3.0	0	0	0	0	0	0	0	1.1	0	0	0	0	0	0	0	0	0	0		0
新疆 Xinjiang	0.4	0	0	0	0	0	0	0	0	0	0	0	0	0	0	0	0	0	0	0	0	0	0	0	0	0	0	0	0	0	
合计 Total	100	100	100	100	0	100	100	0	100	100	100	0	100	0	100	100	100	100	100	100	100	100	100	100	100	0	100	0	0	0	100

图 8-6-28 2017—2018 年全国各省份儿童肿瘤监测机构省外就医肝癌患儿来源分布 /%

Figure 8-6-28 Distribution of provincial-level regions of origin of children with liver cancer going outside their provincial-level regions for medical treatment in 2017-2018/%

6.4 全国儿童肿瘤监测机构肝癌患儿住院费用医疗付费方式构成

6.4.1 全国肝癌患儿住院费用医疗付费方式构成情况

全国肝癌患儿住院费用的医疗付费方式中,占比最高的前 3 种类型分别为全自费(31.68%)、新型农村合作医疗(23.82%)和城镇居民基本医疗保险(23.81%)(图 8-6-29)。

6.4.2 六大区肝癌患儿住院费用医疗付费方式构成情况

六大区的医疗付费方式所占比例各不相同,西南地区、华东地区和东北地区均以全自费占比最高,分别为 52.03%、36.25% 和 23.97%;华北地区和西北地区均以城镇居民基本医疗保险占比最高,分别为 38.34% 和 24.14%;中南地区以新型农村合作医疗占比最高,为 38.31%(图 8-6-30~ 图 8-6-35)。

6.4 Composition of medical payment methods for hospitalization expenses of children with liver cancer in pediatric cancer surveillance sites in China

6.4.1 Composition of medical payment methods for hospitalization expenses of children with liver cancer nationally

Among the medical payment methods of children with liver cancer nationally, the top three methods were 100% self-pay (31.68%), new rural cooperative medical system (23.82%) and basic medical insurance for urban residents (23.81%) (Figure 8-6-29).

6.4.2 Composition of medical payment methods for hospitalization expenses of children with liver cancer in the six regions

The proportions of medical payment methods in the six regions were different, and the proportion of 100% self-pay was the highest in Southwest China, East China and Northeast China, which were 52.03%, 36.25% and 23.97%, respectively. In North China and Northwest China, the proportion of basic medical insurance for urban residents was the highest, accounting for 38.34% and 24.14%, respectively. In Central and Southern China, the proportion of new rural cooperative medical system was the highest, accounting for 38.31% (Figure 8-6-30~Figure 8-6-35).

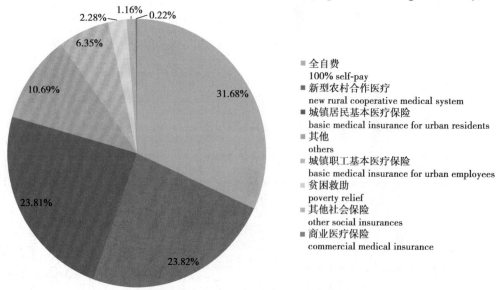

图 8-6-29 2017—2018 年全国肝癌患儿住院费用医疗付费方式构成

Figure 8-6-29 Composition of medical payment methods for hospitalization expenses of children with liver cancer nationally in 2017-2018

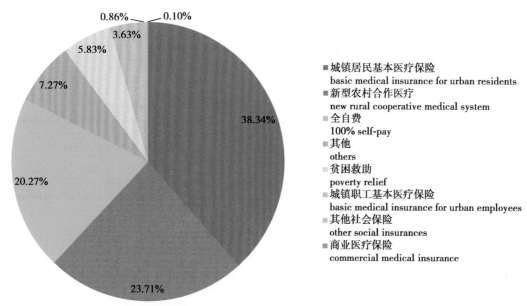

图 8-6-30　2017—2018 年华北地区肝癌患儿住院费用医疗付费方式构成

Figure 8-6-30　Composition of medical payment methods for hospitalization expenses of children with liver cancer in North China in 2017-2018

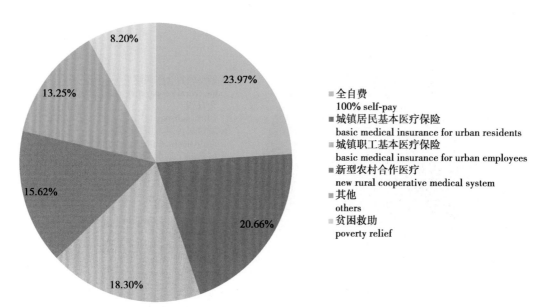

图 8-6-31　2017—2018 年东北地区肝癌患儿住院费用医疗付费方式构成

Figure 8-6-31　Composition of medical payment methods for hospitalization expenses of children with liver cancer in Northeast China in 2017-2018

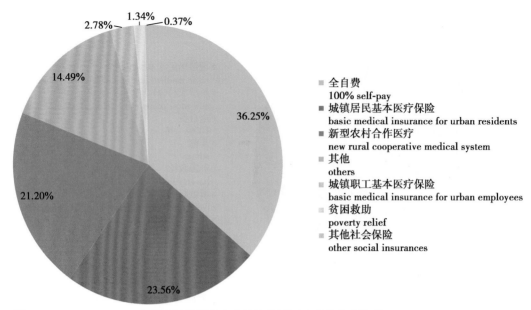

图 8-6-32　2017—2018 年华东地区肝癌患儿住院费用医疗付费方式构成

Figure 8-6-32　Composition of medical payment methods for hospitalization expenses of children with liver cancer in East China in 2017-2018

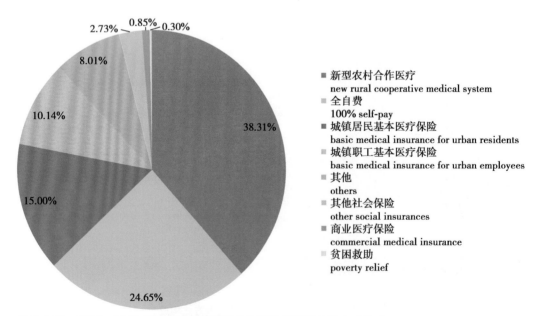

图 8-6-33　2017—2018 年中南地区肝癌患儿住院费用医疗付费方式构成

Figure 8-6-33　Composition of medical payment methods for hospitalization expenses of children with liver cancer in Central and Southern China in 2017-2018

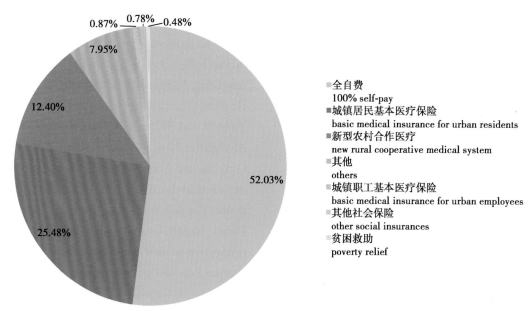

图 8-6-34   2017—2018 年西南地区肝癌患儿住院费用医疗付费方式构成

Figure 8-6-34   Composition of medical payment methods for hospitalization expenses of children with liver cancer in Southwest China in 2017-2018

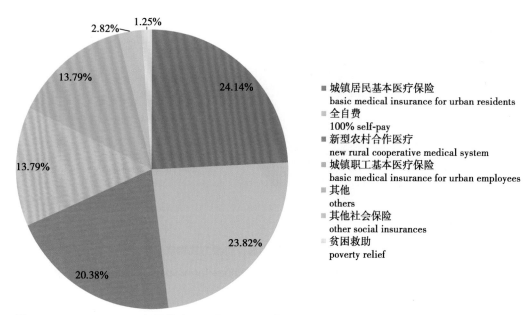

图 8-6-35   2017—2018 年西北地区肝癌患儿住院费用医疗付费方式构成

Figure 8-6-35   Composition of medical payment methods for hospitalization expenses of children with liver cancer in Northwest China in 2017-2018

6.4.3 各省份肝癌患儿住院费用医疗付费方式构成情况

黑龙江、江苏、安徽、福建、江西、山东、湖南、广东、海南、四川、贵州、云南和陕西13个省份均以全自费所占比例最高。北京、天津、山西、内蒙古、吉林、上海、浙江、重庆、青海和宁夏10个省份的城镇居民基本医疗保险占比最高。河北、河南、广西和甘肃4个省份的新型农村合作医疗占比最高（图8-6-36~图8-6-66）。

6.4.3 Composition of medical payment methods for hospitalization expenses of children with liver cancer in each provincial-level region

The proportion of 100% self-pay was the highest in the following 13 provincial-level regions: Heilongjiang, Jiangsu, Anhui, Fujian, Jiangxi, Shandong, Hunan, Guangdong, Hainan, Sichuan, Guizhou, Yunnan and Shaanxi. Beijing, Tianjin, Shanxi, Inner Mongolia, Jilin, Shanghai, Zhejiang, Chongqing, Qinghai and Ningxia had the highest proportion of payment by basic medical insurance for urban residents. The following four provincial-level regions—Hebei, Henan, Guangxi, and Gansu—had the highest proportion of new rural cooperative medical system (Figure 8-6-36~Figure 8-6-66).

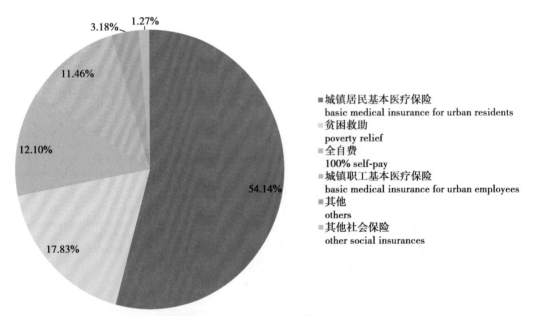

■城镇居民基本医疗保险
basic medical insurance for urban residents
■贫困救助
poverty relief
■全自费
100% self-pay
■城镇职工基本医疗保险
basic medical insurance for urban employees
■其他
others
■其他社会保险
other social insurances

图 8-6-36　2017—2018 年北京肝癌患儿住院费用医疗付费方式构成

Figure 8-6-36　Composition of medical payment methods for hospitalization expenses of children with liver cancer in Beijing in 2017-2018

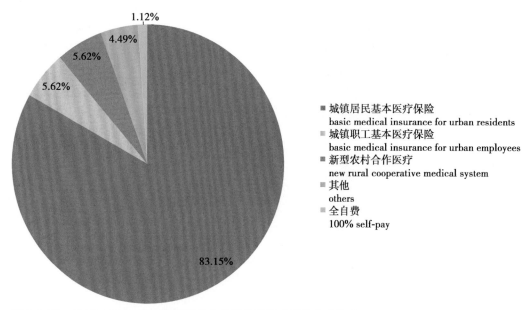

图 8-6-37   2017—2018 年天津肝癌患儿住院费用医疗付费方式构成

Figure 8-6-37   Composition of medical payment methods for hospitalization expenses of children with liver cancer in Tianjin in 2017-2018

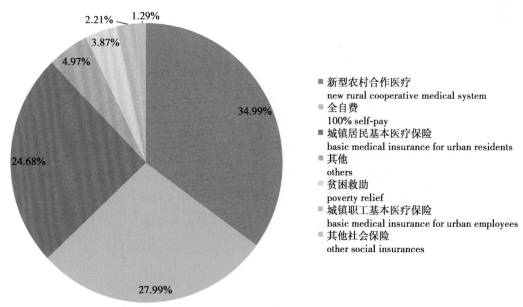

图 8-6-38   2017—2018 年河北肝癌患儿住院费用医疗付费方式构成

Figure 8-6-38   Composition of medical payment methods for hospitalization expenses of children with liver cancer in Hebei in 2017-2018

411

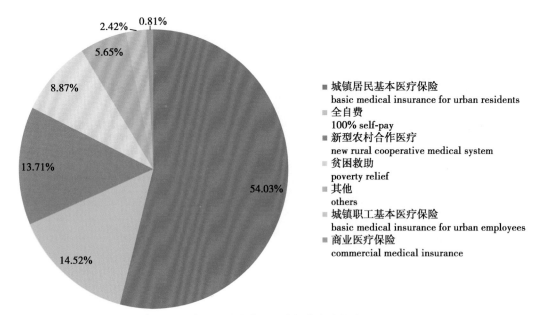

图 8-6-39　2017—2018 年山西肝癌患儿住院费用医疗付费方式构成

Figure 8-6-39　Composition of medical payment methods for hospitalization expenses of children with liver cancer in Shanxi in 2017-2018

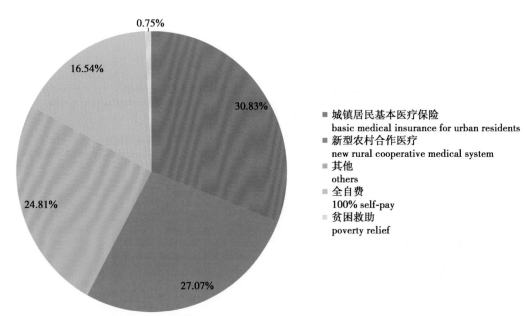

图 8-6-40　2017—2018 年内蒙古肝癌患儿住院费用医疗付费方式构成

Figure 8-6-40　Composition of medical payment methods for hospitalization expenses of children with liver cancer in Inner Mongolia in 2017-2018

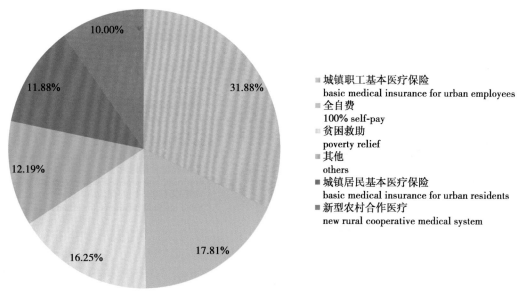

图 8-6-41   2017—2018 年辽宁肝癌患儿住院费用医疗付费方式构成

Figure 8-6-41   Composition of medical payment methods for hospitalization expenses of children with liver cancer in Liaoning in 2017-2018

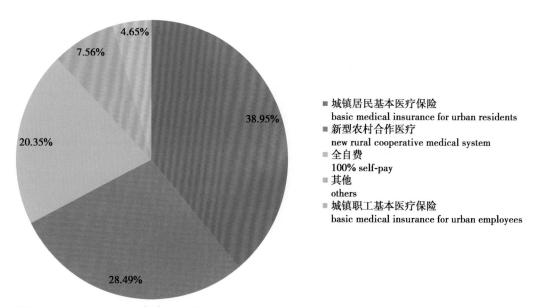

图 8-6-42   2017—2018 年吉林肝癌患儿住院费用医疗付费方式构成

Figure 8-6-42   Composition of medical payment methods for hospitalization expenses of children with liver cancer in Jilin in 2017-2018

413

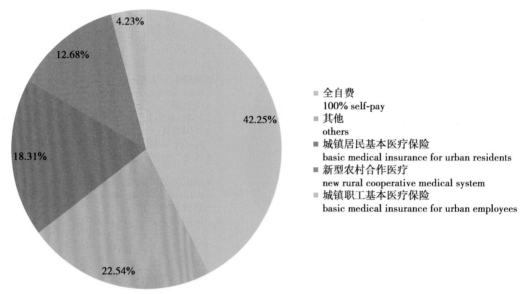

图 8-6-43 2017—2018 年黑龙江肝癌患儿住院费用医疗付费方式构成

Figure 8-6-43 Composition of medical payment methods for hospitalization expenses of children with liver cancer in Heilongjiang in 2017-2018

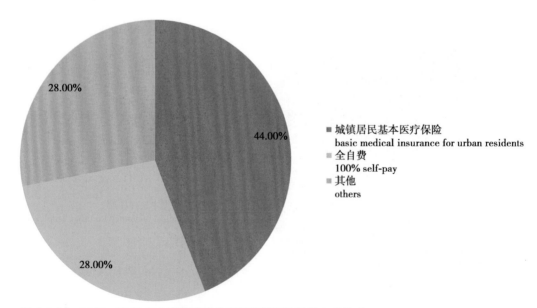

图 8-6-44 2017—2018 年上海肝癌患儿住院费用医疗付费方式构成

Figure 8-6-44 Composition of medical payment methods for hospitalization expenses of children with liver cancer in Shanghai in 2017-2018

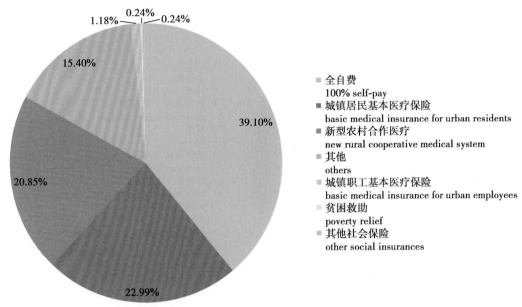

图 8-6-45　2017—2018 年江苏肝癌患儿住院费用医疗付费方式构成

Figure 8-6-45　Composition of medical payment methods for hospitalization expenses of children with liver cancer in Jiangsu in 2017-2018

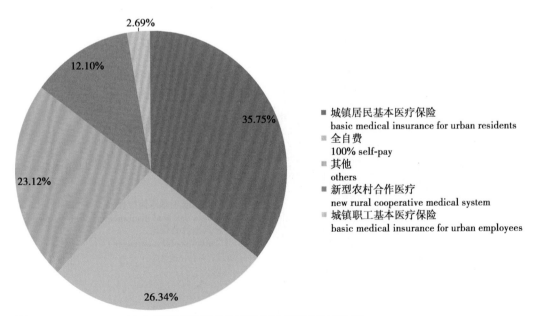

图 8-6-46　2017—2018 年浙江肝癌患儿住院费用医疗付费方式构成

Figure 8-6-46　Composition of medical payment methods for hospitalization expenses of children with liver cancer in Zhejiang in 2017-2018

415

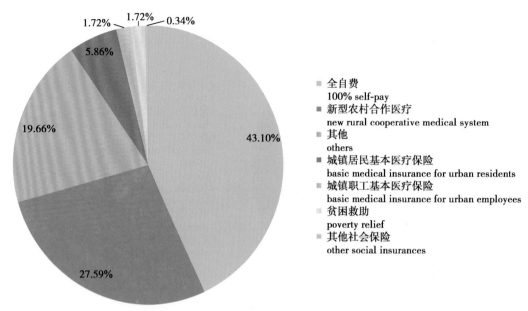

图 8-6-47 2017—2018 年安徽肝癌患儿住院费用医疗付费方式构成

Figure 8-6-47 Composition of medical payment methods for hospitalization expenses of children with liver cancer in Anhui in 2017-2018

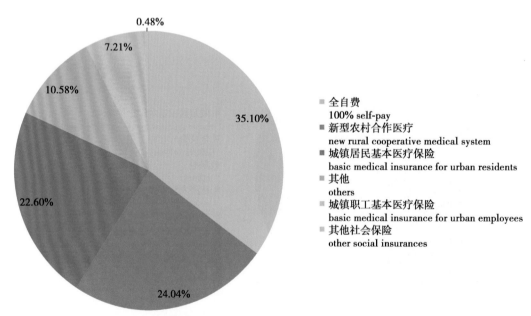

图 8-6-48 2017—2018 年福建肝癌患儿住院费用医疗付费方式构成

Figure 8-6-48 Composition of medical payment methods for hospitalization expenses of children with liver cancer in Fujian in 2017-2018

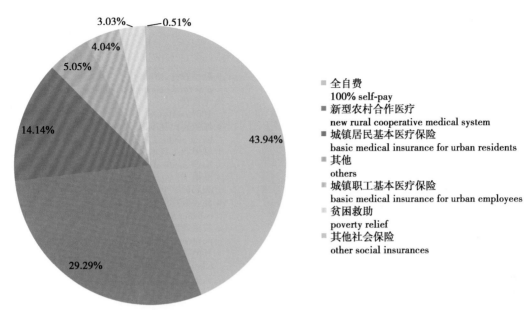

图 8-6-49　2017—2018 年江西肝癌患儿住院费用医疗付费方式构成

Figure 8-6-49　Composition of medical payment methods for hospitalization expenses of children with liver cancer in Jiangxi in 2017-2018

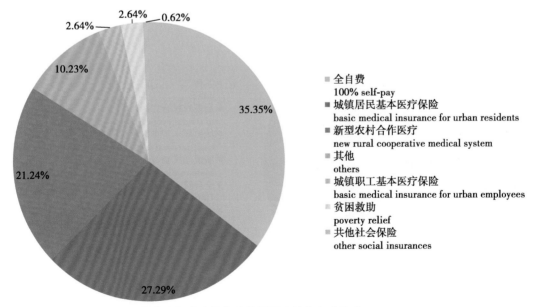

图 8-6-50　2017—2018 年山东肝癌患儿住院费用医疗付费方式构成

Figure 8-6-50　Composition of medical payment methods for hospitalization expenses of children with liver cancer in Shandong in 2017-2018

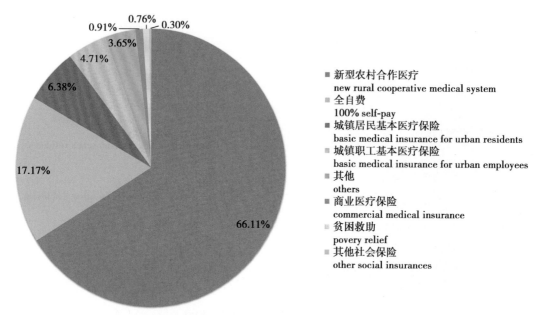

图 8-6-51　2017—2018 年河南肝癌患儿住院费用医疗付费方式构成

Figure 8-6-51　Composition of medical payment methods for hospitalization expenses of children with liver cancer in Henan in 2017-2018

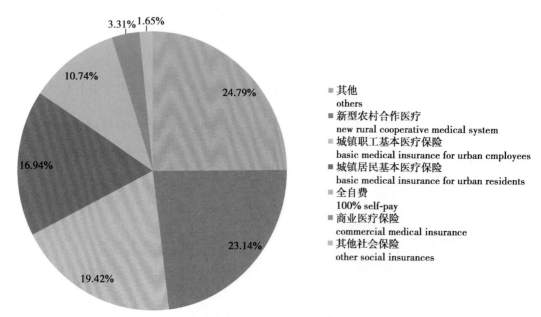

图 8-6-52　2017—2018 年湖北肝癌患儿住院费用医疗付费方式构成

Figure 8-6-52　Composition of medical payment methods for hospitalization expenses of children with liver cancer in Hubei in 2017-2018

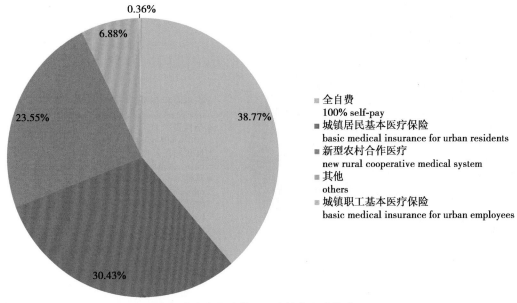

图 8-6-53　2017—2018 年湖南肝癌患儿住院费用医疗付费方式构成

Figure 8-6-53　Composition of medical payment methods for hospitalization expenses of children with liver cancer in Hunan in 2017-2018

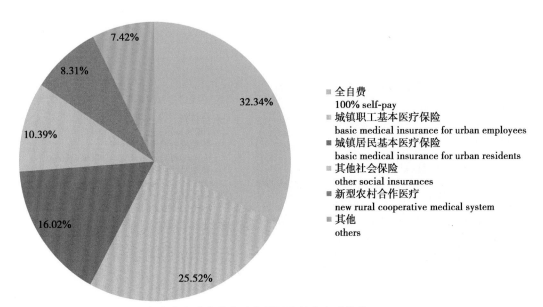

图 8-6-54　2017—2018 年广东肝癌患儿住院费用医疗付费方式构成

Figure 8-6-54　Composition of medical payment methods for hospitalization expenses of children with liver cancer in Guangdong in 2017-2018

419

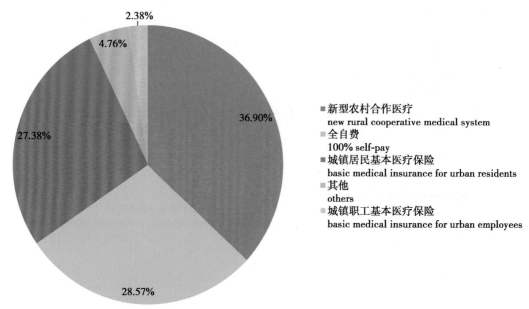

图 8-6-55　2017—2018 年广西肝癌患儿住院费用医疗付费方式构成

Figure 8-6-55　Composition of medical payment methods for hospitalization expenses of children with liver cancer in Guangxi in 2017-2018

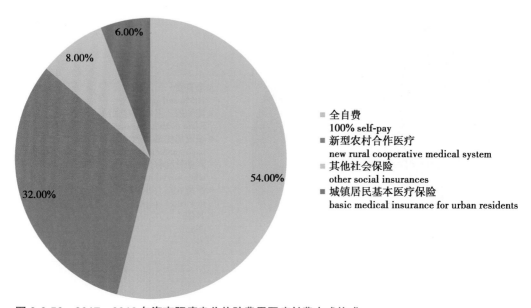

图 8-6-56　2017—2018 年海南肝癌患儿住院费用医疗付费方式构成

Figure 8-6-56　Composition of medical payment methods for hospitalization expenses of children with liver cancer in Hainan in 2017-2018

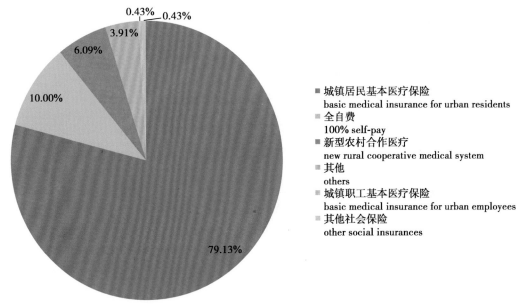

图 8-6-57   2017—2018 年重庆肝癌患儿住院费用医疗付费方式构成

Figure 8-6-57   Composition of medical payment methods for hospitalization expenses of children with liver cancer in Chongqing in 2017-2018

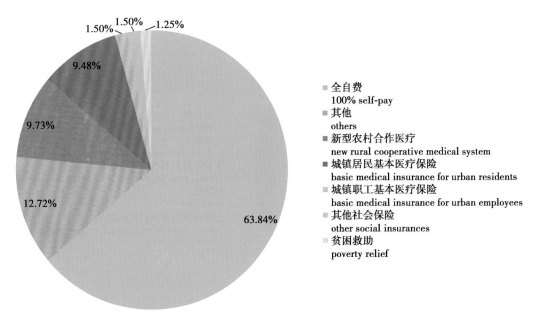

图 8-6-58   2017—2018 年四川肝癌患儿住院费用医疗付费方式构成

Figure 8-6-58   Composition of medical payment methods for hospitalization expenses of children with liver cancer in Sichuan in 2017-2018

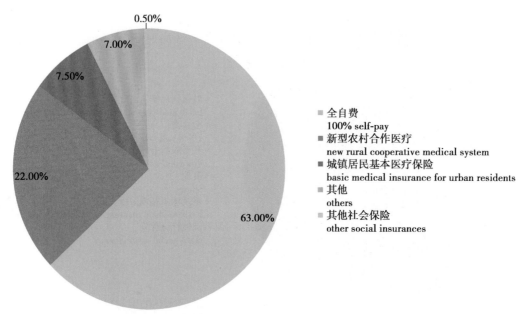

图 8-6-59　2017—2018 年贵州肝癌患儿住院费用医疗付费方式构成

Figure 8-6-59　Composition of medical payment methods for hospitalization expenses of children with liver cancer in Guizhou in 2017-2018

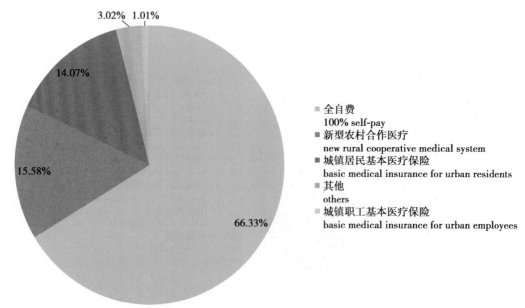

图 8-6-60　2017—2018 年云南肝癌患儿住院费用医疗付费方式构成

Figure 8-6-60　Composition of medical payment methods for hospitalization expenses of children with liver cancer in Yunnan in 2017-2018

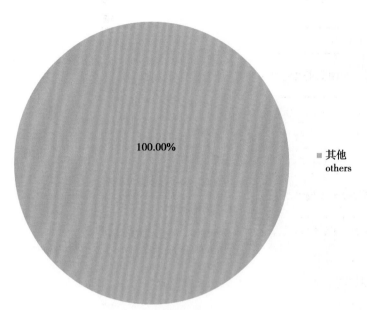

图 8-6-61　2017—2018 年西藏肝癌患儿住院费用医疗付费方式构成

Figure 8-6-61　Composition of medical payment methods of children with liver cancer in Xizang in 2017-2018

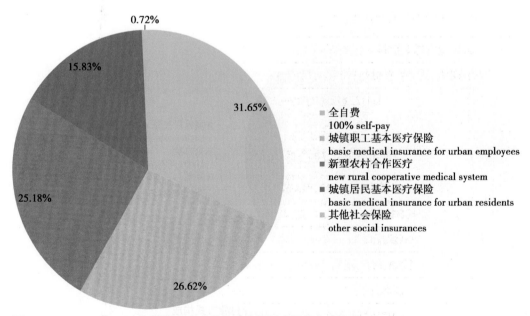

图 8-6-62　2017—2018 年陕西肝癌患儿住院费用医疗付费方式构成

Figure 8-6-62　Composition of medical payment methods of children with liver cancer in Shaanxi in 2017-2018

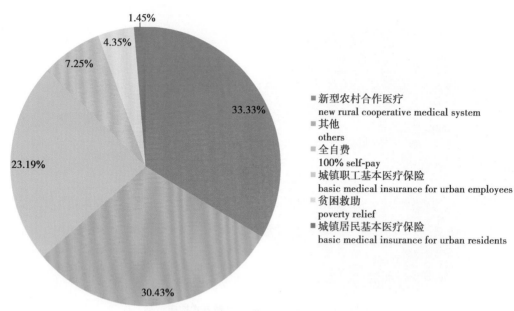

图 8-6-63　2017—2018 年甘肃肝癌患儿住院费用医疗付费方式构成

Figure 8-6-63　Composition of medical payment methods of children with liver cancer in Gansu in 2017-2018

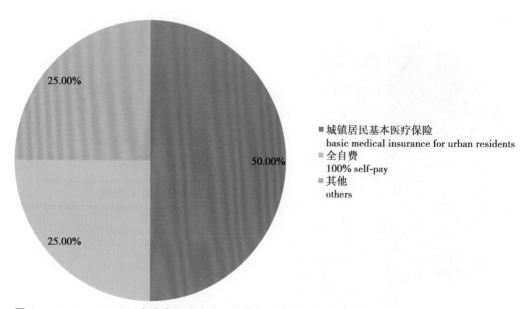

图 8-6-64　2017—2018 年青海肝癌患儿住院费用医疗付费方式构成

Figure 8-6-64　Composition of medical payment methods of children with liver cancer in Qinghai in 2017-2018

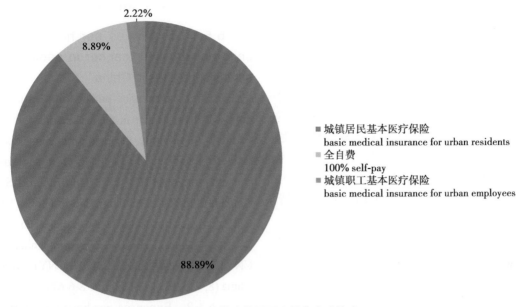

图 8-6-65　2017—2018 年宁夏肝癌患儿住院费用医疗付费方式构成

Figure 8-6-65　Composition of medical payment methods of children with liver cancer in Ningxia in 2017-2018

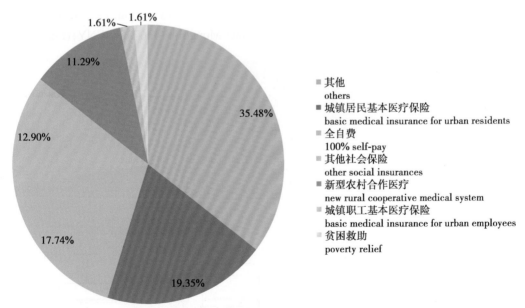

图 8-6-66　2017—2018 年新疆肝癌患儿住院费用医疗付费方式构成

Figure 8-6-66　Composition of medical payment methods of children with liver cancer in Xinjiang in 2017-2018

6.5 全国儿童肿瘤监测机构肝癌患儿住院费用分析

6.5.1 全国儿童肿瘤监测机构肝癌患儿次均住院费用情况

6.5.1.1 全国及六大区肝癌患儿次均住院费用情况 全国肝癌患儿次均住院费用(中位数)为 9 118.67 元。高于全国中位数水平的地区分别为中南地区(10 857.49 元)和华北地区(10 722.56元),低于全国中位数水平的地区分别为西南地区(5 580.07 元)、华东地区(5 617.97 元)、西北地区(7 347.87 元)和东北地区(8 715.85 元)(图 8-6-67)。

6.5.1.2 各省份肝癌患儿次均住院费用情况 根据肝癌患儿次均住院费用(中位数),前 3 位的省份分别为广东(21 119.54 元)、贵州(16 210.19元)和黑龙江(15 571.58 元),后 3 位分别为上海(3 397.60 元)、广西(4 536.30 元)和内蒙古(4 673.97元)(图 8-6-68)。

6.5 Analysis of hospitalization expenses of children with liver cancer in pediatric cancer surveillance sites in China

6.5.1 Expenses per hospitalization of children with liver cancer in pediatric cancer surveillance sites in China

6.5.1.1 Expenses per hospitalization of children with liver cancer in the six regions and the whole country Nationally, the median expenses per hospitalization was 9, 118.67 CNY. The regions above the national median were Central and Southern China (10, 857.49 CNY), and North China (10, 722.56 CNY), while those below the national median were Southwest China (5, 580.07 CNY), East China (5, 617.97 CNY), Northwest China (7, 347.87 CNY) and Northeast China (8, 715.85 CNY) (Figure 8-6-67).

6.5.1.2 Expenses per hospitalization of children with liver cancer in each provincial-level region In terms of the median expenses per hospitalization of children with liver cancer, the top three provincial-level regions were Guangdong (21, 119.54 CNY), Guizhou (16, 210.19 CNY) and Heilongjiang (15, 571.58 CNY), while the last three were Shanghai (3, 397.60 CNY), Guangxi (4, 536.30 CNY) and Inner Mongolia (4, 673.97 CNY) (Figure 8-6-68).

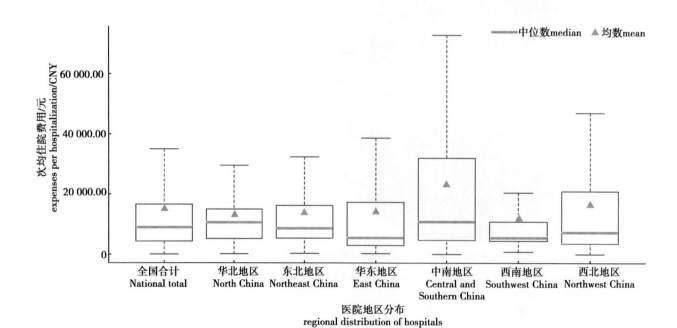

图 8-6-67 2017—2018 年全国及六大区肝癌患儿次均住院费用

Figure 8-6-67 Expenses per hospitalization of children with liver cancer in the six regions and the whole country in 2017-2018

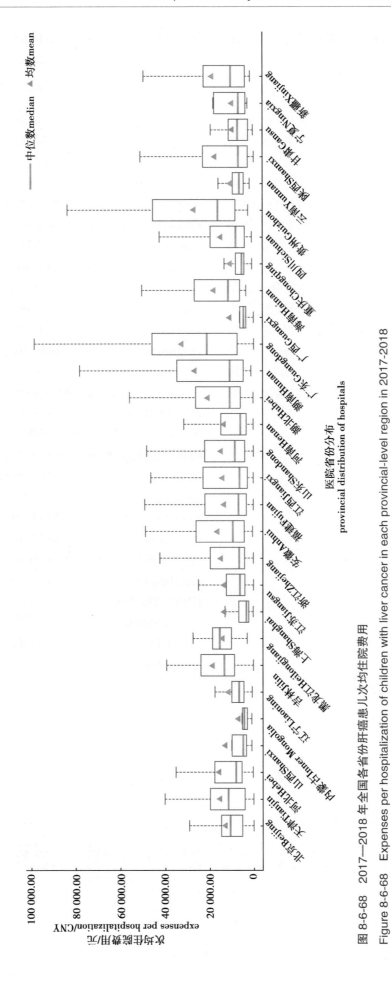

图 8-6-68　2017—2018 年全国各省份肝癌患儿次均住院费用

Figure 8-6-68　Expenses per hospitalization of children with liver cancer in each provincial-level region in 2017-2018

6.5.2 全国儿童肿瘤监测机构肝癌患儿次均住院分项费用情况

6.5.2.1 全国及六大区肝癌患儿次均住院分项费用情况 根据全国肝癌患儿次均住院分项费用(中位数),前3位分别为西药类费用(1 794.02元)、综合医疗服务类费用(1 500.14元)和诊断类费用(1 241.00元)。六大区分项费用中位数的顺位与全国相比略有不同。如华东地区,次均住院分项费用(中位数)前3位分别为诊断类费用(1 460.50元)、综合医疗服务类费用(1 069.00元)和西药类费用(877.39元)(图8-6-69)。按均数统计的结果详见图8-6-70。

6.5.2.2 各省份肝癌患儿次均住院分项费用情况 根据各省份肝癌患儿次均住院分项费用(中位数),以西药类费用为例,前3位的省份依次为湖北(3 894.92元)、贵州(3 627.18元)和海南(2 982.87元),后3位依次为内蒙古(404.86元)、上海(668.59元)和天津(820.21元)(图8-6-71)。按均数统计的结果详见图8-6-72。

6.5.2 Expenses of each item per hospitalization of children with liver cancer in pediatric cancer surveillance sites in China

6.5.2.1 Expenses of each item per hospitalization of children with liver cancer in the six regions and the whole country In terms of the median expenses of each item per hospitalization of children with liver cancer, the top three items were western medication expenses (1, 794.02 CNY), comprehensive medical services expenses (1, 500.14 CNY) and diagnostic expenses (1, 241.00 CNY). The rank of the median expenses of each item in the six regions was slightly different from the national median. For example, in East China, the top three median itemized expenses of each item per hospitalization were diagnostic expenses (1, 460.50 CNY), comprehensive medical services expenses (1, 069.00 CNY), and western medication expenses (877.39 CNY)(Figure 8-6-69). Data by the mean expenses in Figure 8-6-70.

6.5.2.2 Expenses of each item per hospitalization of children with liver cancer in each provincial-level region In terms of the median expenses of each item per hospitalization of children with liver cancer in each provincial-level region, taking western medication expenses as an example, the top three provincial-level regions were Hubei (3, 894.92 CNY), Guizhou (3, 627.18 CNY), and Hainan (2, 982.87 CNY). The last three were Inner Mongolia (404.86 CNY), Shanghai (668.59 CNY), and Tianjin (820.21 CNY)(Figure 8-6-71). Data by the mean expenses in Figure 8-6-72.

医院地区分布 regional distribution of hospitals	综合医疗服务类费用 comprehensive medical service expenses	诊断类费用 diagnostic expenses	治疗类费用 treatment expenses	康复类费用 rehabilitation expenses	分项费用/元 expenses of each item/CNY					
					中医类费用 traditional chinese medicine service expenses	西药类费用 western medication expenses	中药类费用 traditional chinese medication expenses	血液和血液制品类费用 blood and blood product expenses	耗材类费用 medical consumable expenses	其他类费用 others
全国合计 National total	1 500.14	1 241.00	0	0	0	1 794.02	0	73.93	700.24	0
华北地区 North China	1 807.13	776.00	0	0	0	2 404.87	14.44	208.70	926.21	0
东北地区 Northeast China	1 747.37	1 779.14	0	0	0	1 844.86	0	270.00	383.56	799.15
华东地区 East China	1 069.00	1 460.50	60.00	0	0	877.39	0	0	376.82	0
中南地区 Central and Southern China	1 439.00	2 825.00	712.50	0	0	2 548.24	0	0	728.49	104.00
西南地区 Southwest China	1 337.82	1 630.55	0	0	0	1 811.93	0	0	372.97	6.00
西北地区 Northwest China	910.00	2 426.34	32.00	0	0	1 541.51	0	0	271.50	0

图 8-6-69 2017—2018 年全国及六大区肝癌患儿次均住院分项费用（按中位数计）

Figure 8-6-69   Expenses of each item per hospitalization of children with liver cancer in the six regions and the whole country in 2017-2018 (by the median)

医院地区分布 regional distribution of hospitals	综合医疗服务类费用 comprehensive medical service expenses	诊断类费用 diagnostic expenses	治疗类费用 treatment expenses	康复类费用 rehabilitation expenses	分项费用/元 expenses of each item/CNY					
					中医类费用 traditional chinese medicine service expenses	西药类费用 western medication expenses	中药类费用 traditional chinese medication expenses	血液和血液制品类费用 blood and blood product expenses	耗材类费用 medical consumable expenses	其他类费用 others
全国合计 National total	2 151.52	2 796.50	1 344.74	8.06	2.04	3 592.42	189.02	714.95	2 562.42	883.61
华北地区 North China	2 055.30	1 892.23	315.74	0.09	0.29	3 894.78	283.32	827.19	2 230.37	702.85
东北地区 Northeast China	2 206.66	2 744.83	1 547.62	0.27	0	2 584.45	142.62	927.37	2 459.35	1 621.44
华东地区 East China	2 134.73	3 084.75	1 933.38	10.72	1.17	2 569.70	62.70	454.33	2 819.34	646.62
中南地区 Central and Southern China	2 588.04	4 765.73	4 197.53	16.63	8.45	4 951.29	138.99	678.80	4 138.51	2 043.37
西南地区 Southwest China	2 065.15	3 156.96	945.78	33.04	2.02	2 645.73	57.38	609.76	1 646.26	186.02
西北地区 Northwest China	1 707.80	3 590.95	1 334.59	2.22	12.29	4 501.21	187.48	497.40	2 259.54	209.58

图 8-6-70 2017—2018 年全国及六大区肝癌患儿次均住院分项费用（按均数计）

Figure 8-6-70   Expenses of each item per hospitalization of children with liver cancer in the six regions and the whole country in 2017-2018 (by the mean)

省份分布 provincial distribution of hospitals	分项费用/元 expenses of each item/CNY									
	综合医疗服务类费用 comprehensive medical service expenses	诊断类费用 diagnostic expenses	治疗类费用 treatment expenses	康复类费用 rehabilitation expenses	中医类费用 traditional chinese medicine service expenses	西药类费用 western medication expenses	中药类费用 traditional chinese medication expenses	血液和血液制品类费用 blood and blood product expenses	耗材类费用 medical consumable expenses	其他类费用 others
北京Beijing	1 874.80	731.50	0	0	0	2 602.04	28.88	220.00	945.16	0
天津Tianjin	1 925.25	3 493.80	0	0	0	820.21	0	0	1 613.15	0
河北Hebei	747.80	1 720.00	0	0	0	2 074.13	0	20.00	598.51	140.00
山西Shanxi	1 141.75	2 138.00	0	0	0	917.00	90.00	80.00	513.05	0
内蒙古Inner Mongolia	363.00	1 073.00	243.00	0	0	404.86	0	340.00	129.14	385.50
辽宁Liaoning	1 535.51	1 008.87	0	0	0	1 709.76	0	147.86	267.78	1 597.20
吉林Jilin	2 383.25	3 440.51	0	0	0	2 146.67	0	618.51	1 325.83	0
黑龙江Heilongjiang	1 985.50	2 104.50	560.00	0	0	2 034.01	0	225.00	2 293.30	120.00
上海Shanghai	1 065.00	1 017.00	0	0	0	668.59	0	0	315.28	0
江苏Jiangsu	912.00	1 906.00	463.30	9.00	0	1 129.45	31.18	274.30	493.10	120.00
浙江Zhejiang	801.45	1 361.50	176.00	0	0	2 818.87	0	258.50	426.38	0
安徽Anhui	1 678.40	2 596.40	413.40	0	0	1 445.29	64.83	0	697.46	262.50
福建Fujian	1 208.30	1 941.75	10.90	0	0	1 423.72	0	0	91.49	0
江西Jiangxi	710.70	1 940.00	0	0	0	1 134.60	218.40	0	285.83	1.94
山东Shandong	1 584.00	2 313.00	113.45	0	0	948.80	0	0	678.54	24.50
河南Henan	529.00	1 381.80	613.00	0	0	1 541.81	0	0	160.45	160.45
湖北Hubei	1 412.00	2 456.86	44.00	0	0	3 894.92	0	0	0	48.00
湖南Hunan	1 558.00	3 375.50	767.00	49.00	0	2 681.55	0	270.00	1 038.98	56.00
广东Guangdong	2 015.88	4 061.98	4 005.00	0	0	2 589.51	0	230.00	2 414.35	583.44
广西Guangxi	529.05	1 714.20	51.50	0	0	919.67	0	0	247.83	0
海南Hainan	1 300.50	2 462.21	50.00	0	0	2 982.87	0	0	1 784.52	0
重庆Chongqing	1 335.79	1 470.25	0	0	0	1 864.46	0	0	375.78	6.00
四川Sichuan	1 452.60	1 845.50	500.00	0	0	1 286.39	0	0	705.54	233.59
贵州Guizhou	3 894.12	4 627.96	253.30	0	0	3 627.18	0	323.80	313.83	79.38
云南Yunnan	1 212.00	2 226.00	225.00	0	0	2 330.77	58.70	460.00	151.87	0.09
陕西Shaanxi	842.00	1 568.00	0	0	0	1 229.55	0	0	436.81	0
甘肃Gansu	1 539.50	2 565.00	7.50	0	0	941.57	6.90	0	0	0
宁夏Ningxia	1 074.60	2 426.34	115.60	–	–	1 833.98	–	–	847.40	–
新疆Xinjiang	830.00	3 178.00	283.00	0	0	2 581.00	0	0	33.45	62.00

图 8-6-71　2017—2018 年全国各省省份肝癌患儿次均住院分项费用（按中位数计）

Figure 8-6-71　Expenses of each item per hospitalization of children with liver cancer in each provincial-level region in 2017-2018 (by the median)

省份分布 provincial distribution of hospitals	综合医疗服务类费用 comprehensive medical service expenses	诊断类费用 diagnostic expenses	治疗类费用 treatment expenses	康复类费用 rehabilitation expenses	中医类费用 traditional chinese medicine service expenses	西药类费用 western medication expenses	中药类费用 traditional chinese medication expenses	血液和血液制品类费用 blood and blood product expenses	耗材类费用 medical consumable expenses	其他类费用 others
北京Beijing	2 064.30	1 796.06	248.76	0.01	0.27	3 935.73	302.68	830.09	2 213.60	651.96
天津Tianjin	3 568.60	4 047.45	1 759.62	0	0	1 957.83	0	530.42	2 559.54	168.06
河北Hebei	1 563.25	2 375.81	662.81	0.19	1.05	4 207.83	69.53	923.56	2 271.44	1 595.56
山西Shanxi	1 701.10	2 891.93	546.89	22.22	0	2 374.29	434.86	608.32	4 811.88	4.33
内蒙古Inner Mongolia	497.73	2 277.36	1 206.84	0	0	936.39	33.83	570.00	1 213.01	747.09
辽宁Liaoning	1 827.78	1 672.44	1 899.77	0	0	2 152.38	46.23	538.48	1 517.05	2 285.53
吉林Jilin	2 828.86	4 529.46	1 177.61	0.53	0	3 198.67	240.19	1 429.97	3 946.89	600.00
黑龙江Heilongjiang	2 276.67	2 551.59	1 493.11	0	0	4 013.48	126.05	268.93	3 632.41	567.34
上海Shanghai	2 199.82	2 917.57	1 758.13	0	0.50	1 650.44	3.68	88.17	3 788.08	446.52
江苏Jiangsu	1 549.27	2 949.30	1 992.09	77.64	5.48	2 253.13	89.25	956.49	2 589.60	787.83
浙江Zhejiang	2 112.65	2 760.11	2 053.76	9.56	0	4 776.19	21.45	629.15	2 049.46	494.54
安徽Anhui	2 448.06	3 553.50	2 449.15	34.05	18.75	2 742.93	342.44	837.58	3 373.40	417.62
福建Fujian	3 136.62	2 923.06	1 903.52	1.14	0.31	2 651.63	23.69	506.83	724.83	721.06
江西Jiangxi	2 053.39	2 844.57	2 480.48	15.63	1.76	3 177.51	952.55	205.00	2 699.62	28.73
山东Shandong	2 272.64	3 741.98	1 914.52	1.53	0.77	2 791.58	22.39	693.19	2 324.45	1 151.69
河南Henan	1 415.23	2 377.77	1 783.25	0.95	4.78	3 708.57	42.48	325.14	251.63	1 197.17
湖北Hubei	2 270.95	4 137.75	2 387.74	26.24	8.05	6 112.35	370.98	297.60	3 451.81	791.00
湖南Hunan	2 113.71	6 899.73	4 607.12	95.68	0.52	5 250.19	93.06	837.46	6 671.08	126.96
广东Guangdong	3 320.57	5 741.76	5 858.70	3.84	6.77	5 054.98	93.38	964.00	5 395.34	3 274.99
广西Guangxi	1 553.97	3 104.44	1 008.26	0.74	4.00	2 272.25	6.21	826.35	1 076.71	105.31
海南Hainan	1 875.47	3 423.03	2 888.64	0	97.46	4 750.98	93.84	101.63	4 080.59	105.74
重庆Chongqing	1 951.95	3 048.16	557.82	30.43	0.87	2 408.40	25.43	566.78	1 485.61	14.70
四川Sichuan	2 748.22	3 069.58	2 515.76	18.76	7.08	2 430.17	107.95	501.85	2 479.69	869.66
贵州Guizhou	3 641.15	5 689.84	3 195.93	27.50	9.77	5 489.08	411.58	900.29	4 785.89	1 480.27
云南Yunnan	1 608.65	3 207.13	715.29	287.13	0	3 293.01	130.21	1 306.07	950.16	152.74
陕西Shaanxi	1 393.03	2 675.18	1 358.49	0	0	4 255.96	42.69	467.33	2 940.55	5.29
甘肃Gansu	1 775.79	3 551.91	708.71	25.64	131.08	2 046.07	42.38	581.18	472.02	268.20
宁夏Ningxia	1 142.67	3 089.44	1 088.73	-	-	1 277.12	-	-	-	-
新疆Xinjiang	2 420.99	4 891.75	1 648.14	0	0	6 359.56	470.32	516.69	1 745.69	475.20

分项费用/元　expenses of each item/CNY

图 8-6-72　2017—2018 年全国各省份肝癌患儿次均住院分项费用（按均数计）

Figure 8-6-72　Expenses of each item per hospitalization of children with liver cancer in each provincial-level region in 2017-2018 (by the mean)

431

6.6 全国儿童肿瘤监测机构肝癌患儿平均住院日分析

6.6.1 全国及六大区肝癌患儿平均住院日情况

全国肝癌患儿平均住院日的中位数为 7 天。高于全国中位数水平的地区为东北地区（9 天）和西北地区（8 天），与全国中位数水平的地区相同的地区为华北地区（7 天）、中南地区（7 天）和西南地区（7 天），低于全国中位数水平的地区为华东地区（6 天）（图 8-6-73）。

6.6.2 各省份肝癌患儿平均住院日情况

根据各省份肝癌患儿平均住院日的中位数，肝癌患儿平均住院日最长的省份是海南、贵州和宁夏（11 天），其次是辽宁（10 天）、安徽（10 天）、黑龙江（9 天）、广东（9 天）和四川（9 天），最短的是上海、浙江、江西和广西（5 天）（图 8-6-74）。

6.6 Analysis of the average length of hospitalization of children with liver cancer in pediatric cancer surveillance sites in China

6.6.1 Average length of hospitalization of children with liver cancer in the six regions and the whole country

Nationally, the median of average length of hospitalization was 7 days. Noutheast China (9 days) and Northwest China (8 days) were above the national median. North China (7 days), Central and Southern China (7 days) and Southwest China (7 days) were the same with the national median. East China (6 days) was below the national median (Figure 8-6-73).

6.6.2 Average length of hospitalization of children with liver cancer in each provincial-level region

In terms of the median of average length of hospitalization of children with liver cancer in each provincial-level region, the provincial-level regions with the longest hospital stay were Hainan, Guizhou, and Ningxia (11 days), followed by Liaoning (10 days), Anhui (10 days), Heilongjiang (9 days), Guangdong (9 days) and Sichuan (9 days). The shortest were Shanghai, Zhejiang, Jiangxi and Guangxi (5 days) (Figure 8-6-74).

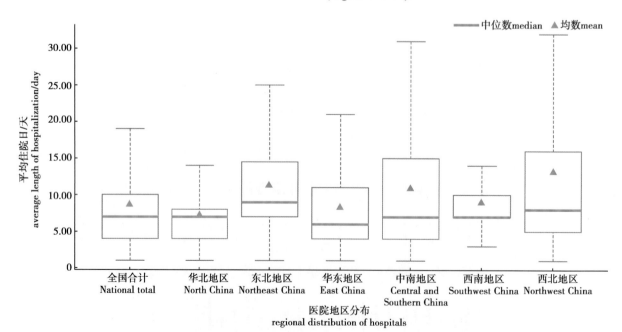

图 8-6-73 2017—2018 年全国及六大区肝癌患儿平均住院日

Figure 8-6-73 Average length of hospitalization of children with liver cancer in the six regions and the whole country in 2017-2018

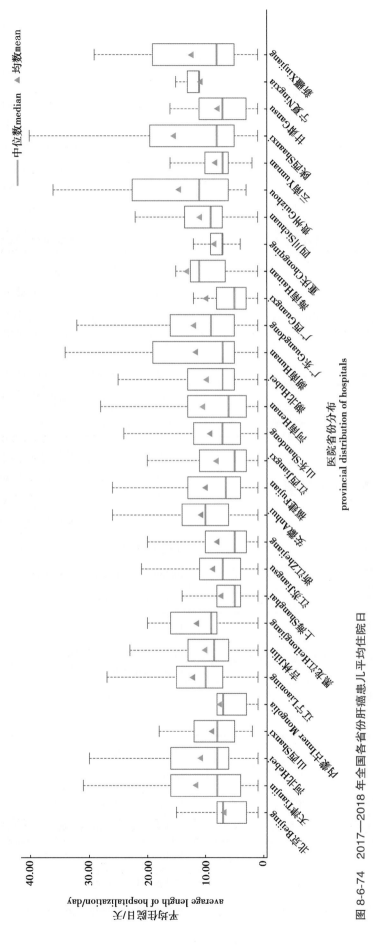

图 8-6-74　2017—2018 年全国各省份肝癌患儿平均住院日

Figure 8-6-74　Average length of hospitalization of children with liver cancer in each provincial-level region in 2017-2018

ICD-10	疾病名称	Name of disease
C00	唇恶性肿瘤	malignant neoplasm of lip
C01	舌根恶性肿瘤	malignant neoplasm of base of tongue
C02	舌其他和未特指部位的恶心肿瘤	malignant neoplasm of other and unspecified parts of tongue
C03	牙龈恶性肿瘤	malignant neoplasm of gum
C04	口底恶性肿瘤	malignant neoplasm of floor of mouth
C05	腭恶性肿瘤	malignant neoplasm of palate
C06	口其他和未特指部位的恶性肿瘤	malignant neoplasm of other and unspecified parts of mouth
C07	腮腺恶性肿瘤	malignant neoplasm of parotid gland
C08	大涎腺其他和未特指的恶性肿瘤	malignant neoplasm of other and unspecified major salivary glands
C09	扁桃体恶性肿瘤	malignant neoplasm of tonsil
C10	口咽恶性肿瘤	malignant neoplasm of oropharynx
C11	鼻咽恶性肿瘤	malignant neoplasm of nasopharynx
C12	梨状窦恶性肿瘤	malignant neoplasm of pyriform sinus
C13	咽下部恶性肿瘤	malignant neoplasm of hypopharynx
C14	唇、口腔和咽其他和部位不明的恶性肿瘤	malignant neoplasm of other and ill-defined sites in the lip, oral cavity and pharynx
C15	食管恶性肿瘤	malignant neoplasm of oesophagus
C16	胃恶性肿瘤	malignant neoplasm of stomach
C17	小肠恶性肿瘤	malignant neoplasm of small intestine
C18	结肠恶性肿瘤	malignant neoplasm of colon
C19	直肠乙状结肠连接处恶性肿瘤	malignant neoplasm of rectosigmoid junction
C20	直肠恶性肿瘤	malignant neoplasm of rectum
C21	肛门和肛管恶性肿瘤	malignant neoplasm of anus and anal canal
C22	肝和肝内胆管恶性肿瘤	malignant neoplasm of liver and intrahepatic bile ducts
C23	胆囊恶性肿瘤	malignant neoplasm of gallbladder

ICD-10	疾病名称	Name of disease
C24	胆道其他和未特指部位的恶性肿瘤	malignant neoplasm of other and unspecified parts of biliary tract
C25	胰恶性肿瘤	malignant neoplasm of pancreas
C26	消化器官其他和不明确的恶性肿瘤	malignant neoplasm of other and ill-defined digestive organs
C30	鼻腔和中耳恶性肿瘤	malignant neoplasm of nasal cavity and middle ear
C31	鼻旁窦恶性肿瘤	malignant neoplasm of accessory sinuses
C32	喉恶性肿瘤	malignant neoplasm of larynx
C33	气管恶性肿瘤	malignant neoplasm of trachea
C34	支气管和肺恶性肿瘤	malignant neoplasm of bronchus and lung
C37	胸腺恶性肿瘤	malignant neoplasm of thymus
C38	心脏、纵隔和胸膜恶性肿瘤	malignant neoplasm of heart, mediastinum and pleura
C39	呼吸系统和胸腔内器官其他和不明确部位的恶性肿瘤	malignant neoplasm of other and ill-defined sites in the respiratory system and intrathoracic organs
C40	四肢骨和关节软骨恶性肿瘤	malignant neoplasm of bone and articular cartilage of limbs
C41	骨和关节软骨其他和未特指部位的恶性肿瘤	malignant neoplasm of bone and articular cartilage of other and unspecified sites
C43	皮肤恶性黑色素瘤	malignant melanoma of skin
C44	皮肤其他恶性肿瘤	other malignant neoplasm of skin
C45	间皮瘤	mesothelioma
C46	卡波西肉瘤	Kaposi's sarcoma
C47	周围神经和自主神经系统恶性肿瘤	malignant neoplasm of peripheral nerves and autonomic nervous system
C48	腹膜后腔和腹膜恶性肿瘤	malignant neoplasm of retroperitoneum and peritoneum
C49	其他结缔组织和软组织恶性肿瘤	malignant neoplasm of other connective and soft tissue
C50	乳房恶性肿瘤	malignant neoplasm of breast
C51	外阴恶性肿瘤	malignant neoplasm of vulva
C52	阴道恶性肿瘤	malignant neoplasm of vagina
C53	宫颈恶性肿瘤	malignant neoplasm of cervix uteri
C54	子宫体恶性肿瘤	malignant neoplasm of corpus uteri
C55	部位未特指的子宫恶性肿瘤	malignant neoplasm of uterus, part unspecified
C56	卵巢恶性肿瘤	malignant neoplasm of ovary
C57	女性生殖器官其他和未特指的恶性肿瘤	malignant neoplasm of other and unspecified female genital organs
C58	胎盘恶性肿瘤	malignant neoplasm of placenta
C60	阴茎恶性肿瘤	malignant neoplasm of penis

ICD-10	疾病名称	Name of disease
C61	前列腺恶性肿瘤	malignant neoplasm of prostate
C62	睾丸恶性肿瘤	malignant neoplasm of testis
C63	男性生殖器官其他和未特指的恶性肿瘤	malignant neoplasm of other and unspecified male genital organs
C64	肾（除外肾盂）恶性肿瘤	malignant neoplasm of kidney, except renal pelvis
C65	肾盂恶性肿瘤	malignant neoplasm of renal pelvis
C66	输尿管恶性肿瘤	malignant neoplasm of ureter
C67	膀胱恶性肿瘤	malignant neoplasm of bladder
C68	泌尿器官其他和未特指的恶性肿瘤	malignant neoplasm of other and unspecified urinary organs
C69	眼和附器恶性肿瘤	malignant neoplasm of eye and adnexa
C70	脑脊膜恶性肿瘤	malignant neoplasm of meninges
C71	脑恶性肿瘤	malignant neoplasm of brain
C72	脊髓、颅神经和中枢神经系统其他部位的恶性肿瘤	malignant neoplasm of spinal cord, cranial nerves and other parts of central nervous system
C73	甲状腺恶性肿瘤	malignant neoplasm of thyroid gland
C74	肾上腺恶性肿瘤	malignant neoplasm of adrenal gland
C75	其他内分泌腺和有关结构的恶性肿瘤	malignant neoplasm of other endocrine glands and related structures
C76	其他和不明确部位的恶性肿瘤	malignant neoplasm of other and ill-defined sites
C77	淋巴结继发性和未特指的恶性肿瘤	secondary and unspecified malignant neoplasm of lymph nodes
C78	呼吸和消化器官的继发性恶性肿瘤	secondary malignant neoplasm of respiratory and digestive organs
C79	其他部位的继发性恶性肿瘤	secondary malignant neoplasm of other sites
C80	部位未特指的恶性肿瘤	malignant neoplasm without specification of site
C81	霍奇金 [何杰金] 病	Hodgkin's disease
C82	滤泡性 [结节性] 非霍奇金淋巴瘤	follicular [nodular] non-Hodgkin's lymphoma
C83	弥漫性非霍奇金淋巴瘤	diffuse non-Hodgkin's lymphoma
C84	周围和皮的 T 细胞淋巴瘤	peripheral and cutaneous T-cell lymphomas
C85	非霍奇金淋巴瘤的其他和未特指类型	other and unspecified types of non-Hodgkin's lymphoma
C88	恶性免疫增生性疾病	malignant immunoproliferative diseases
C90	多发性骨髓瘤和恶性浆细胞肿瘤	multiple myeloma and malignant plasma cell neoplasms
C91	淋巴样白血病	lymphoid leukaemia
C92	髓样白血病	myeloid leukaemia
C93	单核细胞白血病	monocytic leukaemia
C94	特指细胞类型的其他白血病	other leukaemias of specified cell type
C95	未特指细胞类型的白血病	leukaemia of unspecified cell type

续表 Table（Continued）

ICD-10	疾病名称	Name of disease
C96	淋巴、造血和有关组织其他和未特指的恶性肿瘤	other and unspecified malignant neoplasms of lymphoid, haematopoietic and related tissue
C97	独立(原发)多个部位的恶性肿瘤	malignant neoplasms of independent (primary) multipe sites
D00	口腔、食管和胃原位癌	carcinoma in situ of oral cavity, oesophagus and stomach
D01	消化器官其他和未特指的原位癌	carcinoma in situ of other and unspecified digestive organs
D02	中耳和呼吸系统原位癌	carcinoma in situ of middle ear and respiratory system
D03	原位黑色素瘤	melanoma in situ
D04	皮肤原位癌	carcinoma in situ of skin
D05	乳房原位癌	carcinoma in situ of breast
D06	宫颈原位癌	carcinoma in situ of cervix uteri
D07	生殖器官其他和未特指的原位癌	carcinoma in situ of other and unspecified genital organs
D09	其他和未特指部位的原位癌	carcinoma in situ of other and unspecified sites
D10	口和咽良性肿瘤	benign neoplasm of mouth and pharynx
D11	大涎腺良性肿瘤	benign neoplasm of major salivary glands
D12	结肠、直肠、肛门和肛管良性肿瘤	benign neoplasm of colon, rectum, anus and anal canal
D13	消化系统其他和不明确部位的良性肿瘤	benign neoplasm of other and ill-defined parts of digestive system
D14	中耳和呼吸系统良性肿瘤	benign neoplasm of middle ear and respiratory system
D15	胸腔内器官其他和未特指的良性肿瘤	benign neoplasm of other and unspecified intrathoracic organs
D16	骨和关节软骨良性肿瘤	benign neoplasm of bone and articular cartilage
D17	良性脂肪瘤样肿瘤	benign lipomatous neoplasm
D18	血管瘤和淋巴管瘤,任何部位	haemangioma and lymphangioma, any site
D19	间皮组织良性肿瘤	benign neoplasm of mesothelial tissue
D20	腹膜后腔和腹膜软组织良性肿瘤	benign neoplasm of soft tissue of retroperitoneum and peritoneum
D21	结缔组织和其他软组织的其他良性肿瘤	other benign neoplasms of connective and other soft tissue
D22	黑素细胞痣	melanocytic naevi
D23	皮肤其他良性肿瘤	other benign neoplasms of skin
D24	乳房良性肿瘤	benign neoplasm of breast
D25	子宫平滑肌瘤	leiomyoma of uterus
D26	子宫其他良性肿瘤	other benign neoplasms of uterus
D27	卵巢良性肿瘤	benign neoplasm of ovary
D28	女性生殖器官其他和未特指的良性肿瘤	benign neoplasm of other and unspecified female genital organs
D29	男性生殖器官良性肿瘤	benign neoplasm of male genital organs
D30	泌尿器官良性肿瘤	benign neoplasm of urinary organs

ICD-10	疾病名称	Name of disease
D31	眼和附器良性肿瘤	benign neoplasm of eye and adnexa
D32	脑脊膜良性肿瘤	benign neoplasm of meninges
D33	脑和中枢神经系统其他部位的良性肿瘤	benign neoplasm of brain and other parts of cnetral nervous system
D34	甲状腺良性肿瘤	benign neoplasm of thyroid gland
D35	内分泌腺其他和未特指的良性肿瘤	benign neoplasm of other and unspecified endocrine glands
D36	其他和未特指部位的良性肿瘤	benign neoplasm of other and unspecified sites
D37	口腔和消化器官动态未定或动态未知的肿瘤	neoplasm of uncertain or unknown behaviour of oral cavity and digestive organs
D38	中耳、呼吸和胸腔内器官动态未定或动态未知的肿瘤	neoplasm of uncertain or unknown behaviour of middle ear and respiratory and intrathoracic organs
D39	女性生殖器官动态未定或动态未知的肿瘤	neoplasm of uncertain or unknown behaviour of female genital organs
D40	男性生殖器官动态未定或动态未知的肿瘤	neoplasm of uncertain or unknown behaviour of male genital organs
D41	泌尿器官动态未定或动态未知的肿瘤	neoplasm of uncertain or unknown behaviour of urinary organs
D42	脑脊膜动态未定或动态未知的肿瘤	neoplasm of uncertain or unknown behaviour of meninges
D43	脑和中枢神经系统动态未定或动态未知的肿瘤	neoplasm of uncertain or unknown behaviour of brain and central nervous system
D44	内分泌腺动态未定或动态未知的肿瘤	neoplasm of uncertain or unknown behaviour of endocrine glands
D45	真性红细胞增多症	polycythaemia vera
D46	骨髓增生异常综合征	myelodysplastic syndromes
D47	淋巴、造血和有关组织动态未定或动态未知的其他肿瘤	other neoplasms of uncertain or unknown behaviour of lymphoid, haematopoietic and related tissue
D48	其他和未特指部位动态未定或动态未知的肿瘤	neoplasm of uncertain or unknown behaviour of other and unspecified sites
D60	后天性纯红细胞再生障碍［幼红细胞减少症］	Acquired pure red cell aplasia [erythroblastopenia]
D61	其他再生障碍性贫血	other aplastic anaemias
D66	遗传性因子Ⅷ缺乏	hereditary factor Ⅷ deficiency
D67	遗传性因子Ⅸ缺乏	hereditary factor Ⅸ deficiency
D68	其他凝血缺陷	other coagulation defects
D69	紫癜和其他出血性情况	purpura and other haemorrhagic conditions
D76	涉及淋巴网状组织和网状组织细胞系统的某些疾病	certain diseases involving lymphoreticular tissue and reticulohistiocytic system

52检